I Was Blind But Now I Can See

by
Vendon Wright

authorHOUSE

1663 Liberty Drive, Suite 200
Bloomington, Indiana 47403
(800) 839-8640
www.AuthorHouse.com

This book is a work of non-fiction. Unless otherwise noted, the author and the publisher make no explicit guarantees as to the accuracy of the information contained in this book and in some cases, names of people and places have been altered to protect their privacy.

© 2005 Vendon Wright. All Rights Reserved.

No part of this book may be reproduced, stored in a retrieval system, or transmitted by any means without the written permission of the author.

First published by AuthorHouse 10/06/05

ISBN: 1-4208-9101-4 (sc)

Printed in the United States of America
Bloomington, Indiana

This book is printed on acid-free paper.

Editor: Lynne Sykes

To Lady Florence

Film Star

&

Super Model

Best Wishes

This book is a tribute to the loving memory of Colette Lynch, who passed away on Thursday 3 February 2005, aged 24.

INTRODUCTION

My name is Vendon Aston Wright. I was born on the sixth of August 1966 in a small town called Rugby in England, where I attended Fareham High School. Generally, people think that the most interesting aspect of the town is that it is the home of the game Rugby Football.

I have two children named Michaela and Jasmine. Their ages are fifteen and ten respectively and they are both very helpful to me in dealing with my disability. When I'm with them they always take my disability into consideration and are always looking out for me. I'm one of eleven children consisting of six girls and five boys. I'm registered blind and so is my brother, Brian. We have a rare genetically developed eye disorder called Retinitis Pigmentosa (RP) and at present there are no known cures. So far one in three thousand people suffer from RP. My brother has found a way to overcome his disability by concentrating his every thought on education. I'm very proud to confirm that he passed his Degree at Oxford University with the highest standard, being a 1st Degree. He went on to become a Doctor of Psychology and now lectures in a local University. He became my mentor and inspired me in pursuing my goals despite my disability. My full-time job is a Computer Technician in a local school. I teach a Martial Art called Taekwondo, which is a sport that is featured in the Olympics, and am also a Personal Fitness Trainer.

I attained a 4th Degree Black Belt Master of Taekwondo and I was the first registered blind person in England to achieve this level of excellence. After studying Taekwondo for over twenty years, I now teach many classes of my own to help inspire others and at present have twenty Black Belts. I hope that I can show others that disabled people can still achieve great things. This book shows some of the challenges that visually impaired people have to overcome to live a normal life. I explain what it feels like to see the world through a blind person's eyes. Hopefully it will motivate people to see a positive side to their problems and it may also encourage people not to take what they see for granted.

Several character names have been changed to protect the privacy of the people involved.

A GUIDE TO RETINITIS PIGMENTOSA

You may have been told recently or you have known for some years that you have Retinitis Pigmentosa (RP). This diagnosis could well help to explain the months or years of not being able to see properly in the dark – called night blindness, and of falling over objects which you did not see. You will possibly have been told that, at present, there is no cure for RP and that you have to face the prospect of slowly deteriorating sight. Slow loss of sight is a difficult disability to live with, especially as you may not receive the immediate sympathy and understanding usually shown to the totally blind. Indeed many people will not believe that you have a loss of sight because you have no obvious sign of visual impairment. The first and hardest step towards living positively with a disability is accepting it. If you have RP this means knowing the limitation of your vision and learning to use intelligently the visual clues you still receive. Accepting that you have RP will not be easy. You may go through periods of despair and of feeling resentful, bewildered or even angry. All these reactions are understandable, especially as the very nature of this disorder makes adjustment difficult but the way in which you deal with it determines the type of life you and your family will share from day to day. RP can manifest itself in many ways since it is not one disorder but many with similar symptoms. For some, the loss of sight is slow and there may be only a small loss over perhaps ten years or more. Others have periods of rapid loss, often with years in between with no apparent decline. A person experiencing the early stages of RP may have almost perfect day vision but at night, in brilliant sunshine or in rapidly changing light conditions, the same person may react as if they are almost totally blind. Retinitis Pigmentosa is a group of hereditary disorders whose common feature is a gradual deterioration of the light sensitive cells of the Retina. The symptoms of this group of disorders usually become apparent between the ages of 10 and 30, although some changes may become apparent in childhood. There are many syndromes associated with

RP, which result in multiple loss, such as Usher syndrome, in which sight and hearing are both affected.

For more information on RP
www.brps.org.uk

Contents

INTRODUCTION		vii
A GUIDE TO RETINITIS PIGMENTOSA		ix
CHAPTER 1	THE DISAPPEARING WORLD	1
CHAPTER 2	I CAN SEE GHOSTS	11
CHAPTER 3	OPEN YOUR EYES	27
CHAPTER 4	THE ART OF GUESSING	39
CHAPTER 5	DRIVING ME CRAZY	49
CHAPTER 6	LET THE FIGHT BEGIN	59
CHAPTER 7	CAN YOU SEE TO SKATE?	71
CHAPTER 8	GUESS WHO!	89
CHAPTER 9	THE ART OF WINNING	103
CHAPTER 10	A VISION OF MY FUTURE	117
CHAPTER 11	GIVING UP THE GHOST	133
CHAPTER 12	HAVING TO ADAPT TO COPE	143
CHAPTER 13	THE THICKENING FOG	157
CHAPTER 14	MY GROWING OBSESSION	171
CHAPTER 15	LIVING WITH MY DISABILITY	185
CHAPTER 16	SUFFERING IN SILENCE	203
CHAPTER 17	THROUGH MY EYES	215
CHAPTER 18	CREATING A HABIT	227
CHAPTER 19	THIS IS MY STORY, THIS IS MY SONG	243
CHAPTER 20	YOU ARE BLESSED	253
CHAPTER 21	RETURN OF THE GHOSTS	267

CHAPTER 22	I'M NOT A ROBOT	279
CHAPTER 23	CRYING FOR RECOGNITION	293
CHAPTER 24	DOWN BUT NOT OUT	305
CHAPTER 25	CHARLIE'S ANGELS	319
CHAPTER 26	THE FADING SUN	335
CHAPTER 27	FACING YOUR FEARS	355
CHAPTER 28	BUMP IN THE NIGHT	373
CHAPTER 29	I'M BLESSED TOO	389
CHAPTER 30	NOW I CAN SEE	407

CHAPTER 1
THE DISAPPEARING WORLD

When I was six years old I started wearing glasses to correct my short sightedness. My perception of my low vision changed when I was twenty years old and found out that my brother had suddenly gone blind. He was told that he was suffering from Retinitis Pigmentosa (RP), which is an eye disorder that slowly kills the pigment cells in the eyes. There are three different strains of RP and the one my brother has runs in the male line of a family. So far, there are no cures. My brother's eyes deteriorated quickly which confused us all. I soon became curious and persuaded myself to arrange an eye examination to determine whether there was more wrong with my eyes than just being short-sighted.

I was born on the sixth of August 1966 in a small town called Rugby. It is the home of the famous game Rugby Football. The school I attended was called Fareham High School, and it closed down soon after I left. (It couldn't survive without me!) At school I was not great at reading, but I could read and write. I was very good at most subjects especially maths and I used to help others during the maths lessons. The only subject that I struggled with was English. I remember my English teacher saying to me that I needed to concentrate on reading a great deal more because I sometimes seemed to be skipping a lot of lines, and it would then take me a long time to find where I was if I lost my place in a book. Sometimes I complained that words seemed to have missing letters and that was why it took me so long to build up words, but nobody listened. Little did I know what was in store for me. I really thought that I was just badly short-sighted and extremely clumsy. When I was young I was too immature to realise that there was something seriously wrong with my eyes.

My eye appointment finally came through when I was twenty-one years old. (What a great 21st birthday present I was about to receive!) I couldn't help thinking how my brother Brian had gone blind overnight. One minute he was out on bike rides, the next he was blind. I thought, like a lot of people, that he was cursed or did what 99% of men do at some time in their lives. I was young; I didn't know that he had a genetic eye disorder called RP. I also didn't realise that genetic meant that the rest of our family was also at risk. Brian and I both wore glasses for most of our lives, from the tender age of six. We are both short-sighted, and my prescription was stronger than his. He wasn't even registered partially sighted, but he was experiencing sight problems. Suddenly, out of the blue, he woke up one morning and complained to my parents that he couldn't see. They took him to a specialist at Birmingham Eye Hospital and they said that he was blind. It shocked us all.

My appointment was at the same Eye Hospital. None of my other brothers and sisters were interested in finding out whether they had any serious eye problems so I travelled alone. Birmingham was just thirty minutes from Rugby by train. Before I got to Birmingham I began to get quite emotional. Tears trickled out of my eyes in sadness for my ambitious brother who I was so close to. I remember saying that I wished that I had the eye disorder instead of him because he was in the middle of studying at college. There is an old saying, 'Be careful what you wish for'; I was about to find out that it is good advice.

Despite his visual impairment, my brother went on to pass all his exams with flying colours and received a 1st Degree in Psychology after attending Oxford University. His ambitious manner continued and he is now a lecturer of Psychology at a local University. From his positive teachings, two of his children have followed in his footsteps. One attends a University and the other has just won a full scholarship to one of England's top schools. His positive attitude towards life despite his disability inspired me to achieve greater goals.

While I was on the train to my eye appointment, I looked at the other people and observed their habits. They all appeared to be looking around in different directions as if they were too scared to look at anyone else, avoiding eye contact with their fellow travellers. When I got to Birmingham I looked at my ticket to see which one to give to the ticket collector. Although it was a little difficult, I managed to see which one said 'Out' and which one said 'Return'. In a short while I would find out how important little bits of information are. As I was walking out of the train station I thought that I would be really organised and look at the train timetable. Although a little hard to read, I managed to find out what time my train would be returning to Rugby. I then set out to find my destination.

The Eye Hospital wasn't far from the train station, so was not too hard to find. I loved shopping in Birmingham so I decided I'd have a look around the shops on my way back. Dodging around a few boulders and crossing two roads, I finally found the hospital.

Whoops! Tripping up a few steps, I entered the hospital clumsily. After finding the reception and registering myself in, I sat down to wait for my name to be called. It seemed ages before I heard my name so I had time to look around. Was I in the right place? Most of the people waiting were old. Many thoughts started to race around my mind.

"Imagine if I end up like them when I get old. How difficult it must be to get around. I bet most of them can't even find the toilet. Anyway, I'm lucky, I'm only 21."

"Vendon Wright to Room Two please."

"I've been called to Room Two," I thought to myself.

I found the room quite easily (on this occasion). "Wow! That's a big sign. Easy to read," I whispered.

"Can you cover up your left eye and read the letters on the board please?" the doctor asked.

"Here we go," I thought.

"A" I pronounced confidently.

"Well, that was easy to see," I thought to myself. "It's one big letter, hard to miss all on its own. I would have to be blind not to be able to read that big thing."

I then proceeded to read the first line with no problems; the second one I struggled with, and I only just finished the third one.

"Three lines, not too bad," I thought.

I was then asked to do the same with my left eye. I did, but was not really sure whether a letter was an 'O' or a 'D'.

"Thank you Mr Wright, you may return to your seat to await the next test."

I thought for a moment; "Maybe it's time you asked some questions about the tests you're going through."

So I prepared myself.

"Was that good?" I asked.

"That's fine," he said.

"Where should I be able to read to?"

I was a little shocked by the answer.

"All the way to the bottom of the chart."

At this point I was on my feet.

"All the way to the bottom!" I thought, walking towards the chart on the wall.

The writing was ridiculously too small for me to read.

"I thought that the last few lines were for people who are long-sighted," I said.

I stood right next to the board, looking at the last line in amazement.

"How are people supposed to read that?"

I took a long look at it and then left with more questions starting to rush around my head.

"Why don't my glasses correct my sight enough to see everything?"

More and more questions filled my mind and before long I was called for my next test.

I was put in a dark room with what looked like a satellite dish in the middle.

"Cool, I'm going to watch TV!" I thought.

I was asked to take my glasses off and a sticky patch was put on my left eye. I sat with my chin on a chin rest looking into the centre of the dish. It was about the same size as a satellite dish and was white with a black dot in the middle. I later found out that it was not a black dot; it was a small lens so they could see my eye movements in the test that the doctor was about to start. He then explained what he was going to do. He said that he was going to shine a small light onto the dish, and I had to keep looking at the centre while clicking a little beeper whenever I could see the light.

"This sounds like fun," I thought to myself.

For the next ten minutes I played the game, pressing the beeper every time I saw the light. I noticed though that on several occasions the doctor stopped and asked me to make sure that I was pressing it *every* time I saw the light. He also swapped the little light for a bigger one so that I could see it a little more clearly.

We went on to test my left eye. When we had finished he asked me if I was okay. I replied that I was, but that I needed him to explain why the light kept disappearing on certain parts of the dish. Maybe I would have been better off not asking questions.

"The light was disappearing where your eye has blind spots," he said and continued to explain that the light was always there.

"Blind spots?" I asked.

"Yes Mr Wright, there are parts of your eyes that cannot see anything."

"Blind... spots?" I repeated.

"That dish is like your field of vision. If you were outside, it means that if there was something in the field of your blind spots you physically would not see it."

"Is that a tear coming out of your eye?" I thought to myself. "I am a big, tough Martial Arts expert. We don't cry, do we?"

He then put some eye drops in my eyes to dilate the pupils.

"The drops will open up your eyes so that we can take a good look into them," the doctor explained.

He also said that he had to put extra in because I had dark eyes. Then he asked me to wait in the waiting room for the eye drops to take effect.

More questions, more thoughts raced around my mind while I was in the waiting room, waiting for my eyes to fully dilate.

"I wonder, is this why the football and cricket ball kept disappearing like magic when I was at school? Is this why the tennis ball seemed to travel at different speeds almost like it had a mind of its own? Could this be why things on the TV screen seem to appear from nowhere? What's happening to me?"

My thoughts escalated.

"Could this be why words in books seem to become invisible just after I've read them?"

Question after question went around my head. It seemed to take forever to be called in for the next test. I noticed that everything around me slowly became more and more blurred. The room also seemed to be getting brighter as if I could see more in places where I thought there were shadows.

The next test was upon me. The doctor looked into my eyes with a bright light called an ophthalmoscope, asking me to look left, look right, up and down. He even held my eyelids open with his fingers because at this stage the light was really hurting me and I was struggling to keep my eyes open. Tears were also now streaming down my face. I was given a tissue to wipe them and then he continued with his tests. Did I dare to ask any more questions at this stage? I mean, how much worse could this get? It struggled to come out but I finally asked.

"Can you see anything?"

Maybe I shouldn't have asked, but I was here and I wanted to know what was going on in my eyes.

"Yes, I can see," he replied. "The backs of your eyes seem to be scarred – dark spots where pigments of your eyes have died."

"Died? Dark spots? Blind spots?" I asked.

"Maybe I've died, or maybe I wish I was dead," I thought to myself.

He then put my chin on another chin rest without my glasses on and a machine put a small lens really close to my eyes. It was fluorescent blue and looked just like a colourful contact lens.

"Was that just touching my eyes?" I asked.

"Yes," he replied. "I held your eyes open so that you couldn't blink while this was testing the pressure of your eyes."

"I take it that everything is fine in there?" I asked sarcastically.

"No," he replied.

"Well there's a surprise," I answered.

He said that there was a bit of pressure on my eyes and that I would have to use special eye drops to control it. He went on to ask me if I did anything that involved straining myself.

"Yes," I replied.

"What do you do?"

"I do weight training quite seriously. I lift up very heavy weights two or three times a week."

"I strongly recommend against doing that," he stated.

"Why?"

"It puts too much pressure on your fragile eyes. It will damage your eyes faster."

"What are you saying?" I asked. "I love doing weight training, love it to bits," I said, the disappointment clear in my voice.

"You'll have to do light training only, cardiovascular; that is if you want to extend the life span of your eyes," he replied.

I went out of the room to wait for the final test.

"One more to go," I thought. "If this gets any worse I think I'm going to have a heart attack," I moaned.

A vivid thought came to me.

"Something is wrong, I can feel it, I can sense it."

I sat and waited.

"Something's not right. How can someone who is just short-sighted have so many problems? How could I have so many problems without..."

And then it came to me.

"Unless I have RP."

I sat bolt upright in my seat. "Does that mean I'm going to go... blind?" I cried.

The thought overpowered me.

"My God, what have I done to deserve this punishment?" I asked but no answer came from above.

"Am I cursed... is our family cursed? Is it because of the 99% of men thing?" I moaned.

"Did I do wrong to someone? What am I going to do if I *have* got RP and... wait a minute... didn't I say that I wished that I had it instead of Brian?"

A single thought came out of my clouded mind.

"So does that mean that he can see again?"

"If not then life sucks!" I bellowed inside.

At long last I was called into the room for my last test. At this stage I was bumping into everything. The eye drops had fully dilated my pupils and everywhere looked ridiculously distorted. I became dizzy and disorientated. One of the doctors had to lead me into the room like I was an invalid.

"I'm a young, fit man," I thought to myself.

"How could a young, fit, good-looking, tough man need help and assistance like a seventy year old? I'm forty years too soon. Forty years of not seeing," I thought.

"Maybe fifty years," I amended.

The final test was the worst test of them all. Well, they had to save the best till last! They put a big contact lens in both of my eyes. They were so big that they prevented me from closing my eyelids. Also, to prevent me from blinking, they administered some different eye drops to slow down my automatic reaction of blinking. I felt like my eyes were permanently prized open and were going to explode. I kept feeling as though I should be blinking, but nothing happened; my eyes just stayed open. Then I had to sit there for ten minutes or so while they flashed all sorts of lights and colours into my eyes. I wanted to blink so badly, but obviously it was just not happening.

"Lucky I don't suffer from epilepsy!" I thought as I continued to observe the bright and colourful lights.

My eyes were now hurting really badly as if someone had punched them, or like I hadn't slept for days or I had been crying for a very long time, but being punched would have been easy compared to this. The pain in my eyes was getting too much and the tears were now streaming. I wanted to blink so badly. It was like having cramp but not being able to straighten your joints to relax your muscles.

"I can't bear this any more," I thought to myself.

I could feel my eyes reacting to some of the different contrasts of light, but was still unable to blink. The test seemed to go on forever, but finally it was over and the room lights came back on. I could still see the colours like a rainbow before my eyes. For a while afterwards I still couldn't blink properly. My eyelids still felt too heavy and when I did manage to blink it was slow and sluggish.

"I bet I look like a big baby, sitting here crying," I thought as I wiped my eyes with a tissue and wondered how fast the lights had been flashing.

I returned to my seat to await the results.

The doctor called me into his room. I sat there for a few minutes while he observed the results on the sheets of paper laid out before him. He got up and asked if he could look into my eyes with yet another light.

"Yeah, why not? Everyone else has," I replied as he turned off the overhead light.

After a few more minutes he switched the lights back on and returned to his seat.

"Give me the good news then," I pleaded.

"Well, I'm afraid it's not good news Mr Wright."

"Really," I replied patronisingly.

"I'm afraid that you too have RP."

"Surprise, surprise," I replied with a little humour that I squeezed out of a crying body.

He went back through all the tests and explained how they came to their conclusion. He explained that the last test with all the different flashing lights was to determine which colours I could see in different shades of light.

"Your eyes are struggling with some colours," he said. "They're not responding to many colours in the dark; this means that you suffer from night blindness."

This was all too much for me now. I was overwhelmed with information so I just sat there in silence as he read out my death sentence.

"You and your brother have a rare eye disorder called Retinitis Pigmentosa – RP," he continued. "You inherited it from your father or mother and unfortunately there are no known cures. It will get worse as you get older and you will probably go blind."

"What a great future I have to look forward to," I thought to myself.

"We will have to monitor you on a six month basis. This will also help us to understand your condition more and maybe in the future we will develop a cure."

I plucked up some courage to speak.

"There is no way I can go though that test every six months."

"It's for your own good," he replied gently.

He then asked me a few questions about my job. I told him that I was a computer technician working in front of a computer screen all day.

"That's great," he said. "It's the perfect job to be in."

"Why?" I asked waiting for some good news.

"Because you'll be able to see your eyes getting worse so you can monitor them yourself."

"Great," I responded with whatever sarcastic strength I had left.

I sat in anticipation of any more news.

"I have a little good news," he muttered as he reached into his desk. "I'm going to register you as partially sighted so that you can start getting the help that you will need."

He reached over and showed me where to sign.

"Are there any more questions?" he added.

"No," I replied.

I had an information overload. I just wanted to get out of there as quickly as possible. I wanted to crawl under a stone and stay there… forever.

CHAPTER 2
I CAN SEE GHOSTS

The stairs had gone. On the way to my appointment things came naturally so there wasn't much thought to steps and signs. Suddenly I wished that I had memorised my surroundings because with the drops in my eyes that dilated them, I was getting a sneak preview of what it's like to be blind.

Everywhere was blurred, or should I say, more blurred than before.

"Let me think," I thought to myself. "The bright parts are probably the walls so that dark spot must be the stairs."

Luckily I was right, but that was just the beginning of my tortuous journey home. I got to the stairs and looked, and then looked again.

"Who's taken away the steps? How am I supposed to get back down?"

I slowly moved my foot to where I thought the stairs started until I felt the floor disappear.

"I guess this is the first step then," I hoped.

I was right so continued on my way carefully down the stairs. I got to the bottom and then thought to myself, "Why haven't these steps got light strips on them so that a person with poor sight can see the difference between each step?"

My next task was to try and find the right way out. From where I was standing all the doors looked the same with no obvious sign of which way to go, so I just walked close to the doors until I could hear the traffic a little louder through one. As I got closer to being outside again I remembered that there were some more little steps that I tripped up on the way in. They were gone too and only a smooth block was left. Using my hands to hold on to the sides of the doorway, I slowly walked to the edge. One of my feet felt the edge of the first step so all I had to do now was walk down them until I ran out of steps. I eventually found my way outside to the street only to find my next challenge.

As I stepped outside I was met by the blinding bright light of the sun. It was incredible, so bright, and it was hurting my eyes so much that I could hardly keep them open.

"What have they done to my eyes?" was my first thought.

I stood there for a short while contemplating what to do. I first took off my glasses to see if the view was any better, but was shocked to discover that everything looked the same with or without my glasses on. I checked once more, first putting them on and then taking them off again, but the images I saw were the same. I decided to leave my glasses on and think of another solution. I looked down at the ground that now looked smooth without any cracks or potholes, and realised that I could withstand the light that was beaming down from the sun. I took a moment to look around and see what the world looked like through my temporary eyes. People looked like ghosts with the sharpness of their images distorted. It was as though they were walking around with masks on their faces. Their faces had no eyes. There was no sign of eyelids, eyelashes or glasses. I couldn't tell if someone had a big nose or a small one and their lips were an occasionally distorted line of red without a distinct difference in shape. If anyone had spots or blackheads then they were invisible to me.

"I bet people would be happy that I can't see their imperfections. I can't tell whether someone is good looking or not," I thought to myself.

Their bodies were a long line of untouched colour but of slightly different thickness. The shoes on their feet blended in with the bottoms of their trousers. I could just make out their hair so I could sometimes guess whether they were male or female, but at this stage I didn't really care. I just wanted to go home and cry. I did think about going back into the Eye Hospital, but this was new to me. I was used to being independent. I also thought that it might be just as hard trying to find someone to assist me. Imagine having to rely on others to get around, having to ask them to do everything for you and putting your trust in them. I was not ready to accept that I was disabled.

"How do other blind people get around? They must be amazing, or mad. This is very difficult. Now I realise why you don't see many blind people out and about. If I could only see like this I'd probably stay at home."

Then I thought once more about asking for help, but felt as though I had to go through this by myself. "No, I'm going to do it."

I started on my way on this narrow pavement that appeared to be very uneven walking in the direction that I thought was the right way to the train station. I bumped into a signpost that seemed to jump into my way. "Who put that there?" I asked myself. "Why don't people think a little longer before they put signposts up?" I slowly walked on, being even more cautious. Nothing was clear, not people, buildings, roads or cars.

"Have they moved the pavement?" I wondered. I stopped to observe the entire mass of blob-like shapes that had taken over my horizon. I kept trying to make some sense of what I was seeing.

"I guess those big moving blobs that look like huge stones are cars and buses," I imagined.

The sound of the rushing traffic got louder and louder so I knew I was coming to the point where I would have to cross the road. There was no crossing here so I waited very patiently. I stood for a while studying the movement of the traffic in my new world. I knew this was going to be a test of life or death. I began to rely more and more on my hearing, or what hearing I had left anyway. I'm totally deaf in my right ear so it was incredibly difficult to concentrate on hearing traffic from my right side. It felt easier to judge the traffic when I turned my head to the right so my left ear was to the road. My timing of the cars was also getting better, but I struggled with the silent ghosts. These were people on bicycles. They almost seemed to be coming out of nowhere.

"Do I take the risk and cross?" I thought as I watched the movement of the traffic once more.

I saw a ghost crossing, but by the time I had plucked up the courage to ask for help, they were gone. Most people looked like they were in too much of a hurry so I decided that I was going to have to do it by myself. I waited for a big enough gap between the blobs. At one point it almost went silent and nothing was moving apart from a small blob in the distance. I timed it and it was silent for about eight seconds before the rush of cars and buses came past me. I decided that I was going to go on the next silent gap. The time came and I held my breath as I crossed hesitantly. The blobs became bigger quite fast so I quickened my pace across the road. When I got to the other side I quickly took a guess where the pavement started and almost leapt onto it.

"I made it!" I cried out with astonishment. "I must have been mad to take that risk. I could have been knocked over and killed and it was very scary."

I then got ready for my next challenge.

Once again I stopped and looked around and tried to make some sense of what I was seeing. I saw a dark patch, then some green, a white patch then another green patch, finished off on the other side with a much bigger dark patch. All this may not appear to hold much substance, but that really was what I saw. Nothing was clear, no details, just different coloured blurred objects in different sizes. It was like a painting that a two year old would do. The dark patch on the left was a building; the green was the grass (that's an easy one); the white patch was a path with small stones and grass to the right; then the bigger dark patch was a church. There were also lots of ghostly figures rushing around, but I quickly worked out that they were people because I had already bumped into a few so they were certainly not ghosts! This place sounded like where I had come from originally, but without details. The building to the left was a bank with advertisements in its windows. The door had framework around the glass and a block handle with a space for the key; it was brown in colour with large old-fashioned type brickwork that had lots of small indentations. There were also people moving around inside and out, but in my eyes it appeared as a smooth dark grey block with no sign of any such detail that normal blessed people could see. The long and short blades of green grass were waving in the slight breeze; some parts beautifully preserved and others worn as a result of being trampled on by the many people who passed that way. Some sections of the grass were slightly brighter and almost turning light brown from the scattered stones and mud from the path. That too was now invisible to my eyes and only a pure, almost clean section of greenery was apparent.

The path was light brown in contrast with lots of different sized pebbles, each looking almost unique in shape with their own inconsistent colour and all spread out randomly across the path, but these simple pleasures were hidden from me.

The church on the other side of the road was tall with pointed sections on its roof curving down to the rough edged tiles. The graphical windows were amazing with multicoloured paintings of religious artefacts and saints covering the entire surface. The church door was slightly recessed from the outer brickwork that was made up of odd sized bricks. The door had slats covering it from side to side held together with several long brown horizontal metal bars, but again, in my view, it was all non-existent and all I could see was a large dark grey block that appeared almost smooth in texture.

"Was this the place I passed on the way to the hospital?" I wondered.

So I walked onto the pure white patch, quite proud of working it all out, but then I felt a bump.

"What was that?" I wondered while rubbing my right knee.

"It's another post just stuck in the middle of the path! Someone obviously likes to place posts in the middle of paths without considering people with poor vision," I muttered.

I then slapped it with one of my hands like it was a naughty post and walked on cautiously following the path to the end. As I got to the other end, I suddenly stopped as my mind went back to the post I had just bumped into.

"Maybe there's a post on this side waiting to hit me in my groin," I thought as I moved to the side to avoid a confrontation.

I looked carefully and yes, there it was, just waiting to assault me. I walked past it and lifted my leg high to take a big step to meet the road, but was shocked to realise that the road on this side was the same height as the path, so I probably looked stupid lifting my foot up for no apparent reason.

"The way I lifted up my leg I bet people thought that I was going to do a pee, like a dog," I thought, amused at the image I must have created.

I looked down at the road and tried to remember what it really looked like. It was a road that was hardly used by cars so it was covered with small uneven blue slabs similar to block paving. There was a burger van on the left with a sign on the road displaying its deals of the day. Unfortunately, to me it was all very different in appearance. The road looked like a mass of solid blue with no indications of any separations between its stones and a pure white block to the left. The little sign displaying the prices of the burger van's food had disappeared. I listened intently with my one good ear and kept looking closely at the ghostly figures while waiting for almost silence. This indicated to me that there were no cars or motorbikes, but I would have to risk it with the silent ghosts on bicycles.

"Here goes. I must be mad to take such risks. There might be a bicycle, but I have to get home," I thought to myself.

I held my breath as I crossed the road cautiously.

"I made it again without being hit!"

Then I walked along the level path until I met the main road in the City Centre, but not before I was assaulted by yet another post at the end of the path.

"These posts are out to get me. That got me right where it hurts most!" I dealt this offender a slap too.

I was really beginning to hate posts and wondered if they were put there purposely to obstruct my path. Just the thought of the word scared me now.

"I guess I won't be having a look around town after all," I thought, as I looked left and right to try to work out where I was.

There were so many ghosts around to observe. It was like everyone was wearing almost the same outfits – there were no details to pick out. I first looked at the heads of these ghosts and they sometimes had a dark or light patch on their heads that had no sign of individual hair strands or any other defects like the odd grey hair. Dark colours looked black and light colours looked white, but there were no indications of colours in between like redheads or brown hair – no, it was just a pure consistent colour. The ghosts' faces were a cream or black texture with the odd rough edge indicating facial hair. The pupils of their eyes, whatever the colour, were gone; there were no eyelids or white sections of their eyes. I didn't see any long or short noses with any pimples on or big or small lips with unevenly applied lipstick. The ears had gone too with no indication of size or whether they were wearing an earring. Their faces were pure without any scars, glasses, spots, pimples, freckles or any other blemishes that we are so fast to criticize on others. The ghosts' bodies had a few parts where there were two colours blending into one and the sides occasionally moved. There were no moving arms, no clear separation of coats from the tops of their shirts or T-shirts. The lower section of the ghosts moved too, but I couldn't see that they had pockets in their trousers or any labels that are usually easy to notice. The world looked completely different and their movement scared me; just a mixture of light and dark shades with no sign of buttons on clothes or shoes on feet. I took a good look around at my surroundings.

"Everywhere and everything is so blurred that I would be mad to try and walk around town looking in shops."

Then I slowly walked on my way towards the train station, trying to avoid bumping into the mass of ghosts that were obviously in a hurry.

As I came towards the end of the road I decided to have a quick look into the window of a shop where I would normally see posters and other advertisements for food, as I had not eaten since breakfast. I had been at my appointment for hours so thought that I had better eat something. The dazzling light from the sun was still irritating my eyes to such a degree that they were almost closed and streaming with tears of pain. In the window were blank pieces of paper with lots of coloured smudges where there would normally be writing. The door had disappeared and the inside of the shop was shrouded in shadow with more ghosts moving around sporadically. The door blended in with the rest of the shop because it was all painted the same colour. I did think at this stage that it would have been a great help to have the door painted a different colour from the rest of the shop so that poorly sighted people could work out where the door was more easily. I looked again at where I knew posters were displayed and almost broke down with tears of sadness because the small text was unrecognisable. The images that I was seeing now did not correspond at all with what I knew had been there previously. The thoughts of me going blind were beginning to grow once more in my mind.

"What has happened to me?" I cried to myself. "All the beauty of the world has gone and left a view of detail-less images that are so badly distorted that I can't see the point looking at them."

I decided not to risk trying to find the door even though I had become very hungry so I turned around to the road and then continued my quest to get back home.

Shortly I came to a set of traffic lights that appeared to have no lights so I waited with the ghosts. While waiting to cross the road I contemplated on how I would get across.

"I think my best option would be to just trust everyone else and cross when they cross. Surely we won't all get knocked over," I thought as I prepared to hold my breath again.

It worked and I got across safely. The pavement dipped slightly so I didn't trip but I stumbled a bit as I lifted my leg high to get onto a pavement that wasn't there.

"I bet I looked ridiculous lifting my foot high like a horse," I thought as I walked on as if I hadn't done anything unusual.

"I know where to go but I can't see my way."

I stopped and tried to work out what to do.

"I'll follow people who are going in my direction. If I follow in their footsteps then I shouldn't get assaulted by any more posts."

I began to follow a ghost as if I was a stalker, thinking that they would avoid posts so I should be safe walking behind them. I continued in the direction that I needed to go in and when they walked too fast, I just found someone else slower to follow. I looked ahead of me and was startled by the amount of ghosts in my view. On my way I heard someone asking me if I wanted a leaflet so I just put out my hand and grabbed hold of that little white blob that was approaching me. After I took it I said, "Thank you," and had a quick glance at it while still trying not to lose the person in front of me who I was carefully following. The paper no longer looked real. It had lots of large dark blobs of ink that I later found out were photos, but at the time meant absolutely nothing to me. Even the paper itself had no smooth edges, although I knew it was rectangular.

When I got into the bullring where the train station is I hesitated and eventually stopped following people for a while. I became disorientated. The ground looked like it was moving and with the different patterns on the floor it looked like there were small steps everywhere. I stopped to think, but could not remember if there were any little steps. After a while I continued, but kept picking my feet up high as if to go up a step. I looked at the design on the floor carefully as I walked on hesitantly and couldn't help but try to imagine what was going on in the designer's head when he came up with that particular pattern.

"Surely it would have been better to have one all-over colour," I muttered disapprovingly as I approached where I thought the entrance to the train station was. I walked even slower now, observing the large blobs which were shops, until I saw a large space where the blob looked completely different, which I assumed was the escalator that would lead down to the train station. I observed my surroundings for a few seconds while I looked to see where all the ghostly figures were going. Over to my right I saw them disappearing downwards so I guessed that must be the escalator I was looking for. I walked even slower towards it knowing that at any second I too could be on it, but if I wasn't prepared for it I would surely trip and have a nasty fall.

"How am I going to step onto an escalator that I can't see and has no separations between the steps?"

They were all the same colour so looked like one continuous blur. Once again I thought that I must be mad to attempt this, as I edged forward even more. I know that I was wrong to feel this way, but I felt too embarrassed to ask for assistance because this was all too new to me and I was used to doing things for myself, so I got ready to take the risk.

"I'm going to take a big step like when I was going onto the pavement and also hold on for good luck!" I thought (well actually it was just in case I fell flat on my face). I picked up my foot to get ready then hopped slightly forward to ensure that I got on. It worked and I was on, but now the steps began to separate quite fast and I think my feet were on two steps so I had to choose really quickly before I slipped down a step or two. It was a little shaky, but I was safe for a moment as the long escalator continued its journey downwards.

"I lost my balance for a second or two, but I did it. Now when do I get off?" was the next thought that came to me.

My heart began to beat faster as I became more nervous.

"I'll take a big step and almost jump as the escalator begins to straighten again."

After a moment I felt the steps beginning to straighten so I got ready and...

"I made it again!" I thought with happiness.

Then I looked up at the large notice board, but I couldn't make anything out. This notice board is huge with all the different train arrivals and departures on, yet I couldn't manage to read anything so I decided to go and look at the same timetable on the wall that I had read when I arrived in Birmingham earlier. I first had to work my way over to a ticket collector. I followed some ghosts that were going in the right direction and observed what they were doing. I saw them stop at a post and move their arm towards it. However, as I got closer I realised that it wasn't a post, it was a ticket collector, but when I reached into my pocket I pulled out several different cards that now all looked the same. "Why didn't I keep it in a separate pocket? I must remember to do that in future," I thought as I looked long and hard for the ticket.

I handed him the wrong card a few times before finding the correct one. It was the one with a thick orange coloured border on the top and bottom. All the information in the middle of the card had miraculously disappeared just like everything else seemed to be doing. I then walked around to the left to find the timetable on the wall. This time there was nothing to even indicate that there was any writing there to read so I took my glasses off, but I still couldn't see anything despite the fact that my nose was literally touching the board.

"I'll have to make my way over to the information desk and ask someone for the right time and the platform that my train will be leaving from," I thought as I turned back around in disappointment.

After receiving the correct information about my train without asking for more assistance in *finding* the train, I made my own way over to the platform. I still felt uncomfortable asking for help – I wasn't ready to be labelled as disabled. I walked to the far right of the train platforms to find Platform 3a. I walked up close to where the number of the platform was displayed and was happy to be able to read it. I still had to almost touch it to read it, but I didn't care. It felt great to be able to read something again. The numbers were about a foot in height. I must say here (just in case I forget to later on), that they have now replaced them with new small numbers that I cannot read so they have obviously not taken visually impaired people into consideration.

When I got to the steps I was happy to see that they were bright with dark strips on the edges of each step, so even though I was feeling dizzy from the unexplainable blurred vision, I was able to hold onto the side and walk carefully down to the train platform. Now

I was in a little bit of trouble because I could not read the TV screen that displayed where each train was going and how many stops there were before Rugby. This was difficult to do, but I managed to pluck up enough courage to ask someone to read it for me. I then stood around waiting for my train to arrive. While taking a glance around I noticed that the seats had disappeared so I continued to stand and not take any more risks trying to find invisible seats. The walls looked like pure silk, white with no pictures, cracks or any other defects. Everything seemed calm apart from some ghosts rushing around – like they could get anywhere without a train! The ground was dark grey and looked consistent in colour. I looked over to where there used to be a series of train tracks crossed with rough slats running in the other direction and little odd shaped stones that were all unique, but all I could see now was a dark brown mist.

A train was coming towards me. I wondered if this could be my train. It stopped with a loud screech and I peered up to see what the train looked like. It was shaded black with a long white strip on the side. There was a part of it that was bright and rectangular in shape and there was also a short white strip on the side. I worked out that the long white strip were the windows that appeared to blend in with each other. The short white strip was the name 'INTERCITY' and the rectangular shape was the door. I approached the door with caution. I had vivid flashes of a large gap between the train and the platform and the last thing I wanted to do was fall at this stage when I was nearly home. I looked at the edge of the platform and a blob that I hoped was the floor of the train and once again took a big step up. Success! I was now on the train and attempted to look for a seat. Many of the other ghosts had already boarded the train with no mercy for others like me or for people with pushchairs. I began to walk to the left passing what looked like empty seats. I will never be sure whether they really were empty, but that is what I thought at the time. The seats were light blue with a dark blue background and made up of tiny squares – that's not what I saw though. I walked and I stopped, then I walked again until I felt confident enough to sit down. I wouldn't have minded sitting on a young lady's lap, but luckily for her I sat in an empty seat! I stared out of the window watching more and more ghosts entering the train and slowly filling it up. It felt unreal how they walked up to their seats, sat down and then vanished out of sight. The only people I could visually make out were the ones who were directly surrounding me. The other people blended into their seats.

The train eventually started on its journey and I continued to watch people. There was not much detail to make out, but some of them appeared to have big bright grey bodies that seemed to change shape slightly every time they moved their blurred arms. After listening closely and hearing the rustle of paper I concluded that these people were reading a newspaper. I then quickly turned to look out of the window for a while because I felt myself staring too long at people, trying so hard to bring them into focus.

Everything outside was rushing past at great speed. Trees blended in with bushes, and bushes blended in with the grass. Everything looked all as one. The train was starting to slow down for my stop. I had counted the two previous stops and knew mine was the third one. I stayed in my seat until the train came completely to a stop.

"How am I going to open a door when I can't see any handle? I hope that someone else is getting off too."

My next worry was how to get to the door. I decided to look out for someone else getting off at my stop first then follow them. They could then open the door that appeared to have no handle. I was lucky, someone opened the door so I followed them, slightly bumping into seats on the way out. At the entrance to the door I noticed that it seemed much higher than the platform outside.

"Not steps again. I hope that I don't fall between the gap," I thought as I prepared myself to jump once more.

I leapt off the train and landed on the platform.

"I can't believe it! I made it back to Rugby!" I thought with relief.

Some people rushed this way, and some rushed that way.

"Where am I on this platform though?" I asked myself.

Nothing was clear so I guessed left and started walking. Then I stopped and decided to go to the right for a while. I followed someone and soon found that I was on my way out of the station.

When I got to the exit I waited for a while before, yes, following someone elsc in the new direction that I needed. I didn't live more than five minutes from the station so I thought that I would be fine!

After a while my guide went straight on where I wanted to go right, up a slight hill to my house. I was now on my own.

It was very important that I slowed down and concentrated on the pavement and all the obstacles that were on it. Memory of my surroundings became top priority.

"Was there a lamp post coming up soon?" I kept thinking to myself.

Suddenly I stopped, thinking that I was about to get hit. I did this on several occasions, but was let off. No posts wanted to take me on and I was glad. Once again from memory, I had to work out how far along this road I lived. I stopped and turned to prepare myself to cross one more road, my last road! I stood and waited, and waited a little more. The traffic was passing me with great speed. I waited and listened for that gap, that silence. The only worries I had now were those silent ghosts on bikes.

"Here goes," I thought as I held my breath and prayed.

I crossed hesitantly and reached the pavement on the other side. With a large step I was now safe.

"Thank you God," I repeated several times.

As I walked along looking for my home I noticed that most of the houses had no gates.

"This house looks like mine, I think! My house seems to have no gate either."

I felt around with my hands until they stumbled on what felt like a gate.

"Now to open it, where's the lever, and which side is it on?"

Eventually I found it and entered my garden. The shed at the side seemed to have disappeared. My bike looked like a red intertwined mountain of junk (then again, that sounded almost right). The wheels had gone along with the spokes and large framework. The swings in the garden were a mass of multi-coloured plasticine, the grass and the path looked smooth and the door was a blob of brown.

"Where's the door handle?" I thought as I struggled to find it.

Eventually my hand stumbled on the handle and I entered my home. I walked into the sitting room and looked to find an empty seat.

"Hello and how was your appointment?" my dear mother said.

I relived the whole dramatic experience in my head for a few seconds and then replied; "Fine thanks."

My brother and sister entered and joined in the conversation.

"Have you got what Brian's got?" asked my mother.

"Yes," was my reply.

There was a short silence as we all tried to come to terms with what had happened. My sister then made me some food because I was also complaining of hunger. She made sausage, chips and beans, which was one of my favourite meals. Eating it with a knife and fork turned out to be quite a challenge. The chips had lost their individual appearance and now looked like a clump of potato that was all mixed together. The sausages were as one and the beans were like red soup.

"How am I going to eat this?" I thought anxiously.

"I'll just have to use my fingers," I answered myself.

Feeling very embarrassed, I began using my fingers; first each of the chips and then the sausages. Without looking I continued to feel around the plate for my food before placing it in my mouth. I almost felt like a baby needing assistance to eat. When I thought that all the chips and sausages were gone I used my fork to scoop up the beans. My fingers were wet and sticky from feeling around the plate for chips and coming across beans but I didn't care. I was hungry!

Something sounded interesting on the TV so I began to watch it.

"Where is everyone?" I wondered as I looked around.

All I could see was a series of lines that varied in colour and size. Every time I heard someone speak the shaded lines would change their order. I knew that there were people on the TV somewhere because their voices were so clear but I couldn't see anyone. This all became too overwhelming so I gave up watching the scrambled screen and went to my bedroom.

As I lay there on my bed I struggled to stop the vivid thoughts rushing through my mind.

"Am I going to go blind? Is this how some visually impaired people have to see? What would be the point of trying to watch TV or struggling to go out and enjoy myself? What am I going to do if this really happens to me?"

The thoughts continued as I began to cry, tears streaming down my face as I wondered what hell my poor brother must be going through.

"Maybe he's cured now that I've taken his curse away from him? I'm going to be an invalid, disabled for the rest of my life with no cures and no tablets to help."

I lay there that awful depressing night and I cried and cried until I finally fell asleep.

CHAPTER 3
OPEN YOUR EYES

The next morning I opened my eyes to see more blurred images around the room. Nothing was in focus. My poster of Bruce Lee was jumbled and was just a mass of intertwined shades and colours. Then I looked over at the door and realised that the handle was nowhere to be seen. It had vanished as if it had never been there and what was left was a smooth looking shape with no sign of detail. There was a Martial Arts magazine on my hi-fi, but as I tried to focus on the words I had no luck. It just looked like someone had smudged all the writing and pictures so that nothing was recognisable. My world was still very distorted in an unimaginable way.

"What am I going to do, will I ever see again?" I thought hysterically. "The Eye Hospital has damaged my eyes and speeded up the process of not being able to see."

I sat there for a moment almost bursting into tears and feeling sorry for myself. It was as though my whole world had ended. Without sight I would be no good to anyone.

"I'll have to give up all my hobbies," I thought miserably. "How will I be able to do Martial Arts without sight? Why should I bother going out to try and enjoy myself if I can't see anyone? Nobody will want to take me out if they know that they'll be guiding me constantly."

The thoughts continued and I felt as though I was going out of my mind.

"Well I won't be able to roller skate any more and how will I ever read a book or write? I felt much better before I went to the Eye Hospital – I wish I'd never gone. How can anyone enjoy life seeing like this? I just want to curl up and die."

Then it hit me. I suddenly realised that I hadn't put my glasses on yet. My heart began to race again and I became excited. Feeling for my glasses and unable to visually see where they were, I continued to use my hand and not my eyes to find them. My hands touched a few things and I had to quickly think of what they felt like until finally

I found them and placed them on my face. The world became clear again.

"I can see!" I shouted ecstatically.

The smile came back to my face as I looked through my glasses and felt blessed by having the privilege of being able to see. The difference was incredible. Plain blue curtains turned out to have pretty little patterns on them with a mosaic of colours. My plain brown blanket transformed to show small squares in different colours. The wallpaper that had looked like a solid bold blue broke up into light and dark blue stripes. The difference between my two worlds, with and without my glasses was like looking through a pair of binoculars and slowly turning the adjustment so that the images would turn blurred and unrecognisable. It was almost impossible to describe.

The poster of Bruce Lee on the wall was clear again. His muscles were standing out in great detail. The difference that my glasses made was incredible, so I removed them and then replaced them once more to see the amazing transformation again.

"I'm back," I mumbled as I proceeded to read the magazine. "I can read again."

The words were quite clear and the photos looked sharp. Looking around I also saw the door handle. It was amazing how many things were almost reappearing before my eyes.

While I was in the bathroom freshening up, I couldn't help but notice the definition of everything, from my toothbrush hairs to my face in the mirror. In the mirror I could see my eyes and their colour, facial hair and a few spots! The name of my toothpaste stood out and I could read some of the labels on the bottles of shampoo. It felt wonderful to be able to see again. I felt lucky and started to appreciate having this precious gift. I really felt blessed and was very grateful.

When I walked down the stairs I noticed each step; how they stood out so distinctly from each other and even the pattern on the carpet. Our wallpaper had shape and life shone from its pattern. The glass in the front door was clearly visible as were the numbers on the phone. My mother's flowers in the vase had leaves and a few different colours, but when I removed my glasses to look, it was as though the leaves had disappeared into a mist, leaving an image that had one plain colour with no leaves. It didn't even look like a flower; it was like someone had mixed all the different colours in a paint pot. These are the beauties of life that we all take for granted.

"I didn't realise how beautiful flowers are. They are so colourful and hold great detail. I guess it's time for me to appreciate everything because the ability to see things might be taken away from me at any time."

I walked into the kitchen to find something to eat.

"What should I have for breakfast?" I thought to myself as I looked at the Corn Flakes and Weetabix boxes.

The Corn Flakes seemed to jump out at me, so I had a bowlful. While I was eating I studied the food, admiring the way I could see each individual flake, and comparing it to what I would have seen the day before. Slowly I started to relive a few depressing moments before my mother called me.

She wanted to know a little more about what had happened and what had been said at the Eye Hospital. Trying not to get too emotional I began to explain, but missed out some information that made me feel depressed. She seemed very concerned and asked me why I went by myself.

"I suppose that I was expecting the best. I didn't know that they would put eye drops in that would cloud my vision to the extent that I wouldn't be able to see. I've been to Birmingham by myself before and thought nothing of travelling alone. Maybe I should have asked Brian what to expect, but I really didn't think that I would end up with RP."

My mother also said that I must have been mad because I could have been knocked over by a car or a bus. I tried to explain that I was more scared of bicycles because they were silent and invisible to my eye, but she kept on at me. Then I asked her a few questions about her sisters and brothers. I was trying to find some logical reason why this had happened to both my brother and me.

"She must know something about it," I muttered to myself. "I bet she's hiding the truth."

She told me that she didn't know how this could have happened to first my brother and now me.

"None of my family went blind," she said. "My eyesight is poor, but the doctors said that it's to do with my diabetes."

"Are you quite sure?" I asked her.

"Yes, quite sure," she replied. "I always thought that Brian lost his sight because when he was about nine he was playing in the house with a friend and got something stuck in his eye, but now that you have a problem too, I realise that it must be something you both have."

She thought for a moment before continuing, "When Brian was young, I always thought that he had the clearest eyesight out of all of you. He could find a small pin easily when it fell on the floor."

I sat and listened.

"Maybe it's all that hard physical training you both do. Maybe you're straining yourselves too hard," she concluded.

"No, there's more to it than that," I answered. "I think that it's a coincidence that we're both short-sighted," I said.

My mother was a great believer in superstition and kept trying to convince me that it was someone trying to curse our family.

"There are plenty of people back home in Jamaica who would want to do harm to our family you know," she said.

"What do you mean?" I asked.

"When your father left Jamaica back in the 1960s he came here to look for work, but many people didn't like his ambition and tried to stop him coming to England."

I listened and took it all in, but I wanted a medical reason, not a mystical one.

Then a warm thought flashed through my mind.

"Now that *I've* got it, Brian should be cured," I thought as I prepared to phone him.

He answered the phone and I told him about my experience at the Eye Hospital. Then I waited for the good news; for him to tell me that miraculously his sight had been restored overnight, but by the end of the phone call I knew that we both had a degenerative eye disorder that was going to get worse. At this point I felt like my whole life had ended.

"So I could go blind too?" I cried. "I could wake up blind any time. How am I going to live happily with this problem? I'm young with many years ahead of me, but now I could be knocked over because I can't see cars."

My mother was watching the television so I joined her after putting the phone down. It was amazing how clear the television was compared to what I had seen last night. Many thoughts came to my mind while I sat there admiring the clear picture.

"Do people realise how lucky they are to be able to see this?" I thought. "People are so blessed to be able to read the writing on the adverts or to be able to look at people on the screen in great detail. I wonder how other people would cope without their sight. Would they still be so outgoing? Or would they just stay in and cry themselves to sleep like I did last night? How would people feel if their independence was taken away and they had to rely on other people every moment of the day?"

I gazed around as my thoughts continued. "Look at everything; it's so clear and beautiful. Normal sighted people are so lucky and they really are blessed because if God took away their eyesight, their lives would crumble. We use our eyes for nearly everything. I only know one person who's blind. He has glaucoma; I wonder how he copes because he doesn't go out that often."

I concentrated on the pictures on the television once more, feeling increasingly sorry for blind people. It was a lazy day for me; I had nothing planned.

"I think I'll take a walk into town and look at hi-fi equipment," I mumbled as I got up and walked outside.

As I closed the front door behind me, I remembered what I could, or should I say couldn't, see yesterday. The door handle was back. My red bike had wheels and spokes, but it still looked a mess! The swings were clear and colourful again; the blue, the yellow and the red were so easily distinguishable from one another. On my way to town I began to admire everything that I saw and thanked God for my sight. No longer would I take my vision for granted. It was time I cherished every moment because I was now beginning to worry about that morning, that day, when I would wake up and think that my eyes were still closed because I would be blind.

In the distance I saw some friends approaching. I could see their eye colour, their noses, lips and a few spots! Rather than picking faults on their faces I was just glad to be able to see them. They were so clear and in focus, and for the first time I was grateful to be able to see them.

"Hello John, hello Fred," I cried out.

We stood and chatted for a few minutes and talked about general things like our jobs. John then went on to ask me how I'd got on with my appointment and I explained it in detail. Talking about it made me feel depressed and worthless. He refused to accept that I, his best friend, could go blind.

"How can you be partially sighted when you look fine to me?" he asked.

"That's what the doctor said so that's what I'm going to have to accept," I told him emotionally. "I'm going to try and enjoy my life to the full now. Appreciate every moment of every day."

"Maybe you should learn to drive now then?" he suggested. "Would you like me to teach you?"

"Why not, that sounds like a great idea," I answered as a smile came back to my face.

"How does one Sunday morning sound?" he asked.

"That sounds great," I replied as we parted company.

Learning to drive was one of my biggest dreams at this stage of my life. I was a young boy and all young boys learn to drive! The thought of the independence and the freedom excited me. My imagination ran wild as I made my way to the hi-fi shop.

"How cool I would be if I had my own car!" I mused. "I could take my parents out any time or drive to work instead of catching the bus every morning. Maybe I could be a taxi driver; no, that's not very ambitious, but I know I'll love driving."

I entered the shop, the thoughts still coursing through my mind, "What car would I like to drive? This is so exciting!"

The shop sold TVs, hi-fi equipment and videos. I visited regularly to consider which equipment I would buy in the near future. My favourite brand was Technics; most of their products were of good quality. I browsed around the shop, seeing the individual buttons, numbers, LED screens and their colour codes quite easily. After having a good look I decided to go and speak to my dad.

He lived at 128 Murray Road, in our family home on his own. The property was in need of some desperate home improvements. My dad was a great believer in God and went to church on a regular basis. On the way to the house a few memories came to me. I remembered that everyone used to call me 'Daddy's son'. This was because my dad had tried to teach us all how to save money in a bank account and read the Bible regularly. Although most of us read the Bible, it seemed that I was the only one who continued to listen to him and save money regularly. From the time when I first started working at seventeen years old I gave my dad money every week after I got paid to save up for me. I used to get twenty-five pounds per week and I would give twenty pounds to him and have a mere five pounds to spend on myself. At the time I felt rich. Five pounds was loads of money! This teaching has stayed with me and I'm now well known to be great with money. He also used to give me a few treats if I went to the shop for him without complaining. He would give me a small drink of QC sherry, something that I still drink in moderation today. My brothers and sisters said that he spoilt me and favoured me, but that wasn't true. I just did more for him than they did so although they gave me the nickname through spite, I've kept it in my memory out of respect for my father.

Another great memory was being smacked for something by my mother! In order to get less punishment I cried hard and loud like I was in a lot of pain. When my mother stopped and left my room, I opened the window and began to laugh to my brothers outside.

"It didn't really hurt!" I shouted.

I laughed to my brothers, but my mother was still outside my door and came in to continue my punishment. The pain was real this time so I cried for real.

I also remembered the time when I dropped my nephew Dyonn just a few years earlier. He was only a few years old and I was spinning him around in my hands. As I spun him upside down I accidentally dropped him on his head. He has never forgiven me for it up to this day, but we laugh about it!

As I came out of my reverie I realised that I was on Murray Road and just needed to cross over to get to my home. As I stood there on the kerb I relived the tense moments that I had experienced the day before when I had needed to cross a road without being able to see properly. Now the cars were plain to see, their colours and shapes so easy to distinguish. I crossed with ease. As I stood there ready to go up to the door, I thought about the fact that we were in a temporary house with my mother waiting to come back home, but my father was going slightly senile and refused to have any of us back until it was redecorated. He had worked for the Ford Car Company for many years before he was made redundant a few years earlier. Things were not going quite right financially and I think that it had damaged his self-esteem and pride. He was so lonely and I felt sorry for him, but he refused to let us help him get back on his feet. I missed my home and missed seeing my dad on a daily basis. Then I began to get a little tearful so I tried to think of something happy to cheer me up.

A few years earlier I had been escorted home from the Rugby Sports Centre one day by a lovely young lady friend of mine called Doreen. We stood outside my home for about an hour, talking about what might happen in the future if we got together. She liked me and I liked her, but she had a child with a friend of mine and we somehow controlled our feelings and never got romantically involved. She was very pretty and sexy, and I kissed her on the cheek when she went home. She used to work in the town centre and on many occasions I met her after work and we talked intimately, but although we still see each other occasionally, we have never taken it further. That memory made me smile as I knocked on my dad's door. He answered and let me in.

It was a five-bedroom house. We were lucky to have the attic converted into two rooms and when I was very young I used to share them with my two brothers, Brian and Fergus. There were nine of us living there plus my parents so we all had to share rooms – my two eldest sisters live in Jamaica with their aunt. When I got a little older and some of my older brothers and sisters had moved out, I had a bigger bedroom at the back of the house by myself. This room used to belong to my dear sister Carline who has now unfortunately passed away. I had a double bed all to myself and the room was so big that I could train in there. I used to do press-ups, sit-ups, use a weapon called a nunchaku and do my Martial Arts training.

After a few moments of chit-chat with my dad, I finally got to the subject of our eyes. The questions I asked him were the same as those I had asked my mother and most of his answers were the same. He was just as superstitious as my mother and went on to say that one of his brothers had gone blind when he was quite young and had then suddenly died. He said that his brother had been quite a ladies' man and many men had hated him, so he always believed that some other jealous man had cursed his brother. Even though it was very sad about the loss of his sight, I was just as worried about why and how he had died suddenly. My father stuck to his story to the end of his days. He was a positive man and started to give me some advice.

"Don't worry about your eyes," he said. "You won't go blind because nothing can harm you. Now drink some Guinness and you'll be fine."

I had a drink as I listened some more.

"God will open your eyes and you will see people more clearly," my dad said.

"How can I see more clearly if my eyesight is going to get worse?" I asked, wondering what he meant.

"Don't worry, you will see," he replied.

We spoke for a short while longer then I left to go to the post office to get a provisional driving licence form to send off.

The next day I went to work as usual at the Rugby College. My job was an Audio Technical Assistant working with two other people for a company called 'The Talking Newspaper'. Amazingly this was compiling and developing all the information in the local newspapers onto an audiocassette for the visually impaired. The job involved working in a recording studio with the microphones and other recording equipment. We then had to reproduce hundreds of copied-on cassettes each week after first erasing the information previously recorded the week before. It was an interesting job and I enjoyed it, but it was temporary and was coming to an end very soon. I then put out my CV to most schools in Rugby for Audiovisual Technicians or IT positions. I eventually got a job in a local school as a Computer Technician. It was quite remarkable that I got this job because when I attended school, I didn't even like computers. I didn't understand all that 8bit business. Why couldn't they work one bit at a time! In our days there was only one computer in the whole school and that was a BBC computer.

This new position involved assisting both students and teachers with all their computer needs. It was an interesting and challenging job. When I attended college I trained with the old BBC computers, but now they were IBM so I used to stay behind after work to learn how to use every piece of software that they had in the school. I was a keen worker. I managed to use the standard keyboards and 14-inch screens. When students needed help I would go to them and look at their screen, then sometimes talked them through the step-by-step procedures or corrected whatever the problem was for them. Sometimes they had produced colourful drawings and just wanted the yellow section to be moved so I would assist them. Part of my job was to work in 'Dos mode' and correct programs that didn't work properly or write small programs called 'Batch files'. Working with the teachers was always a highlight of my day because it felt like I was teaching the teachers and that always made me feel extra special. The students were easier to teach because the teachers panicked like big babies! One of the teachers who I often helped used to teach me at my old high school. Imagine how good it felt to tell someone off who used to tell me off ten years earlier!

On an average day at work I would first switch on all the computers in the school. When a class came to use one of my rooms I would assist the teacher with the lesson. If they were told to open a document, but couldn't find it, I would help those students while the teacher continued to deliver the lesson. Sometimes there would be a class in another computer room at the same time and some of the students would be struggling to keep up. I would then literally put on a pair of roller skates and zoom between the two rooms. This is why I used to teach the teachers how to use the software that they wanted the students to use. Most IT teachers were fine and very competent; but the English or Science teachers who had to incorporate IT into their curriculum didn't have the faintest idea how to use the software. I actually enjoyed these busy days.

At break time I would have a group of people come in and reserve computers for lunchtime. Then there would be more classes and I would be doing the same thing, assisting, especially during troubleshooting tasks. A typical troubleshoot was when a student couldn't find a document. I would have to use my computer and go into their files to see if they had accidentally (on purpose) saved the document under the wrong name. It was quite easy because I would first ask them what date they had saved it and then look for any files under their username that had been saved on that particular day. Some kids were naughty and instead of saving a document as, lets say, 'English 1', they would save it as 'Danny's stuff', or even a swear word! It was also my job to show pupils how to cut and paste work while their teachers continued to deliver their lesson plan.

At lunchtime we had fun. It became a major part of the students' day because I used to put on a few games and pupils loved to play and let their hair down. They loved it so much that most of them showed me great respect only because they knew that I could ban them from using the games or computer room at any time. We did give priority to any students wanting to do serious coursework because that was more important than playing games!

Another great attraction was the 'Intranet'. It was the school's version of the Internet that hadn't become worldwide yet. I suppose that the pupils knew that the Internet would become a hit and look how often it's used now. I was the Intranet nanny so I could check if pupils were sending any other pupils nasty messages and believe me they did! I had a few favourite students who would always come at lunchtime to see me even if they hadn't reserved a computer. Some of them started training with me and after more that fifteen years they still train. Other students used to offer to get my lunch, but I soon found out that they were enjoying my lunch too! My favourite student was Tanya. She used to buy me two sausage rolls and come back with one. The other one would be in her tummy. Other times I would leave a sandwich on my desk while I went to help another pupil. When I got back I would notice that there was a bite taken out of it. I knew that it was her because food only disappeared when she was around. She added fun to lunchtimes but at a cost – my food!

Students were allowed to change their passwords and yes, they sometimes forgot them, but I always saved the day because I had the master computer that overrides all the others. It was great, I felt loved and needed at that school. Even my boss was great and you can't say that about many bosses. She trusted me and gave me a lot of power to change things whenever I thought that they needed changing. I designed the desktop for all the students to use. After the lunch break I would have my lunch, but most of the time I ate it during students' lunchtime so that I could help the next group in my computer room. Throughout the afternoon I would continue to assist the teachers. There were some days when I had no classes and during these periods I would search the main computer for files that were either old or not needed and there were usually hundreds that would keep me busy. Just like your computer at home, when the hard drive is loaded with files the processing speed slows down. When you have hundreds of computers trying to access one main computer, speed does matter. After the students had left school for the day, I would continue deleting old files, check and repair loose wires or clean the computers. Once a week I would back up all the students' work and on a few occasions the value of this process asserted itself because it was necessary to retrieve information from back-up disks.

Another part of my job was to input all the books in the school library onto a database. It was the beginning of the barcode system that is now used at libraries. This took a very long time because I had to input the title, author, fiction or non-fiction, what year it was published and key words of each book. I admit that I did struggle to read the barcodes but I managed somehow. Networking was something else that I learned to do. I used to assist another floating technician who worked in many schools. He would stay in each school for a few hours to sort out any troubleshooting problems that we couldn't deal with. I watched and studied him closely and soon learned his job. I used to drill holes in walls and set cables through them to connect more computers together, this is networking. I also struggled with this part too. Sometimes I would find it difficult to find the holes that I had previously drilled. The end of my working day seemed to come quickly. I was kept busy and the days just flew by.

CHAPTER 4
THE ART OF GUESSING

About three times a week I headed to the Rugby Leisure Centre for my regular Martial Arts training. I'd been doing Martial Arts for five years and I trained about three times a week at this local class. I pursued several different sports and hobbies, including weight training and roller-skating, but Martial Arts was my favourite. I practised a lot at home, where I would train at least five times a week for about an hour each time. My life revolved around my training to which I gave serious dedication. During this period I was training to become a black belt and I was just one belt away from achieving that.

I originally started when I was sixteen years old. My friend John was already a black belt in Wing-Chun Kung-Fu and was teaching me regularly. He also taught me how to use a weapon called a nunchaku and I must say that he was very fast. When he was spinning them around his body he would go so fast that you would struggle to see them – he could use two just like the great legend, Bruce Lee. He'd taught me a few times after college before he said that I needed to train more regularly and advised me to join a club. He encouraged me to learn in a local Martial Arts School, but there were no Wing-Chun schools at this time so we went around to have a look at a few different schools. The best one we saw was the Tae Kwon Do School called the R.I.F.F.S. It was a large class with quite a few black belts so I enrolled. At my first lesson I had to fight some of the black belts because I had a big build (I wish), but that didn't help. After applying all the techniques that John had taught me, I was beaten to the ground. That was when I made my first goal and decided that I too would become a black belt one day to be able to beat someone else, and to beat that black belt who had battered me!

During the class, while I was warming up, I remembered an interesting episode that had happened to me a year or so before.

When I was a blue belt I entered a competition with several other fellow students. After winning a few fights, I was observing the techniques of other competitors in my group when an instructor came to speak to me. I was sitting on the floor minding my own business when he approached me and said, "Do you see that guy over there?"

"Yes mate, why?" I answered as I weighed him up.

"Well, he's a kickboxing champion and you've got him next," he bellowed confidently.

As I looked over at him I started to prepare a plan of attack. Unfortunately for this guy I was trained to fight full contact and this fight was semi-contact, so I thought about hitting him a little harder. He was a heavyweight with quite a big stomach so I knew it was going to be a hard-hitting fight. Trying to be tactical, I left it to the last moment to stretch off so that he could not work out how I would fight. This is a common strategy at competitions to see what techniques people were good at.

The time finally came for the big fight so I took my glasses off. The world was again a strange place through my eyes without my glasses on, but I could work out what the blurred images would have been if they had been in focus. It also helped that there were no bits missing off the people who I could see. Through my eyes without my glasses people still had a head with eyes, nose and mouth. It was no longer clear and focussed but I could still see them. Their eyes were there, but the detail of eye colour, eye lashes and the whites of their eyes had disappeared. Their nose was there, but all skin blemishes had faded away. Lips looked like a solid block of colour but the indentations were gone. I could distinguish hair from face and ear; what I couldn't see was the individual strands of hair or inner ridges of their ears. The only time I could see facial hair was when they had a full-blown beard. I could see that they had a Martial Arts suit on, but I could no longer see the badges or separation between their suits and their skin, unless they were of dark complexion. Each set of pads that they had to wear had a logo on, but without my glasses the logo had also faded away. It really was like living in a magical world where objects would disappear then reappear when I placed my glasses back on. The images that I saw were blurred, but I somehow worked out what they would be if they were clear and in focus.

We bowed to each other and the fight began. I bounced around for a while like a boxer, blocking most of his techniques. He rushed in with his fists and punched my body every time I dropped my guard to perform a kicking technique. Unluckily for him, after about a minute of fighting I felt that I had already worked him out. It was time for me to prepare to attack. I dropped my guard on purpose and waited eagerly. My best leg was in front and itching to be used. The time came quite quickly as he began to move forward. He rushed forwards to punch me a few times. I leaned back and put all my weight on my right leg, then picking up my left leg as fast as I could, I thrust it out straight into his stomach. My body was facing to the side as I hit him with a side kick that sunk into his bulk before lifting him off the floor. He seemed to almost fly as he eventually fell to the mat on his back. He had to take a few seconds out to compose himself before continuing the match. He then backed off for the rest of the fight as he attempted to regain his breath, but I continued to attack, not giving him a chance. First, switching legs quickly I performed a turning kick and spun around to do a reverse turning kick, which landed on the side of his head. He came in straight away and we exchanged a few punches before he continued to back off. After I repeated the same kicking techniques, I timed another side kick to his stomach that caught him perfectly as he tried to move in. Although I couldn't see his fingers or eyes without my glasses, I had no problem seeing his arms, legs and big stomach. He came back in with a series of kicks and I moved back and then timed a back kick to his chest. We were into the last few seconds so I pressured him once again with a series of hop side kicks to his chest. This forced him to put his guard down and just at the right time I lifted my leg high to give him a hop side kick to his face. The whistle went and the match was over. I knew that I had won and the judges gave the right decision. There were four judges sitting at the corners of the ring, each with a white and a red ribbon in their hands. They lifted their arm up with the appropriately coloured ribbon that the winner had on the back of his belt. They were a little too blurred for me and I could not quite see them so I looked to the floor and waited for them to raise my arm of course!

 The next round was the semi-final and unfortunately I was against one of my fellow students. Looking around at the other competitors I felt that I had a great chance of winning the following fight. My problem was my fellow student.

 "Should I let him win?" I thought.

I knew that I could beat him; he was not as strong as me, so I decided to let him win. "You better win the final or I'll never give you another chance again," I told him.

"Yes, I'll win," he replied.

So I purposely lost the fight against him, but I easily won my next fight for third place. He did go on to win the final so we were both happy with the results and our instructor was ecstatic.

I returned my attention to the class. The warm-up was over and my instructor asked me to take part of the class. This was standard procedure when you get to my level so by now I felt comfortable teaching them. My progression from the beginners row at the back of the class to the front row, right next to the black belts seemed quite quick, and there I was, teaching. There were about ten lower grades to teach. They would copy the techniques I was showing them and then I would look at their posture to make sure they were following correctly. I would observe their hand positions, wrist angles, whether or not they had their thumbs outside their fists and if they had their fists on their hips. It was important to see the exact position of a student on every move. The students would then punch and it was my job to check whether their two big knuckles were positioned correctly. It's important that they punch with two of their knuckles and not all five or they would not be able to generate their power to its full potential. It was also important to see whether their hands were clenched tight or not. The students would then perform a series of kicks and, as their teacher, I had to check that their feet were positioned correctly so as not to damage their feet or toes. To be able to see students clearly was very important especially when they performed the patterns. After about half an hour my instructor relieved me from my duty and said that it was now my turn to be taught.

In just a few weeks I would be taking my black belt grading exam and my instructor wanted to go through a few important sections that he thought I needed to improve. Although I felt confident, I trusted the experience of my instructor. The first section was self-defence. He told me that my timing was slightly slow when I took my glasses off. After explaining my difficulty focussing without my glasses and that I had recently been registered as partially sighted, he told me to work even harder to perfect the skill of being able to recognise unfocused images quickly and accurately. I had a great respect for my instructor, Shahid Yusaf, so I followed his guidance. He told me to use my mind as well as my eyes. Over and over I would go through the same moves trying to improve my timing to a speed and accuracy that was acceptable. Without my glasses the images I could see became a multitude of intertwined contrasts. It was difficult and very frustrating, but I had to do it if I was to be allowed to go for my black belt. It wasn't easy with my glasses *on*, so now that they were removed it was very difficult indeed. My instructor was happy with my standard when I was wearing my glasses, but he said that if they were accidentally knocked off, I had to be able to defend myself confidently without them.

At last I found a technique that worked. Instead of concentrating on trying to focus on their fingers or the knife in their hand, I had to judge where they would be from the ends of their sleeves that I could just about see – the knives were almost invisible to me. Next I had to do the same thing with their feet and toes. It was easy to see the different sizes of feet with my glasses on, but without them it was almost like looking at an empty suit. The way that I conquered my problems was by guessing. If I thought that someone had a knife in their hand, I would assume that it was quite long and block accordingly. When my instructor was happy he moved me onto the next section, which was breaking boards.

He concentrated on reverse techniques, which are techniques executed after turning around. He told me that my problem was that I appeared to delay for a split second before attempting to break the board. The crux was that I only had a split second to break a board especially when I jumped off the ground. After feeling frustrated by my failed attempts I felt that I was again at a crossroad where I could admit defeat and remain at this grade, or keep trying until I was finally able to move onto the next belt. That split second delay while I was attempting to refocus on the board made my accuracy look poor. The kick that I struggled with the most was my jump back kicks. After jumping off the ground and turning in the air, I looked for the board, but after I saw it I was too late to execute a kick.

"I can't believe it, I missed it again," I muttered in frustration.

"How badly do you want this black belt?" I asked myself. "The black belt doesn't mean anything. I just can't focus quickly enough," I argued silently.

"This is embarrassing; I'm going to give up. Nobody can do everything so it's time to admit defeat and quit."

Then I remembered what had happened two years ago when I failed my blue belt grading exam. At that stage breaking had only just been introduced so it was not a major part of the exam. It was clear to my instructor that I was very confident with most of my techniques, but needed to work on breaking. At that grade I wouldn't say that I was confident, cocky is the word that I would use to describe me! During the practice session before my grading exam I thought confidently; "My techniques are good enough, who cares about breaking? Everything else that I need is as good as everyone else so there's no chance that he can fail us all. I'll help the others."

My instructor was looking over, but he never said anything to me. All the other blue belts were practising hard, concentrating on trying to improve their moves just that little bit more and there I was helping some lower grades. I was so confident (cocky!) that I even helped a few higher grades brush-up a few of their techniques. That day, I don't think that I practised at all.

"Why do I need to practise when I know everything already?" I thought again.

Soon it was my turn to perform and in most sections I did well. When it came to my breaking I missed quite a few and on some occasions I didn't even try and my accuracy was very poor.

"Missed another board?" I thought to myself. "It shouldn't matter because I still did as well as those other blue belts there."

In our next lesson after the exam my instructor read out the results of all the different belts.

"Peter, you've passed... congratulations," he said. "Andrew and Donna have also passed."

"Well at least I know that I've passed now because I performed better than them," I boasted confidently to myself.

"Vendon... sorry but you failed."

"Did I just hear that I failed?" I cried to my instructor.

"Sorry, but yes, you did fail," he repeated. "Can you see me after the lesson so that I can explain your result to you in private?"

"Yes... sir," I mumbled.

After the lesson my instructor took me to a quiet corner and explained his decision to me. Most of the other students had gone and only a few keen ones remained to do a little more work.

"Do you know the real reason why I failed you?" he asked.

"No sir," I replied courteously.

"You have amazing potential and could have performed much better, do you agree?"

"Yes sir."

"I failed you because you showed me a lack of effort. You're quite capable of doing much better than the others, but they tried as hard as they could. You are instructor material, would you agree?" he continued.

"Yes sir."

I respected my instructor too much to argue with his decision so I kept quiet, but I felt like a failure and wanted to quit. I couldn't help thinking about what he had said.

"Me… an instructor?" I thought.

This was the first time I had ever thought about being an instructor. When I started, all I had wanted was my black belt; that was my only goal. That was my only goal – until now. After a while of arguing with myself over the decision, I finally agreed and knew that I could have done much better so rather than quit after three years, I chose to continue.

For the next few months it was hard living with a failure under my belt, but it was probably the best thing that could have happened to me. It inspired me to do better and I never repeated that attitude again. At the next grading exam, I put in so much effort that I jumped two belts higher. This is called a double grade and only the elite achieve them. Few people carry on when faced with a tough situation because it's easy to quit, but hard to succeed. Failure is hard to accept, but I was determined now, because I had a new goal. I was determined to become an instructor.

Now here I was, a year or two later, being assessed for my black belt and one of the techniques that I was struggling with was the breaking. It was only a small part, but it felt like so much. I was struggling with the back kick and the jump back kick, and both these two techniques are very fast and need split second decisions.

"I just can't do it," I muttered. "I've been doing the same technique for ages. Maybe it's time to admit defeat."

After remembering that I wanted my black belt to open my own class and become an instructor, I became more determined to succeed. It took a while and several poor attempts, but my breaking improved dramatically. By repeating the same techniques over and over again I became very accurate at board breaking and very good at guessing.

When I broke a board with a reverse technique I concentrated very hard and then turned and kicked without looking. The technique that I guessed the most on was the jump reverse back kick. That technique has now become my best and I'm well known for that kick. Guessing is also something that I have incorporated into my fighting to improve my timing.

Once the lesson was over the instructor asked the people who were going to take their black belts to stay behind for some extra tuition. Over the previous few months he had been concentrating on a great deal of breaking techniques using our hands. We were about to find out why he had been so determined to toughen up our hands. He pulled several bricks out of his bag of tricks. They were real house bricks. He got down on his knees and started to set them up; one brick on its side on the left and one on the right with another one suspended in the middle like a bridge. This last brick had the flat part on top. He measured a few times while concentrating very hard. His arm slowly touched the brick and then he brought it right up high into the air only to repeat his actions. When he was confident he swung his arm high and then in a fast swoop chopped the brick with the outside of his hand between his little finger and wrist. The brick smashed in two and then he said; "And now it's your turn."

One by one we took turns at smashing the brick. There were five of us being assessed and I was the third one to have a go. They all took several attempts but eventually they broke it to pieces. Then it was my turn.

The bricks were placed before me in a pile of mess. Trying to be smart I decided to use one of the side bricks from the previous person's attempt as the one that I would break. It had been crushed by the other bricks so I was hoping that it had been weakened. I knelt down and began to set the bricks up. When I had placed the bridge brick on top I began to slide the other two further apart. The bricks slid slightly too far apart and the bridge brick that I was going to break fell.

"How embarrassing," I muttered to myself.

"Concentrate and try again."

The bricks were set up again and I had put the other two bricks as far apart as I could without making the central one fall.

"The wider apart they are, the less power needed to break it," I thought as I sat there meditating.

The time had come to start measuring so I put my right hand onto the centre of the brick. Then I made sure that the knife-edge of my hand was on the brick as though I was going to chop it. At this point I curled my four fingers slightly and touched my thumb against them. This made my hand hard and firm enough so that when I finally did try to break the brick, my fingers wouldn't clash together, as that could quite easily cause my fingers to be damaged. With my hand on the brick I just sat there. It felt a little uncomfortable so I picked my left leg up and put the sole of my foot on the floor. This felt much more comfortable and it also felt like I could generate more power from this position.

"Take your time," my instructor hinted.

My hand was back on the brick and I proceeded to bring my right hand up high and then straight back down. My left hand was touching the brick to stop it from moving when I repeatedly touched it.

"Concentrate," I said to myself as I began breathing more heavily.

I had touched the brick several times now and I knew that it was time to break it. After placing my hand on the brick for the last time I paused… and then I brought my hand up high and down again to hit the brick with a thud. It had not broken and my hand began to tingle.

"I don't believe it," I thought in disappointment.

The brick had not broken and it was there, just staring at me.

"Well, I think I chose the wrong brick," I muttered.

"Would you like to try again?" my instructor asked.

"Sir!" I shouted as I checked the position of the bricks.

The bricks were set up and I prepared for my second strike.

"Is your hand hurting?" my instructor asked.

"Just a bit sir," I replied.

"Then break it this time and it won't hurt," suggested my instructor.

"I *will* break it this time sir," I cried in determination.

This time I swung my hand in a slight circular action like you would use to chop a tree with an axe. It felt a bit uncomfortable for a while, but then I got used to it. My concentration was back.

"Concentrate," I repeated several times.

"This feels good. You can do it, go for it!" I finally thought as I paused on the brick.

With an almighty thud and a shout I had hit the brick, but I didn't feel much pain. When I looked down the brick was lying in two. I had broken a brick for the first time and was now ready to take my black belt exam.

CHAPTER 5
DRIVING ME CRAZY

It was a fine Sunday morning. The sun was out and I was ready for my first lesson on how to drive a car. I had received my provisional driving licence and I was eager to get in a car and actually drive. My friend John was outside in his car ready and waiting for me to get in and go. This was my biggest goal and I had to prove that I could do it. The previous day, on the way to the shop, I began to read car number plates. It was easy so I kept trying to read them further and further away. The letters on the number plates seemed clear.

"My eyesight is fine!" I thought. "Maybe I'll try that blue car over there."

So I blinked a few times to clear my eyes and I proceeded to read the number plate. That seemed fine too.

"Now to find one that is twenty seven point five feet away. That's what I was told is the given distance required to drive."

As I walked I saw a parked car that looked like it was far enough away.

"That looks like the correct distance," I thought.

It was too far and the number plate was out of focus. Again I tried and strained as I attempted to read it once more.

"Maybe I should take a few steps forward because I think that must be too far," I thought cunningly.

As I stepped forward and closer to the car I kept trying to read it, but I was still struggling. I took several more steps, several large steps! Maybe five or so, but I could read it now. Things were looking good and I was happy with my accomplishments, even though deep down I knew that I was a little too close. I then rushed home from the shop full of excitement and ready for my big day.

John stood there waiting for me as I confidently walked out of my house.

"Are you ready?" he asked.

"I was born ready," I replied.

He drove a red Ford Fiesta, which is a small car. We sat in it for a while as he asked me a few questions from the Highway Code book.

I'd been reading it for quite some time and answering questions from it so I was pretty successful with his quiz. He was happy that I had got most of the questions right so he began to explain what some of the things in the car were.

I looked around and recognised that I could see most things, but they were not very clear. There appeared to be lots of small drawings everywhere on the dashboard and on the levers on the steering wheel. The buttons on the dashboard were visible but hard to make out.

"How can you see those buttons on the radio?" I asked.

"It's easy, can't you see them?" he asked.

"Yes of course," I replied sarcastically.

"Here are the lights: full beam, dipped and off. Can you see the different pictures?" he asked.

As I looked I wondered why anyone would want to draw silly little pictures on the levers that people would find hard to read, but I was just trying to fool myself. As I looked around at other blurred drawings a part of me knew that I was wrong to continue, but the time had not come for me to give up on my dreams and hopes of driving. It meant too much to me.

"The pictures are a bit confusing and a little hard to see," I admitted.

"They are a bit confusing, but you'll get used to them," he replied.

He had not picked up on my careful choice of words. John was referring to the quality of the pictures and had failed to realise that I was struggling to see them.

He continued to question me. "Next is the speedometer. Its use is a bit obvious, but you also have a small dial that shows your miles; can you see it?"

As I looked in the direction he was referring to I saw the dial but could not read it. He would soon want me to respond so I had to think quickly.

"Yes, yes, there are too many numbers. Let's just drive!" I replied craftily.

"I just want to go through a few more things then we can go," he answered.

"Down there are three pedals, one for accelerating, one for braking and the third is called a clutch, do you see them?"

"It's a bit dark, but yes, I can see them," I replied.

"Well an easy way to remember them is A… B… C… from right to left; does that make any sense?"

"It does and I knew that already because I've being going over it in my head," I replied.

"These are your mirrors; can you see the cars in them?"

"They look a bit small," I answered.

"You get used to it," he responded.

What I saw in the mirror was very different to what John saw. To me, the images were smaller, less detailed and slightly out of focus, but I still wanted to drive. I must have been crazy to carry on despite the difficulties I was experiencing and, to my ignorance, it was also dangerous to others. For a few moments I sat and watched as cars and bikes came past, reflected in the mirrors. Most of the time I could hear them before I saw them. They only appeared for a few seconds before passing our car so I knew I had to time things right. I continued watching until I had finally figured out the timing. With such little vision through the mirrors I had still learnt how to estimate the time it took a car to pass after I had seen it in the mirror.

The next thing he taught me was all about the gears. Again I had strange thoughts about the pictures on the gear stick.

"Some more drawings that are not clear," I thought to myself. "This is going to be hard. I'll have to memorise those too."

At last the basics were over and he stopped asking me questions. He was happy with my progress so he told me that it was now time to drive.

"I'll drive to a more quiet and safe area and then you can have a go," he said.

We set off to his designated area while I watched his actions of driving carefully. Finally we were there and he stopped the car. He then jumped out and we swapped seats. The adrenaline started pumping straight away. The suspense was killing me. Had the moment that I had been waiting for finally come? Would my dream of learning to drive actually come true? John went through his entire checklist again while I sat there with my seat belt on in the driving seat.

"This is so exciting," I thought to myself. "At long last my hopes and dreams of driving will finally come true."

I sat there looking through the mirrors and studied the timing of the cars passing once more. I was really struggling to get used to it.

"The cars really do look small," I thought.

Fear entered my mind and I began to have second thoughts.

"This is too hard; I'm very excited but also scared. Maybe I should tell him that everything seems a little hard to see."

"Are you ready?" he asked.

I thought for a few seconds, still contemplating whether or not I should risk driving under these conditions.

"I'm ready," I replied hesitantly.

The time had come and I started the car, the handbrake was on and I was in neutral. I pressed hard on the clutch and pushed the lever into the position of first gear. He told me to find the biting point and to check my mirrors, which I did without stalling the car.

"Tell me when you think that it's time to pull off," John said.

"It's clear," I replied as I looked through my mirrors.

"Not yet," he said, "there's a car coming."

"There isn't a car… oh yes there is; I see it now," I replied.

"I must be crazy to try this," I thought. "The cars are just not clear enough, but now that I've started I might as well go through with it."

I refused to let my poor eyesight get the better of my burning desire to drive and proceeded to try and drive.

"It's clear and I'm ready," I confirmed as I built myself up for the move off.

"Yup, it's clear, so you can go for it," he agreed.

I'd been practising the routine in my head for weeks and now here I was about to take my first driving lesson. The road looked clear so I signalled, found the biting point again then released the handbrake and we were off and on our way.

"I don't believe this, I'm actually driving," I thought.

"That's incredible; you didn't stall the car!" John bellowed. "You're in the middle of the road now; can you steer a little to your left?"

It didn't feel like I was in the middle of the road so I said; "Tell me when I'm where you want me."

"This is fine now," he said.

At that point I looked around in all directions to measure how high on the window the pavement was and at what part of the bonnet the white line met. I was guessing (again!), but I was driving. It felt very unsafe and dangerous. I needed things to be closer to be able to see them properly.

"Here comes a car from the opposite direction," I muttered as I began to panic.

The car came closer and closer and I drew more and more scared.

"Here goes; hold onto that steering wheel tight," I commanded myself.

I began to get frantic; I just wanted to jump out of the car and run and hide. I slowed right down as it approached us. If it was going to hit us I wanted to be going as slow as possible to minimize damage.

The car passed and I was still going! We had survived our first passing of another car. Feeling a little more confident, I began to speed up again.

"You're going a little too fast; slow down," John said.

"Tell me when I'm at the right speed then," I said as I slowed down.

John still hadn't realised that I couldn't see the speedometer. When we were going at the right speed I listened carefully to the engine noise. The faster we went the higher the pitch of the engine. When the pitch was consistent I knew, or guessed, that we were going at the right speed. It felt like too much hard work having to concentrate on driving *and* watching my position on the surroundings. I continued to guess my speed and position on the road.

"We're coming to a junction and you'll need to reduce your speed," he said.

"Where is it?" I asked.

"Just ahead; slow down."

I reduced my speed gradually, but it wasn't enough for John. He began to panic as he shouted at me to slow down once more. This made me panic too and I slammed the brakes on too hard. The car stopped just over the line. He told me to signal to go right.

"Well done, and you didn't stall it," he said.

"What did you think of that?" I asked boastfully.

"That was good, but now there's a car approaching us from the rear."

Whilst getting confused about what to do I stalled the car. Now it was my turn to panic as my nerves got the better of me. He helped me and put the hazard lights on and the car went around us. We didn't feel too bad because we had learning plates on.

Eventually I restarted the car and I was ready to move off. The only problem was seeing the oncoming traffic. The images of the cars were still too small and as I sat there I wondered if I should call it a day and give up. At this point I really had had enough of guessing.

"You can do it," my friend said encouragingly. "Go after this next car."

The car passed and I felt that it was too late to back out so I persisted and pulled away once more.

"Turn a little more," John said as he assisted me with the steering.

My eyes were darting everywhere. Sometimes it felt as if I was not looking straight ahead but concentrating on my side view. The cars coming from the right were hard to see and hard to hear. This was another problem I had to endure. Being deaf in my right ear, totally deaf from birth, I sometimes experienced difficulties. In many situations it doesn't affect me, but when noises come from the right I struggle.

We were straight and off down the next road. It felt very uncomfortable. I still felt like I was guessing too much and taking too much of a risk, but I just couldn't bring myself to give up. The car was slowly veering to the right again and into the middle of the road and straight towards an oncoming car. The worry of hitting this car head on was overpowering me because in the distance it looked like it was exactly in my target line. John kept touching the steering wheel to straighten me up, and advising me of my speed. It felt so easy to pick up speed and it happened so quickly. My heart began to race as the car drew closer and closer.

"I'm not sure about this," I thought hysterically. "It's not clear where the other car is. The pavement isn't clear, the white line isn't clear, everything is moving too fast and I really am struggling to focus quickly enough. I must be crazy," I concluded.

The car passed and we were still alive and I was lucky because there weren't many cars on the road. Then again, that was why John had brought me here.

"There's another road coming up and I want you to take the next right," John stated.

"Road!" I chuckled nervously. "I can't see any road."

"Stop messing around," he warned. "It's just there on your right. Slow down!"

"How can he see the road from so far away? Something is definitely wrong," I thought as I looked once more for the road. "Well I'd better slow down anyway until I can see it."

After a few more seconds I said; "There it is. I can see the road now." His eyesight must have been amazing to be able to see so far away.

I struggled to find the indicator to signal right as I came to a stop. Eventually I took the right turn. There were no cars coming and I was extremely glad because I went slightly onto the wrong side of the road and if there had been a car waiting to come out of the junction, I would have hit it.

The road dipped slightly and then went back up again, and our car began to go too fast again. He slowed me down and told me to use my mirrors more.

"What's the point?" I thought to myself. "I can't see much in them anyway but I'm not going to tell him that!"

"These mirrors make things too small," I complained.

"They're not that small to me," he remarked. "Stop over there."

I stopped the car but forgot about the clutch and stalled it once more.

"That wasn't too bad but you're parked a bit too wide. Now I want you to do a three point turn," he said.

Looking through the mirrors didn't seem to help so I looked for cars through the windscreen.

"How far am I supposed to turn the steering wheel?" I asked as I began to panic.

He told me and I began my manoeuvre. The road was clear and it seemed like I had plenty of time but as I drove forward and hit the kerb and came to a stop, a car seemed to appear from nowhere. John waved them past and proceeded to instruct me on how to reverse and turn the steering wheel at the same time.

"Which way is reverse?" I asked.

"Look at your gear stick, it tells you," he replied.

I looked… and I looked, but the drawing wasn't clear enough. I still couldn't see it.

"It's too hard to understand," I told him deceitfully.

He instructed me on the relevant direction and I began to reverse while turning the steering wheel, but I didn't have the foggiest how far to go. Everything seemed just out of focus and I wished that it was all closer to the car.

"My eyesight can't be that bad," I thought.

The back wheels hit the kerb and the car stopped.

"Come on, you can do it," John said encouragingly.

I turned the steering wheel the other way and began to turn again. Luckily for me the road that John had chosen was very wide so I managed to complete the turn.

"I don't believe it!" he said. "You did a three point turn first time! Now just stop over there and we'll swap seats and go back home. How did that feel?"

"Should I tell him that I was struggling to see?" I thought to myself. "Maybe there's more wrong with my eyes than I think. I felt like I was going to crash into those cars. Maybe I should get my eyesight checked for the correct driving distance. Maybe I should change my glasses. I suppose I'd better answer him," I concluded.

"It felt great," I said.

"You were quite good for your first time," he complimented. "You should learn to drive with a qualified driving instructor. Would you like that?"

I took a few seconds to answer as I went through the risks and dangers of not seeing clearly enough.

"This could be the best way to finally see if my sight is good enough to drive. I'd know if my calculated driving distance was too far. I have a burning passion to drive so I have to go through with this," I thought to myself.

"Well I might as well learn," I answered.

He drove us home and helped me look for a driving school. He decided on one and we phoned to make an appointment. A few days later I heard a knock on my door and it was the driving instructor.

"This is the real thing," I thought to myself.

I was very excited as I followed him to his car. We sat in there and settled ourselves on the seats and I got ready to go. I buckled my seat belt and waited for him to drive off. The adrenaline was rushing around inside my body and I was almost sick with the excitement.

"This is it! I'm really going to learn to drive. Finally my dreams are going to come true. I'm going to be so lucky being able to drive and go anywhere I want at any time. At last I'm going to own my own car. How cool!" I continued to think. "Let's go! I want to show this instructor how good I am already."

I was ecstatic; over the moon; on cloud nine; this is the moment I had been waiting for.

"Can you read that number plate over there please?" he asked.

"That car all the way over there?" I said as I looked into the distance.

"That red one in front," he replied.

As I looked at the car and tried to focus on the number plate I was astonished that he actually wanted me to read it.

"Are you sure you want that one there?" I asked.

I tried and I tried, but I was struggling to focus on the *car* and the number plate was virtually non-existent through my eyes. It was incredible to finally realise what people who are allowed to drive can see. The car was so far away and so small in my eyes that I was speechless. There was no chance that I could focus on that number plate. It would have been impossible to guess the number so I had no choice but to tell the truth.

"That's two or three times further than I can see. There's no point carrying on. If you're really talking about that car in the distance, then I can't read the plate," I replied despondently.

"Sorry, but if you can't read it then we cannot proceed with this driving lesson. Are you sure that they're up-to-date glasses that you're wearing? The right prescription?"

"They are," I answered.

"Well I can see much further than that car; that's just the minimum distance," he replied.

He left me there on the spot, outside my house. The driving lesson was over before it had started.

"Well, I guess I can't see far enough to drive," I thought sadly. "How embarrassing to be left on my own doorstep. My eyesight must be worse than I thought. I'm never going to be able to learn to drive."

The moment was very emotional and I felt tearful as I thought, "There go my hopes and dreams of ever being able to drive."

CHAPTER 6
LET THE FIGHT BEGIN

I went to the local gym three times a week to do weight training with three other people. I also attended my Martial Arts class three times per week and trained myself at home five times per week. Sport was my number one priority. It was more important than women! When I get serious about something I like to give it my best shot so you could say that I was seriously dedicated to my sports.

At home I would sometimes find anything to use as weights, like picking up a bag of sugar over and over again to build up my biceps. Tins of baked beans and even a chair would also have their uses. I slept, ate and thought fitness. A simple walk down the road would turn out to be a warm-up zone for me. I would regularly jump and kick lamp posts, bus shelter roofs and tree branches. I could easily jump and kick leaves on trees up to eight and a half feet off the ground. My black belt exam was approaching fast and I had to practise whenever I could.

A typical day of exercise for me would be:

- Before work – 15 minutes stretching, kicking, press-ups and sit-ups at home.
- Purposely lifting up chairs during my breaks at work.
- Performing Martial Arts patterns while waiting for my food to cook.
- Warm up for 15 minutes at home before going to a class.
- Take part in Martial Arts class for an hour.
- Go to the gym and have a late weight training session.
- Kick hundreds of times for half an hour before going to bed.

Conditioning my body was just as important as the Martial Arts itself because it had to be tough and ready for any punch that got past my defence. We lifted up some heavy weights to make us tougher and stronger, wearing a special weight lifting belt to support our backs from the strain.

The gym was quite small, about three metres by eight metres. We went to several gyms, but this was our local one that we used the most. It had an exercise bike, treadmill, shoulder press, multi-plex, chin-up bar, calf press, bench press and a bicep curl. There was only one of each piece of equipment apart from the sit-up benches, of which there were two. The gym was small but served its purpose. We usually worked in pairs taking turns at using the same machine and I usually paired off with John. He was fit and strong for his size and always pushed me hard – he was about three stones lighter than me.

We started with the exercise bike and the treadmill and used them for ten minutes each. We then took it in turns on the bicep curl while the other two swapped and began to use the bike and treadmill. We would do some light weights to warm-up then a few heavy sets. We were not interested in much light work or cardiovascular training. The pain of the heavy weights was part of our thrill – almost therapeutic I would say. We did four sets of ten curls and gradually increased the weights. They went up in five kilograms and we would start on thirty kilograms then end on seventy. The numbers are written clearly on the front of each weight.

"Put that weight on thirty please," John asked.

As I looked at the weights from where I was standing I couldn't manage to read the numbers so I moved my head closer and closer until I could see clearly. It felt like I was too close. I hadn't seen my friend bending forwards as much as I was – my head was less than two feet away. As I put the pin in the correct slot I asked John how far away he could stand and still read the numbers.

"It's time to compare what I see with others," I thought to myself. "Let's see how bad my eyes really are when looking at everyday things. I've been curious for a while so let's find out."

"I still can read them from over here," he said as he stood with his back touching the wall nearly three metres away.

"Are you serious?" I asked frantically.

"It's no problem; if the wall wasn't here I could go much further back," he replied.

I went and stood where he had been with my back against the wall and looked in amazement. Through my eyes it was impossible to make out that they were numbers – they didn't even look like numbers. They were not blurred but more like a white dot painted on each weight. As I stood there still staring at the vertical line of white dots I said; "Are you sure you can see that clear?"

He rejoined me at the wall. We both stood there looking around and comparing our eyesight.

"Can you see those three posters on the opposite wall?" he asked.

"Yes I can," I replied.

"Now tell me what the middle one says."

"I can only read the title. What can you read?"

"All of it including the words at the bottom," he confirmed as he began to read it out loud.

"What about the poster on the left?" he asked.

This time I looked long and hard and then finally gave my conclusion.

"There are nine squares but I can't make sense of the writing," I answered. "What do you see?"

"Yes, there are nine squares, but inside the squares are little drawings of the weight bench and machine and the different ways to use it and I can also see the little drawings clearly," he replied confidently.

My emotions started to get the better of me. Here I was trying to have a serious weight training session and I was now struggling to find the strength and confidence to carry on.

"Are my eyes really that bad?" I thought to myself. "It's amazing what John can see. I thought everyone could see what I saw but just a little clearer, but it's almost like there's another visual world out there. I thought that other people had to go a bit closer to posters to be able to read them. Now I know why they said that I'm partially sighted; and it might get worse! I wish I could see what John sees. All this time I've been fooling myself thinking that people see like me and that the doctors were referring to my eyesight without my glasses on."

It was obvious that I was in denial. Trying my hardest to come up with excuses to prove that my eyesight was better than it really was, but the only person I was fooling was myself.

"What about the third poster; what can you see?" I asked.

"I can read all of it; what about you?" he responded.

I paused for a few seconds while I wondered how he could see so much more than me. It was like blurred lines became words and empty spaces suddenly had things in them. It was almost magical, but scary.

"Nothing really; it's all out of focus, but I can see that there are words, I just can't make any of them out," I replied.

It felt like I had just lost a fight. The feelings I was now experiencing were all negative and very stressful. The thoughts continued and I struggled to ignore them, but I had to because they were making me feel more and more depressed.

"Why me?" I wondered to myself. "Why am I suffering like this? What have I done to get such poor eyesight? Are you punishing me God? I used to think that I could see quite clearly but now I'm aware that everything looks completely different to other people who can see clearly. I've been kind to others, so why do I have to suffer like this? Why can't I do what others do and see what others see?"

It felt like someone had taken away my most important ability and I struggled to fight off my emotions.

"Let's continue training," I said.

"Hang on. Look at that wall and tell me what you see," John said.

"It's blue; yes, it's painted light blue and it looks smooth," I answered.

"*Is* it smooth?" he countered.

"Yes, just a plain light blue wall," I replied.

"Why don't you look behind you and you'll see it much closer and clearer on that wall? The wall *is* blue, but it's not smooth; you can see the brickwork through it; you can see where each brick joins the next."

As I turned to have a closer look at the wall he said; "Can you see the bricks now?"

Looking at the wall it was now obvious that my vision was worse than I had imagined. Things looked totally different when I was close up. My face was less than a foot away from the wall and now I could see the details. Feeling so bad and useless, I was now looking to blame my disability on someone else and I began to slowly lose my faith in God.

"Why me God?" I asked my inner self.

As I looked around the room I continued to wonder what it really looked like. I was now feeling sorry for myself. Poor me, like I was the only one with problems. I felt more negative, disappointed and slightly angry at the world than ever before. With all this turmoil going on in my head I attempted to continue training.

"It's time for some sit-ups don't you think?" John said.

The long benches to do sit-ups had hooks at one end. We hooked them on the highest bar on the wall. We were crazy doing sit-ups in an almost vertical position. The strenuous exercise took my mind off the thought of my visual impairment. The pain of the sit-ups felt good, but the angle of the incline was hurting my back so I lay back on the bench. John carried on for a few more seconds before coming to a stop. We rested for a few minutes then continued with our second set of sit-ups. I only managed a few this time. The mixture of back pain and mental pain from not being able to accept the knowledge of the deterioration of my eyesight was upsetting my concentration. Then we put the bench angle lower to make the sit-ups easier and finished another two sets, then sat on the floor and began to stretch.

As I sat there I began to wonder what else I was missing out on.

"This carpet is grey isn't it?" I asked.

"Tell me about the pattern on the carpet," he replied.

"Well the carpet is plain grey and that's it isn't it?"

"No, sorry, but it isn't. You see, there are small bright grey squares on it and I can see almost every woven fibre from here. There are lots and lots of strands that make up the carpet; that's what I can see."

Here I was once again looking at something and admiring it in my own way only to find out that there are more details that I cannot see. Hidden from my view, hidden from my world. As I looked again I became almost fascinated by their world. Thinking to myself that I would give anything to be able to see like him, I looked at our images in the mirror and saw how plain we looked.

"Well at least I can still see us in the mirror," I muttered.

"Describe what you can see," he said.

"Us; our faces, noses and mouths. Your hair, your hands and your t-shirt."

"Describe what you see in more detail," he commanded as he leapt to his feet and began to smile. "Give me some more detail on everything you see in the mirror."

"Well, I can see that you're now smiling and I can see your teeth, but I can't see the separations between them. I see your eyes but I can't quite make out their colour. There's the door in the distance with four sections of plain glass and the exercise bike and sit-up bench. That will do; now what do you see?" I asked.

"I see what you see, but in much more detail. You appear to have a plain view of life. It sounds like you can see fine but you always miss out on the finer details. Like, you see my mouth and teeth; I see my mouth and each individual tooth, my gums and the odd shapes of each tooth. You see my eyes but I can clearly see that my eyes are brown and the centre is darker with some light reflection on part of them. I didn't hear you mention seeing my eyelashes and my eyelids. My face was plain to you, but I can also see my facial hair and each individual drop of sweat. When you said that you could see my t-shirt and trainers, well I can also make out the logo on my t-shirt and trainers, the little hole near the bottom of my t-shirt made from pinning keys to it and also with my trainers I can see the laces. The sit-up benches are there but you failed to mention the individual bars to the side. With the door you saw the four sections of glass but I can also see the little squares in the glass. The wood grain and the keyhole are also visible. I bet you see my fingers but can't see my finger nails."

"No, I can barely see your hands," I replied.

"Can he really see that much more than me? I can't believe my eyesight is that bad. I can hardly see the door in this mirror so how can he see the keyhole so clearly? I can't believe that he can see so much. It all looks so small and dark." The thoughts ran riot in my mind.

It was only a matter of time before I realised that I had been living under false pretences. I'd been hiding from finding out the truth, but with the constant deterioration of my eyesight, it would happen sooner or later. Deep down I knew the truth. Call it an inkling or whatever, but I had felt that there was more wrong with my eyesight than just my short sightedness for a few years. I think the first time I came to this realisation was when I left school and attended college. We had to solder some capacitors onto electronic boards. At first I thought that it was colour blindness because I got a few colours mixed up, but when I saw the colours in bigger bolder objects I managed fine. I wore my glasses, so I thought that either the opticians had incorrectly prescribed the lenses or there was something else wrong with my eyesight. As a teenager I dismissed that theory and tried to cope. At night I was known to be clumsy – I would occasionally bump into things or knock things over but I kept telling myself that many people are clumsy.

When I was at school I put it all down to my very thick glasses. They were about one centimetre thick. I used to struggle with reading. During our English classes the teacher would pick one of us at random to read. We had to stand by her desk with our book on her table so that she could follow it too. For me, trying to read from that distance was difficult. The words appeared to be too small and jumped around the pages. Sometimes words would appear almost from nowhere. When I complained to my teacher she said that I just wasn't very good at reading.

When I sat at the back of a classroom to copy work from the blackboard there was nothing to see. I would still struggle when I was sitting right at the front. Once I remember playing cricket and running after the ball. I remember having to concentrate very hard to keep my eye on the ball, but on this occasion the ball disappeared right before my eyes. When you're young you wouldn't even contemplate that you might have blind spots; no, it was always because I was short-sighted. Well, that's what I thought.

John had opened my eyes to the real world and it is magnificent, or that's what I would think if I had one more chance to see it. The time had come for me to face the truth and learn to deal with my disability. I felt very sad on the inside but continued to hide it and proceeded with our training.

My favourite piece of equipment was the next to use – the bench press. You have to lie down on the bench and push up a bar with weights attached to it. My partner went first and he put the weight on sixty kilograms to warm-up with. Then it was my turn and I wanted to put it on eighty kilograms to warm-up. I took out the pin and looked for the number but once again I had to go really close to be able to read it. My concentration slipped and I began to wonder why I had to go so close. I began to feel a little angry, but then I fought off the thoughts and renewed my concentration. We had finished the warm-up and it was my turn again to move the pin – this time to ninety kilograms. As I struggled to read the numbers I began fighting off the negative thoughts again. My last two sets were on a hundred kilograms, which is about fifteen and a half stones.

In my almost depressed state I managed to lift it up ten times and I noticed that while I was lifting I felt fine and could deal with my mixed emotions. It was mostly when I was doing something visually that I felt at my lowest. I realised that as long as I kept myself busy I felt less insecure.

"Maybe I should just lock myself away," I thought. "I don't seem emotionally disturbed when I do nothing or when I'm busy. Maybe that's why many visually impaired people choose to become a recluse. Should I stay at home or should I fight this continuous depressive state?"

It was very tempting to give up hope, but I chose to persevere and trained on.

Each time we changed equipment and I had to change the weight I felt the same. I kept questioning myself. It was difficult not to compare my visual abilities with others. I was jealous of what they could see. It felt like just a few short months ago I had been able to read the numbers on the weights with no problems, but I could now see and feel the deterioration.

We had nearly finished our training – the only piece of equipment left was the chin-up bar. This was a metal bar about seven feet off the floor. We had to slightly jump off the ground to reach it. It was literally just a bar and we did chin-ups with our palms facing inwards to work our biceps and outwards to work our triceps. We did wide ones and some with our fists touching. My whole body felt tense from all the different exercises I had performed.

After we had finished and stretched off we began to show off and perform some amazing kicks, trying to out rank each other. On a day-to-day basis I would kick hundreds of times with both legs. John then astounded us by jumping back on the chin-up bar and then turning himself upside down so that his feet were perched on the bar. With his hands now dangling near the ground and upside down in a vertical position, he proceeded to perform a series of sit-ups, touching his knees with his head each time. Then he froze in that position, holding his chin firmly against his knees for a prolonged period of time. We looked at each other to see if anyone else wanted to try it. My weight was fifteen stones and I considered that as heavy; so I opted against trying it for fear of damaging my ankles (well that's my excuse). We then set on our way down the stairs.

On the way out of the gym we were fairly quiet so I observed my surroundings. I decided to get that little bit closer to objects like the wall on the way downstairs. At close range I could now see that the bricks were not smooth even though that's what they looked like from my usual distance. They had lots of indents and fault spots. The mortar between the bricks was more visible and didn't have a consistent colour. The clear glass door that I had seen for years as just plain clear glass was now made up of hundreds of tiny squares and I could now see the keyhole. It was as if the glass has taken on a new appearance.

There was a large plant pot downstairs with a bushy plant in it so I walked up to it and peered at the leaves. They were green and fairly irregular in shape with a slightly glossy surface. I was now intrigued by the appearance and detail of everyday things that others take for granted. It was important to me to see the clearer world since I didn't know for how much longer I would have the opportunity. The gift of sight could be taken away from me any day; tomorrow even. I realised that as each morning came I would wonder if that would be the day – that was how my life was going to be. I knew that there was a growing possibility that I could go blind at any time and all I could do was wait. Suddenly everything I saw was of vital importance.

"I want to see a leaf really close," I said to myself as I plucked one off the plant.

It was like magic. A plain green leaf slowly began to look like it had more life. The closer I got to the leaf the more detailed it became. My face was now almost touching it and what I saw fascinated me. The leaf had tiny lines like on the palms of my hands. I wouldn't usually get this close to objects but now I wanted to learn a great deal more about what things really looked like, I wanted to study every detail.

"What are you doing?" one of my friend asked.

"I'm taking a closer look at things to see what they really look like," I replied.

"What for? You're not missing anything!" he remarked sarcastically.

My emotions changed from being overwhelmed to anger and almost hatred. Here was someone with the ability to admire flowers, plants, people, creatures and photos and he was taking it all for granted. He had no appreciation of the gift that had been bestowed upon him.

"Doesn't he realise how quickly it could all be taken away from him? Doesn't he realise how lucky he is? I would give any amount of money to be able to see what he sees. How selfish and inconsiderate he is. Didn't he stop to think how a simple statement like that could affect me?"

My temper began to boil. I now had no consideration for *his* feelings either.

"If you had a visual impairment like mine, if you were partially sighted, if you didn't know how long you would be able to see things in their true beauty, maybe you would appreciate things more and stop taking your eyesight for granted," I shouted angrily.

He never replied to that and continued on his way out.

We passed a notice board and I stopped to observe the different sizes of prints and tried to read the various posters. I was able to read less than half the posters because most of the text was too small. The only reason I could read some of them was because I was less than a foot away. The photos seemed more appealing. Some posters looked like they were just pictures and I became a little confused as to what they were trying to advertise. I would normally just walk along and ignore this kind of advertisement but I was now more interested in finding out what things really were. I wanted to know what I was missing.

"What is this advertising?" I asked another friend.

He stopped in his tracks and took a look. He stood a few feet behind me and too far away from the notice board for me to be able to read anything. He asked me to point to the one I wanted more information about so I did.

"That's advertising wrestling," he told me.

"What colour is the writing?"

"It's red on a black background but it's quite big so I thought that maybe you'd still be able to see it."

"Obviously not," I replied in disgust.

As I stood there looking at the blank black poster I began to think. "Your eyesight is worse than you realise. To me that poster hasn't got any text, yet it's so clear to others. He said the words were quite big so why can't I see them? The words are apparently written in red on a dark background. If the words are big and bold enough to see, then maybe I struggle with the dark more than I realise."

More thoughts entered my mind one after another. "Why am I suffering so much? Why me? Why can't I see the writing if it's so plain and obvious? What else am I missing? I admire wresting and would have liked to read it for myself so why should I have to ask someone else to read it for me? It feels like I can't see and can't read. I'm still young so how am I going to manage the embarrassment of having to rely on others? I feel disabled and hopeless."

As we walked out one of my friends asked me if I was feeling ill because of the expressions on my face.

"Do my thoughts shine through the expression on my face?" I wondered. "Is it that obvious that I'm dissatisfied with myself? Have I made it that obvious? What's happening to me? People don't really want to know how I am. They'd think that I'm going mad if they knew what I'm thinking. They all have their own problems and don't need mine on top. He can't help me anyway unless he has a pair of eyes to lend me."

My head was beginning to hurt and I felt like I was getting a headache from all these thoughts but I knew I had to answer him.

"I'm fine thanks," I replied.

It was amazing that I had so many thoughts rushing around in my head yet that was my reply.

"I will never trust anyone who says that they're fine ever again," I thought to myself.

"Should we have a night out? I bet that would cheer you up," he suggested.

"I think I do need a bit of cheering up at the moment," I replied. "I feel like some changes are about to happen in my life and I need to switch off from thinking about them."

Suddenly I heard my name called in the distance.

"Hello there Vendon, and what are you doing here at the Sports Centre?" a sweet voice said.

She sounded familiar but her image was still out of focus. As she walked closer, maybe six metres or so away from me, I recognised her by sight. It was Doreen and she brought the smile back to my miserable face. As we chit-chatted for a few tender moments, I purposely stood a little closer to her but not for long because I was now in her comfort zone and I didn't want to make her feel awkward. I just wanted to see if she was any different when I was closer and could see her in more detail. My smile grew much bigger as I drew closer and closer.

"She is more beautiful than I imagined," I concluded as I took another peek at her face.

Then I stepped back to my original position as we carried on chatting. She was so clear and so cute!

"So I *am* missing out on something," I thought as we parted company. "How pretty is she? There's a separate world out there – one that I don't get much chance to see. One that soon I'll no longer be able to see at all."

Then my mind drifted off her and back to me. Something else was beginning to trouble me.

"I'm sure something isn't quite right. Usually I would have been able to focus on people slightly further away, but she had to be really close for me to be able to recognise her. How much time have I got left until the lights in my eyes are switched off forever?"

My emotions began to get the better of me. I began to get scared of what could happen and I had no control over it.

"What can I think of to cheer myself up?" I wondered. "I feel fine as long as I'm thinking of something happy or if I'm busy."

The thoughts continued to battle within me until I remembered the planned night out.

"What I need is a drink! That will cheer me up and if it doesn't then it will send me into a deep sleep without the painful thoughts."

CHAPTER 7
CAN YOU SEE TO SKATE?

Every two weeks on a Saturday morning I took part at a local roller skating club. It felt important to work off some energy the morning before my big night out. I went to meet my friends Adam and Peter at the entrance to the skating rink, where people were already queuing up, waiting to be let in. As I looked around at the features of the crowd I was unable to recognise my two friends. I thought that I could pick out a few people who I knew but I wasn't sure that the blurred figures were my friends so I joined the queue and waited patiently. Many people queued up early because they wanted to get the best of the skates that were for hire. We never rushed to get there because we had purchased our own roller skates. My skates had a long black leather boot with yellow wheels and a soft yellow rubber stopper at the front. My wheels were supposed to be good quality and could continuously spin for over a minute. The rubber stopper was soft because this slows you down more rapidly. They were expensive skates and I expected them to perform well. We were so sad and childish that we used to have competitions on whose wheels could spin the longest. The hired skates had a harder rubber stopper and the wheels could only spin for a short while, so people who wore them couldn't go very fast and continually lost energy trying to keep a constant speed. They were also not balanced correctly so sometimes one skate would veer off in its own direction like it had a life of its own.

Skating was important to me, just like all the other sports that I was involved in. It strengthened the muscles in my legs to help me kick harder and was great at building up my stamina. My friends were late so I tried to find things to occupy myself. Reaching into my pockets I found some money and began to count out what was needed to enter the skating rink. Although they were not extremely clear, I was able to distinguish the difference between the coins. Clumsily I dropped a coin and struggled to find it. Searching long and hard I was unsuccessful. I began to panic, knowing that I would need it to be able to enter. It had disappeared right before my eyes.

"Where's it gone?" I thought to myself in embarrassment as I proceeded to turn my head this way and that way.

"It's there by your foot," said a voice kindly.

"Sorry, where?" I asked.

Someone waiting in the queue had tried to tell me where the money was but I still couldn't see it.

"It's right by your right foot; can't you see it?"

I thought for a split second, wondering whether I should disclose my disability and what words and phases to use.

"Should I tell her that I'm registered partially sighted? Or maybe tell her that I've got poor eyesight? Yes, that sounds more gentle and she'll notice by the thickness of my glasses. No, I need to get used to this feeling and tell her the truth."

I prepared myself to respond.

"No, sorry, but I'm partially sighted and can't see very well."

The person in the queue then helped me; she picked the coin up and placed it in my hand.

"Thanks," I replied.

Although I was very grateful, it made me feel extremely uncomfortable and inadequate. I could have coped if I really was just clumsy but now I had a disability I felt incompetent and useless. It felt demoralising and I began to get worried about the number of times I may need to ask for help.

"Are you telling me that I now have to ask for assistance with finding money? Will I need help every time I drop something small? This could be on a daily basis and that would really frustrate me."

Another voice called out to me. I couldn't see them yet and felt uncomfortable while waiting for them to appear.

"Didn't you see us? We were just over there," they said.

My close friends Hanna and Samantha came into view.

"Now I bet I'll have to tell them too!" I thought.

I braced myself.

"Sorry but I'm partially sighted now."

"What! You seem to see me most of the time and you appear to get around all right. I don't believe you," Hanna said.

"What's wrong?" Samantha asked.

"Well, for a long time I thought that I was extremely short-sighted, but now a doctor has told me that I have a serious eye disorder called RP and it may get worse."

"Is it the same thing as your brother?" Hanna asked.

"Yes, it seems so, but no one is sure."

"Can you see me?" Samantha asked.

"Yes."

"Can you see my eyes?" Hanna asked.

"Can you see my smile?" Samantha asked.

"Yes I can see you both."

"You seem fine to me," Hanna said.

"And me, you always see me so how can your eyes be that bad? Why not get a second opinion?" Samantha asked.

"It's quite easy to recognise you both, you talk a lot and once I hear your voices I then know who you are. I can see you but not in great detail. A few of your features are blurred but I can usually recognise *you* Samantha because, well… you were my girlfriend for a while so I've seen you real close! If you were a few metres away from me and you never spoke to me, then I probably wouldn't be able to identify you because I wouldn't be sure it was you. I actually didn't realise that I was using my hearing so much to know who people are."

"Well I'll look after you!" Samantha said as she gave me a cuddle.

It was about a year before when I had been dating Samantha. We only dated for about a month. We met at the skating hall and got to know each other pretty well. Peter told me that he thought Samantha liked me but I wasn't sure (typical man, walking around with my eyes closed!). She was a lovely girl with brown bushy hair and big sexy kissable lips; yes, I think it was her lips that I was first attracted to. I liked her too but was too shy to ask her out straight away.

One day on the way out of skating I stopped to have a private chat to her.

"Samantha, can I ask you something?" I asked nervously.

"Yes, what is it?"

"Well… if I was to ask you out what would you say?"

"Well, why don't you ask me and find out?" she replied.

I paused hesitantly as my heart began to beat hard.

"Samantha… will you go out with me?"

There was a big smile on her face.

"Yes, stupid, I was wondering when you'd ask me. I thought that I'd made it so obvious."

"I'm a man so you have to say it straight, stop playing games, we are a little thick you know!"

We hugged and I got to kiss those sexy lips. They tasted yummy! If I was ever hungry all I needed to do was suck on her juicy lips. I'm not even sure why we split up. We still liked each other but I think that I put my training first and I must have made it obvious to her. Maybe I didn't give her enough attention and concentrated on the Martial Arts too much. After about a month she asked me if I wanted to split up. My mind was somewhere else and I agreed and that was the end of that. (She now lives in another country and we rarely see each other but we're still good friends. I think!)

Then I heard my name being called again. This time I knew who it was. It was Peter – he was an excellent roller skater. At that point I could hear him but couldn't see him yet. It felt very confusing not to know which direction he was calling from. Since I'm totally deaf in my right ear, everything I hear appears to come from my left. Turning around and around I still felt unsure of where to look. Then I asked Hanna if she knew where Peter was and immediately she directed me. She had no problem seeing Peter and he could see me, but I couldn't see him. This annoyed me and began to send more messages around my head.

"This is really embarrassing," I thought. "Why do I have to ask for assistance every time I need to see or talk to someone? Am I going to have to tell him about my latest medical diagnosis too? I feel uncomfortable and emotionally drained."

As he approached within my six-metre radius I clearly recognised him. Then I told him about not being able to see well and being registered as partially sighted and I had a little help from Hanna and Samantha. He was very understanding and sympathetic towards me but I still felt embarrassed.

"This is so humiliating having to tell everyone about my disability. That's four people already today and all I'm doing is explaining the same thing over and over again. This is beginning to affect my self-esteem. We're all talking about me and I hate the attention. Listen to them going on like I'm some sad case. I'm not sure how much more of this I can take."

We moved with the queue and filed into the building. We then handed our tickets in and attempted to enter the hall. The man on the door repeatedly asked me a question, but I couldn't hear him. He was on my right, my deaf side, and the music from the disco was also blaring away which didn't help. I turned my good ear towards him to hear him proficiently. He was asking for my hand to stamp it so I had proof that I had paid if I left the room to go to the toilet. We then found some seats and sat down to put our skates on.

"Here comes Adam," Peter said.

As I looked in the direction of the door I only saw a hazy outline of people. After a few seconds his shape emerged and I recognised his chunky form. He strode towards us confidently as if he had already spotted us from afar and sat down too.

"Everyone sees each other long before I do. Why do I have to be the last to see people, or anything else for that matter, these days? Nobody knows how much I'm suffering inside my head. How will I cope if I really do get worse and being deaf in one ear as well doesn't help."

Adam began to speak to us but the music was too loud and he was sitting on my wrong side. As he spoke I constantly asked him to repeat what he had said. I seemed to hear him more clearly when I looked at his lips, which was strange because I can't lip-read, but it certainly helped. Then he got up and skated around a bit while continuing to talk. His speech sounded muffled when he was on my right but as he skated towards my left his speech became clearer. It felt weird the way I could first hear him then struggle every time he moved from my left to my right.

"Great," I thought, "first I have problems seeing people, now I can hardly hear them. What am I going to do with myself? I can't even have a decent conversation with my friends. Maybe I should have just stayed at home and why can't he stand still while he's talking? It's like he's got ants in his pants! Maybe I'm better off not being able to hear him because he talks mostly nonsense anyway!"

Our skates were on and we were off. Skating around and around I almost felt like I was in my own world where it was almost peaceful not to be able to see or hear people properly. I was struggling even more than I used to. The disco lights were on but the hall lights were off so it was quite dark. We were skating anti-clockwise and I was enjoying the peace. I skated, trying to guess who was who from the frail features I saw. Weaving in and out of people, missing them by a whisker, I dodged everyone. Sometimes I would pass someone at great speed only to be confronted with a mass of people clustered together and forcing me to stop or be diverted. Some people skated on their own and others held hands or skated in groups. It was interesting to see how fast I could work out where to go or what to do with all the obstacles before me. Occasionally I would spot my two friends' outlines and follow them. It was fun and I was a pretty good skater.

I'd been skating since I was fourteen years old. Sometimes I would skate to school, Fareham High School, which was a two-mile journey from where I lived. It was a good way of keeping fit (but I bet I never smelt too good at school). I could skate forwards, backwards and even sideways – called 'spread eagle'. To do this I had one skate facing forwards and the other facing backwards. My feet were in line and my body was facing to the side. I couldn't do this for too long because it hurt my ankles. It took me a few months to become good at skating and I had my fair share of falling to the ground, but now I could speed skate and do acrobatics like jumping over people forwards and backwards, although I noticed that it was becoming increasingly difficult to focus efficiently and my accidents were becoming more frequent. People said that I was becoming very clumsy, but I always blamed it on being short-sighted.

Suddenly I was grabbed by the arm. I looked for a short moment before recognising in the dim light that it was Sally, a girl who I had known for years and somehow had became my skating partner.

"I've been calling you for ages, trying to get your attention. I kept trying to catch you but you skate too fast," she said, panting from her exertions.

"Sorry dear but I never heard you. Remember I'm deaf in my right ear."

Struggling to hear her clearly I turned to face her as we stopped to chat.

"I know you're hard of hearing but you're not blind! I've been waving my hands for ages, sometimes right in front of your face."

"Well…" I stalled for a second while I plucked up the courage to tell her, "actually I have very poor sight and I'm now registered as partially sighted."

At that moment I felt emotionally drained and very sorry for myself.

"This is sapping away all my energy having to tell everyone about my condition and my hearing. It's too much," I thought desperately.

My head was hurting and I could feel myself crying on the inside. She held my right hand and we began to skate.

She enjoyed being with me and loved being my partner at roller-skating.

"How can she trust me in the dark?" I thought. "Doesn't she realise how little I can see in the dark? *I* wouldn't trust me especially at this high speed!"

She suddenly pushed me to the left and grabbed my right shoulder. I turned my head to see if she was saying anything.

"Are you trying to kill me?" she shouted. "I was trying to tell you that we were going to hit someone's feet but you couldn't hear me."

Wearily, I told her once more about my difficulties. Then I spun around so that I was skating backwards and held onto both her hands as we skated along. Dragging her faster and faster I began to accelerate to a breakneck speed. I could feel her clenching my hands tighter and tighter as she became more nervous. Feeling a little sympathetic, I soon slowed back down to a manageable pace. Then she wanted a turn at skating backwards so we swapped places and I pushed her to help as she attempted to skate backwards, but she wasn't very good and we had to go slowly as she clutched my hands tightly. Tired from all the effort she asked to sit and have a rest so I carefully took her to a seat and we sat chatting for a while.

About five minutes later, after explaining to Sally that I would be back soon I sped off to skate solo. Once again I enjoyed the peace and tranquillity skating around, but I couldn't keep the demons out of my head. I wondered why I was seeing obstacles too late these days. I felt sure that things looked different, slightly less clear. Suddenly, out of nowhere, some feet appeared before me. It happened when I was skating too close to a wall to avoid hitting someone and it was too late to stop because I was already touching them with my skates. By the time I realised what was happening I'd bumped into their feet and gone crashing to the floor. I had skated too close to the wall and someone was sitting on the floor with their legs spread out straight and their back against the wall. They laughed as I lay there for a few seconds.

"I should have been able to see that," I thought. "No one else is tripping over their feet. I'm so clumsy. Maybe I need to swap my eyes with someone else. Now I'm sure my eyes are worse. Last month I would have seen that coming."

"You hurt my leg!" a voice shouted.

"I'm not in the mood to explain my difficulties with seeing again," I thought to myself as I sat up.

Slowly I got to my feet and composed myself.

"Sorry, but it was a stupid place to sit," I said angrily.

"Why don't you watch where you're skating?"

I stood there and thought for a second or two. "She's only young. She'd probably believe me if I told her that I can't see very well. A common response would be to get my glasses changed. Maybe she's right; maybe people like me shouldn't be here because I can cause accidents. No, I won't bother to argue."

I skated on casually.

A few minutes later I returned to my seat where I had left Sally. As I sat down I realised that she wasn't there. Taking a good look around I found that she was nowhere to be seen so I sat there waiting and contemplating. I watched as all the other skaters passed by. They were all too far away for me to recognise anyone clearly but I thought I recognised a few outlines. It was difficult to tell whether it was even them, but a few gestures and postures looked familiar.

"Why can't I see anyone? They're only a few metres away from me. Look at that corner on my far right, look how dark it is. It's as dark as the night sky. I see lots of people, some holding hands and groups of boys and girls but nothing is clear. I can't identify anyone. I can only guess."

Then I looked long and hard to see if I could spot anyone by guessing. They all looked so plain, nothing was clear. Then I looked for people's body shape, posture, facial features (if I could make any out) and skating styles.

"That fast one looks like Peter. He's tall, dark... look at the way he skates so well, yes, I would say that's Peter."

I looked to see if I could identify anyone else.

"There's Sally, small, a little nervous… no, hang on, she's got the wrong clothes on. That looks like one of the stewards, tall, skinny, with short black hair. That crazy person looks like Adam. He dresses like him, skates like him and takes risks like him. There's no sign of Hanna and Samantha though."

Just then Sally sat right next to me.

"Where did she appear from?" I thought to myself.

"Why are you sitting alone? I was just there talking to someone else," she said.

"Didn't I just explain to her not half an hour ago about my…? Why do I have to say it all over again? Doesn't she realise how hard this is for me? I'm useless. She was just a few metres away and I couldn't see her. How humiliating," I thought crossly.

This felt very stressful but it had to be done and I desperately needed to get used to it. There were many more years of this feeling to come.

"Sorry, but I can't see very well, remember?"

"Oh yeah; I forgot. I wasn't far and I thought that you'd still be able to see me. Are you sure you weren't just ignoring me?" she said jokingly.

"I really couldn't see you and would not have been able to hear you AND it's beginning to frustrate me."

"Tell me what you *can* see. Can you see those two holding hands or that boy with long hair?"

"Yes, I can see them holding hands and I can see the guy with long hair who's just skated past but that's just their outlines. Their detailed features are missing like the colour of their eyes or contrast of their hair. Everyone has dark eyes. I don't even know if they're brown or black, they're just really dull in this dimly lit room. I don't know what I'm talking about. Sometimes I really think that my sight is fine. It's mostly when I find out what you see and realise the big difference, that's when I know my sight is bad. Let's just sit and chill."

We sat in silence for a few seconds then she asked me to help her once more with her skating so I held her hand and off we went.

There were numerous thoughts whizzing around my head and without realising I began to go too fast for her. We weaved in and out of people, dodging all the obstacles before us. Sometimes I would be going so fast and close to people that I had to skate sideways, backwards and then return to normal skating. I felt her squeezing my hand tightly but I carried on. We continued passing most people and just then someone passed us. His posture looked familiar and after a few seconds I worked out that it was Adam, so I went in hot pursuit to catch him up. Sally was trying to say something but I couldn't hear her properly. Once again she was on my right side, the side of my damaged ear. We weaved in and out of people, dodging crowds as I tried my best to catch up with Adam. Eventually I understood that she wanted to sit down because we were going too fast. She let go of my hand as we approached her usual seat, then I continued chasing Adam. He weaved in and out of people, round and round and he was going extremely fast. He was another experienced skater who I enjoyed being with. He was about my size and build and just as fast and crazy as I was. I followed recklessly as I attempted to copy everything he did. When he turned to go backwards, so did I. He knew I was behind him and he did his best to lose me but for now I kept up. We were fast approaching two people who were skating at different speeds with a small gap between them. He turned sideways and did a spread-eagle and so did I. We both got through the small gap. Then he bent both knees like he was going to sit on the floor, and straightened one leg out horizontally. He was now low to the ground and kept it up for a few seconds while I copied. This was a difficult position to be in because you needed great leg strength and balance. Then we carried on skating at high speed. As he was passing someone another person crossed his path and he swerved violently to miss them. With a great display of agility he managed it, but I was in hot pursuit and couldn't follow him so I slammed my brakes on and lost him in the crowd. Embarrassingly I had to wait for him to circle the hall and come past me once more. It was quite easy to spot him and pick up where I had left off.

"Here he comes now. I'm not positive, but the facial features and body outline look right and it looks like him from the way he skates."

As he passed me I accelerated quickly to catch him up. I was once again copying him and when he spun around to skate backwards I did the same. He carried on and then as we were skating backwards

I recognised Peter from his tall dark figure, and he joined in the game. There were now three of us travelling at great speed backwards through the crowd. First Adam, then me, followed by Peter. We began to pass each other, I passed Adam, Peter passed Adam, then Adam passed us both. It was a fun battle that took a great deal of energy out of us.

After a few more minutes the lights came up and we heard the DJ ask everyone to sit out and let just the fast skaters remain on the rink. It took a short while for people to take their seats; we had all slowed down at this stage. We skated quite slowly down the middle of the hall. I was still travelling backwards when suddenly my back wheel was halted by a small stone (that's my excuse!). I was relaxed and not concentrating at the time and I went flying backwards landing on my back. I lay there feeling stupid for a few seconds.

"This time I was beaten by a stone, maybe I should give up skating," I mumbled to myself.

Just then almost out of nowhere a young lady put out her hand to help me back to my feet. She was beautiful, but then she disappeared out of my focus range.

It was time to skate fast. The floor was clear and only a dozen of us remained. This would be fun racing against the fastest skaters.

"I must be crazy, skating at high speed without being able to see properly. One mistake at this speed and I'll be on my backside, I must be mad," I grumbled.

The music started, the lights were on and we were off. We skated faster and faster for the duration of the record. The music kept speeding up and this encouraged us to go even faster. Travelling at this speed, there was no room for mistakes. Somehow with what little vision I had, I passed most people. It was very scary because skaters sometimes appeared from nowhere and I would then have to think quickly to avoid colliding with them. Sometimes I ended up skating backwards again just to avoid a crash. I enjoyed focussing on people ahead and attempting to catch them. It was a thrill and very tiring but immensely enjoyable. During those exciting moments I hardly thought of my disadvantages and it felt quite therapeutic.

The DJ called for us to stop and then make a chain – a group all holding hands in a line. As we skated towards a corner, the person on the far end would speed up to keep up with the first person. This acceleration is automatic and dangerous for the person at the far end. They can sometimes hit amazing speeds. We all joined hands and Hanna came to join me on my left.

"Didn't you hear me earlier?" she complained. "I've been trying to attract your attention for ages. I even waved my arms in your face but you carried on skating."

"Have you forgotten that I can't see very well? I've got poor eyesight – I'm registered as partially sighted; remember?"

"Hold my hand please," she cried.

It felt humiliating. I felt exhausted from constantly repeating the same depressing things. People were confusing me with their ignorance. I didn't know what to think.

The human chain started and we approached the first corner. The person on the end chickened out by letting go of the linking hand and sat out. The next corner was upon us and we turned hard and fast. The person on the end went flying, straight across the floor and onto their backside. It was now my turn at the end of the chain. There were still about five people left after me. We hit the corner fast. Somehow I managed to hold on but then we headed for the next corner. The momentum was too much for me and I went flying. Being good at skating helped me not end up on my backside but my next challenge was stopping before I hit a brick wall. I slammed on my breaks hard burning some serious rubber. The wall came rapidly towards me and I had to put out my hands to protect myself. My reduction in speed was just enough to stop as my hands hit the wall.

The next game involved stunts. Someone lay on the floor and the DJ asked for participants to attempt to jump over them. Adam and Peter lined up with three other people. I stood back for a moment and wondered to myself.

"I can usually jump that distance, but now I'm not sure it's a good idea with my failing eyesight. Maybe I should sit this one out. They look slightly blurred to me and I'm not sure whether I should risk it."

"Are you going to have a go?" Sally shouted encouragingly.

"It's time to admit defeat. I wouldn't be happy if I hit their legs and hurt them, no I think that I'll sit this one out."

"You can do it; go for it," she replied.

My heart began to beat faster as the adrenaline pumped around my body. This was something I could previously do with relative ease, but as my eyes were deteriorating, objects were becoming more blurred and difficult to focus on.

"Go for it," I muttered to myself recklessly.

"I *will* have a go," I replied to Sally.

I lined up behind Peter and we watched as the first person had a go – he jumped and succeeded. They all did and then it came to my turn. I paused for a short while to try and focus on the person lying on the floor. They were about eight metres away and not clear in my eyes. I couldn't even tell if they were male or female so I thought for a second. "Just skate fast towards them until you see them properly then hopefully you'll have time to jump before hitting them."

A few seconds later I was on the move travelling faster and faster towards them. As I picked up speed the blurred features slowly began to get clearer. It was all happening very quickly as I picked my knees up higher to gain more speed. When I got to about four metres away from them, I felt like I could see them clearly (or what I would call clear). I focussed quickly and had a split second to work out how far away they were, how high I would have to jump and where on the floor I would take off from. In an instant I decided that it was time to jump and so I bent my knees and then straightened them quickly to leap into the air. For that short moment when I was in the air everything went silent as I glided over their feet. As I landed I quickly put my brakes on and turned as I came to a stop. Amazed at my success of jumping over someone without being able to see their features clearly, I began to smile and soon regained my confidence.

Then the person on the floor got into a crouching position. Some of the jumpers dropped out and that only left four of us. The crouching person tucked his head right up to his knees. This time we would have to jump much higher and have a longer take off. The 'jump' was about half a metre up from the floor and now waiting patiently. Everyone stood around waiting and watching in anticipation. Once again Adam succeeded. He made it look so easy, full of confidence he was. Peter made it as did the other participant, but it was now my turn; again.

"If they can do it, so can I. Well I hope I can!" I thought as I prepared myself.

It was the final jump and there was no backing out now. My run began and I picked up speed fast but so far with nothing clear to focus on. I had to travel a little faster this time to be able to get the height needed to clear them. With only a few metres left they came into focus. Thinking fast I decided that it was time to jump so bending my knees low to the floor, then suddenly straightening them, I leapt into the air. Once I was airborne I bent my knees again to make sure that my skates wouldn't hit them and over I went. It was a good jump and I returned to the floor putting my brakes on hard and keeping my balance. Amazingly I had made it. While wearing out some rubber I screeched to a stop. It was another happy moment for me.

The lights were turned back off and the DJ asked us to skate clockwise. As we all began to skate off to do our own things I noticed some people standing around at the side and could vaguely hear them talking. Taking my time, I weaved in and around them, skating closely behind them, crossed my skates to the right to pass them on the inside then leaned to the left to straighten up and skate in front of them. There were lots of blurred people to pass and sometimes they would not leave enough space to pass them straight on so I would spread my skates to do a spread-eagle. After I passed them I skated backwards then forwards again. As I went on I looked around trying to guess who people were. It was very hard unless I could hear their voices too.

It was now the final record before the end of the skating session. After getting my breath back I went looking for Sally, my usual skating partner. She was sitting waiting patiently for me, but she was behind a small group of people. Skating slowly past I eventually recognised her features and posture before being positive that it was her. I grabbed her hand we began to skate away. This time we were skating clockwise as instructed.

"I saw you fall earlier," she said jokingly.

"How embarrassing was that?" I replied.

The difference was amazing. I could hear her very clearly compared to when she was on the other side of me. It would have been great to always skate clockwise but obviously it was up to the DJ to decide so I had to cope. We spoke for a few more minutes before the lights were put back on. I appreciated being able to see and hear again. I no longer felt so humiliated and incompetent. Although nothing was actually clear and focussed, to me it was a blessing to have the lights back on.

We skated outside and waited for the rest of our friends. A few people came out and said that they had seen me and I never spoke to them so I explained my disabilities to them too. As usual it felt uncomfortable to have to repeat it but I managed. I looked around at all the people I thought I knew and observed them closely. It also helped when they spoke to me because I used voice recognition before visually recognising them. As people came towards me I would almost play a game of guess who. Sometimes I would get it right and sometimes wrong but the more I played the better I became. Also the more I played the less frustrated I felt.

"Now that looks like Peter over there," I thought to myself. "His facial features and posture appear to be familiar and he looks tall. I also recognise the way he skates."

As he approached, his face became clearer.

"Yes, it *is* Peter!" I thought to myself in triumph.

We exchanged a few words as we circled around on our skates. My trainers were now tied together by their laces and placed around my neck.

"Who's this? Here comes… Adam. He's dressed like him, skates like him and is a little chubby like him… Yes, it's him!" I mumbled as his features became more apparent.

Our gang was now all there and we were ready to skate home. We moved off and made our way down the slope. Skating outside was different from skating in a hall because the ground was no longer smooth. The tiny stones kept trying to jam my wheels but I would then skate with the other foot. The path beside the park was quite smooth so we began to spin and occasionally skated backwards. Adam was skating on my left but I could see someone walking towards us. As they got closer I noticed that they were in my line of target so I skated a little faster towards them and then swerved to my left in front of Adam. After the pedestrian had passed I leaned to my right to be on Adam's right-hand side again. I could hear Adam as he spoke to me but I struggled to hear Peter who was behind me and a little to my right. Every now and then I would either ask him to repeat what he was saying or attempt to turn my left ear towards him at the same time as skating safely.

We got to the end of the park and were now at the road.

"There're some big trucks," Adam said. "Shall we grab on the back and hitch a lift towards home?"

"You guys are crazy," I answered. "I can't even see properly and you want me to risk getting knocked down?"

"Come on. You've done it before."

"That was before. My eyes are more blurred now and things are beginning to look a little scary."

"Here comes a truck now. Look it's stopping! Let's grab the bar at the back," they urged.

They both skated off and I followed hesitantly, feeling like I was being forced into it (wimp). We grabbed the bar at the back and held tight. What I was worried about was that although the road was quite smooth there were little holes in some parts. If you were not aware of this and your skates went into a hole then you could lose your balance (and your life), as the skate wheels would suddenly become jammed. I just hoped that there were no cars too close behind the truck or it could be disastrous. We held tight as the truck moved off. We didn't actually skate, no; we were at the mercy of the speed of the long truck. It began to accelerate and so did we. I looked behind and saw that there was a car approaching us slowly. At that moment one of my wheels got jammed and I lost my balance slightly. I quickly skated on the other foot while picking the problem one off the road for a few seconds. Then I placed it back down on a smoother part and continued to hitch a ride. My skates began to shake a little from the increased speed but I held on. It was becoming too much for me and I wanted to let go and skate on the pavement. We got to the end of that road and the truck slowed down. I quickly let go and went to the side of the road. My friends soon joined me and that was the end of our adventure.

We had been deposited on one of our favourite roads. It was very smooth and great for skating on. It was quite steep, and as we skated down we used minimal effort, the incline helped us gather enough momentum to almost roll down the hill. My skates went faster and I decided to take another risk by turning and going backwards. It felt great, exhilarating, as I gradually went faster. As soon as I felt a little uncomfortable I turned around to continue skating forwards. My wheels began to shake as our speed increased, first a gentle wobble then a vigorous shake. I knew I would have to slow down soon, if I carried on too long then I could be thrown from my skates, but my friends were still there going fast and experiencing the same problems. I didn't want to be the first to put my brakes on so I was determined to continue. My skates were skidding from side to side as I picked up more speed.

"I have to slow down or I'll fall," I thought frantically. "My skates can't take any more, but I can't be the first to slow down. No, just a few more seconds."

A split second before I gave up and put my brakes on I saw Peter slam his on.

"That will do me," I cried as I burned rubber braking hard.

My skates were still shaking as I slowed down. I needed to slow down quickly before I lost my balance so I dug my rubber stopper hard into the road leaving a trail of burned rubber particles behind. We all slowed to a speed at which the shaking stopped and none of us were hurt.

The next road was level so we skated casually towards home. As we parted company I asked them if they wanted to join me for a drink or two later. They weren't sure and said that they might meet me later. Once I got home I made something to eat and relaxed before my night out.

CHAPTER 8
GUESS WHO!

It was a cold but dry night, perfect for getting dressed up. It was about nine in the evening and almost time to go. We had arranged to meet at the clock tower in the centre of Rugby town. I was dressed to kill (as usual!) and ready to dance. My hair was slightly long in an Afro like Michael Jackson, it took ages to get it ready but I looked cool! It wasn't too windy so I wore a shirt without a jacket. My friend Nigel had arrived and we set out to meet the others for half past nine. On the way we met some other people who we knew but they were going in different directions. They acknowledged us from afar but didn't say their names and in the dark I hadn't recognised them yet so I waited for them to identify themselves. They came closer than my six-metre focus range, but I was still unable to work out who they were. Nigel had already recognised them and began to speak but I was still waiting to recognise some features or voices. Five metres became four, then three but I was still struggling. If it had been bright I would have already guessed who they were but it had become apparent that I struggled more at night. Finally they became clear and after we had exchanged a few words we were back on our way to meet the others. After just a few steps my mind began to wander.

"That took ages to be able to see them. I didn't know who they were until Nigel said their names. How did they see me from so far? Their faces were dark and I never recognised their voices."

We walked on and came to the end of the road. It didn't look safe so I delayed in crossing.

"Come on; it's clear," said Nigel.

"How did you see that it was clear? It's too dark and nothing is clear," I replied.

"I could see clearly," he said.

We walked on towards the town centre.

"It was just a mixture of lights. I could hardly see any cars and they mostly looked black and white. Oh well it must be because it's dark," I thought.

Moments later I bumped into someone in a poorly lit part of town. I apologised and walked on but then I wondered why I hadn't seen them when others didn't seem to have any trouble. It was as though they appeared from nowhere. We finally got to our meeting point and waited for John. I observed my surroundings and watched people go by. There were lots of people walking around; I could see them, their eyes, noses and mouths but not in great detail. Most of them looked like they were wearing black or white clothes and at a distance they looked like they were all wearing masks. There wasn't much colour to be seen. Most of the time I could identify men from women and their ethnic backgrounds, my problem was putting names to faces. Nigel saw John approaching.

"Where is he? I can't see him yet," I said.

He pointed in the direction that John was coming from.

"That's him? He doesn't look clear yet but I can see someone who resembles him."

As he came closer I could see that his posture looked like him but I just couldn't see him clearly enough to know for sure that it was him. Although at about four metres I thought it was John, I still wasn't positive. He only became clear to me at about two metres. That was the distance needed to see enough detail to identify him for sure.

As we walked away from the clock tower, I turned to have a glance at the time on the massive clock face and I could read it. After telling John that he was a fraction late we arrived at a pub. My name was called from behind so I turned to see who it was. There was a group of people approaching us but I was unable to identify them yet. I heard my name again but still couldn't determine which person was speaking. Nigel saw the person speaking and told me which one of the group was calling to me. They were at least ten metres away and I was amazed that everyone could see so well. They must have been able to see me clearly because they recognised me from the back.

The friend asked why I wasn't talking to her and, as usual, I explained in more detail about my disability. It took a few minutes to convince her but eventually she accepted it. We spoke for a short while then entered the pub. While we were waiting to be served I couldn't help but think about this insignificant issue. It began to eat away at my mind.

"Not being able to recognise people earlier makes me feel like a failure. How can they all see each other from such a long distance away? I feel incompetent. Why do I have to explain it all over again to different people? It's like they don't believe me and I have to prove it but talking about it regularly depresses me. It's draining the energy out of me and I think I'm beginning to crack up. I'm not sure how much more of this I can take."

Nigel got the first round of drinks and we then moved to stand by the dance floor and watched people dance. The beer calmed me down (a touch) and I felt a little more relaxed. After a few minutes someone approached me and began to speak. They were on my wrong side and there was also loud music in the pub so I was unable to hear them. It felt very uncomfortable seeing their mouth move but not hearing anything coming out. As I moved my head to my right the words they were saying became less muffled.

"Why is your head facing backwards?" they asked.

"I'm deaf in my right ear so I have to turn my head the other way to hear you. Why not stand on my other side so that I can hear you more clearly?"

He moved to my left and we continued to have our conversation.

"I've been trying to attract your attention for a while. Didn't you see me standing over there on the other side of the dance floor?"

"Well, I have another difficulty too. I can't see very well so I never saw you."

I had trouble convincing him of my disabilities and I was feeling slightly frustrated. As he left another person approached and we had the same conversation about my disability and I informed him too of not being able to see clearly. After he had left I realised that he hadn't asked as many questions about my eyesight as most people did. I'd told him that I couldn't hear in one ear and had poor eyesight, but I'd told the others that I was registered as partially sighted. It irritated me a great deal when I had to go into detail but I never felt as useless when I just stated that I had poor eyesight. The feelings that I felt every time I had to go into detail were embarrassment and hopelessness. This was a constant battle for me because the Martial Arts built up my self-esteem, then the lack of eyesight knocked it right back down.

After a few more minutes Nigel tapped me on my left shoulder.

"There's someone over there and I think they're waving at you," he said.

"Over where?"

He pointed me in the right direction and I could see a hand waving towards me but I couldn't see their facial features or any other detail that would help me identify them. From what I saw they could have just being dancing weird! After a short while of trying to work out who they were from their blurred image, I gave up and just waved back.

"If they want to talk to me then they can come over here. I'm not positive that they were even waving at me. Nigel knows most of the people I know and he didn't recognise them so maybe they were waving at somebody else."

It was my turn to buy the next round of drinks so I went to the bar to be served. As I stood there I heard my name being called. Someone was calling me from the other side of the bar. The voice was not familiar but I could hear that it was another man. I took a good look at everyone standing at the bar. They all looked so different, yet all the same. Through my eyes they had similar hair colour, hairstyles and clothing – most of them appeared to be wearing black. I noticed that I could see a few blond haired people but all the other hair colours just blended in. This made me curious as I heard my name being called once more. I tried my hardest to concentrate and see if I could pick out any features that would help me identity the mystery person. A few of them looked familiar but I still wasn't sure, so I began to smile in their direction as though I had seen them.

"There, now they'll think that I've seen them so if they want to speak to me they can just come over."

Unfortunately I never found out who they were.

The barman asked me what I wanted to drink. Well that's what I assumed because he was standing directly in front of me speaking but I couldn't hear any words being spoken. Behind the bar it was quite bright, nothing was crystal clear but I could see the different bottles lined up along the wall. What I couldn't see were the labels. After informing him of what I wanted, he returned with my drinks and told me the price. I asked him to repeat it while I turned my good ear towards him to try and actually hear what he was saying. Success! I gave him the money. I paid with the loose change I had in my pockets to lighten the load. Although I struggled slightly, I was able to see the difference between the coins. Pushing my way through the crowd of people I returned to my friends.

They were still standing at the edge of the dance floor speaking to some people. It was quite dark and I was really struggling to identify the other people. After a short while of trying to work out who they were from their facial features, they turned and began to speak to me. I immediately recognised their voices and guessed who they were. While talking to them I kept looking at them carefully so that I could remember what they looked like for the next time I saw them.

They moved away and we began to talk between ourselves. Most of the time I had to ask my friends to repeat what they had said because of a combination of loud music and my hearing loss. This was one of the worst times that my hearing loss affected me. It's hard enough hearing in a nightclub at the best of times with good hearing; being deaf in my right ear made it much harder.

Maybe I was a thick child because I don't remember being deaf before I was twelve years old and attending high school. We're not sure how I became deaf, whether I was born that way or whether I blew my nose and burst my eardrum. That was the story my mother told me when she found out that I was deaf. She told me that I used to blow my nose very hard and that she kept saying that I should be careful not to burst my eardrum. For years I've baffled people and myself. Some say that I speak very clearly for someone who is totally deaf in one ear. If I was born with a defective ear then my speech should be affected. People have actually had conversations with me about how most people are easily identifiable when they have a hearing impediment. Then when I've asked them if they think that I have any hearing loss, they always say no. The only time it's obvious that I have a hearing problem is when there's loud music playing. It makes me feel very uncomfortable sometimes but then I have found one fun use for hearing loss. When someone is talking to me who I don't particularly want to talk to, with music blaring, I turn my deaf ear to them so that I can't hear them. Then I keep nodding my head and saying, 'Yes,' as if I can hear them; but really I can't! It's an easy way of switching off from people.

Another problem I have with hearing is when I'm travelling in a car. If I'm in the passenger seat, the driver of the car is on my right, which makes it difficult for me to hear them. Their speech sounds muffled but when there's music playing it's even worse. Sometimes I get sick of asking people to repeat what they've just said and I try not to have a conversation. I just sit there in silence, thinking how wonderful the world is! Sometimes I may grunt and agree with whatever they're saying. Every now and then I will turn my good ear and ask them to repeat what they've said but not often because I can feel that it frustrates some people. After being silent for a while I sometimes ask a question knowing that I won't hear their response but will answer with a grunt, then return to silence. If I'm a passenger in the back of a car then I try to sit on the right, behind the driver, so my left ear is towards the other people. Or I pretend to be looking out of the car window when the driver is speaking; this positions my good ear to get maximum volume.

Now that I've thought about it I've realised that I've learned to adapt myself in so many different circumstances that I've almost forgotten how many adjustments I've made myself! When I'm on a train I automatically sit on the right of people. I try to have minimal conversations so that people don't feel too uncomfortable having to repeat themselves all the time. Sometimes I even close my eyes and pretend to be resting or asleep, so they don't strike up a conversation with me and have to keep repeating everything they say (I am considerate). If I'm travelling on buses and coaches, I use the same methods. When I'm at parties or just having general conversations, people don't even notice that I'm literally always on their right. Even when I'm walking with people, they don't realise that I'm always fighting to walk on their right-hand side.

The most interesting person to talk with is my good friend Kyle. He's also deaf in his right ear and you should hear some of our conversations. We are both constantly trying to be on the right and most of the time we end up slowly walking around in circles! It sometimes looks like we're having a slow dance. Another position we end up in is with Kyle facing forwards and me facing backwards with our left ears closest to each other! Well, you have to see the funny side of it or you would end up crying! Kyle is gay and holds a black belt in Martial Arts. He's no weakling and could quite easily kick some serious ass!

In the distance I saw a tall dark figure heading in my direction. It was time to guess again so I looked for familiar features. He was tall, quite slim, light brown face and approaching us fast. It looked like Peter but I wasn't sure. There were hundreds of people here and I didn't want to make a fool of myself talking to someone who I didn't really know. As he got nearer he stopped to talk to someone else. I couldn't quite hear his voice so was still unsure of his true identity. He finished talking and came up to our group. It was a little dark and I found it hard to make out his features clearly.

"Hello you guys. Hello Vendon, it's Peter."

"Hello Peter and well done for turning up! Would you like a drink?" I asked.

He accepted my offer and we went to the bar.

Peter has always identified himself to me by saying his name. He still does to this day and he has never passed me by without saying who he is, and I appreciate his consideration. If everyone did this I would find it much easier to know who I'm talking to. I've always felt comfortable around Peter and he remains one of my best friends. Unfortunately most people are not so thoughtful and chat away to me without making sure that I know who they are even though they know that I have very poor eyesight. It's not all their fault though; if I could see better then they wouldn't have to.

As we were waiting to be served someone came up to me and started talking. They asked me how I was and we had a few minutes conversation before they left.

"Do you know who that was?" Peter asked.

"No!" I answered with a smile on my face.

Peter laughed and seemed to find me quite amusing. The barman came over, but I wasn't sure whether he was ready to serve us. Peter told me that he was so I gave our order. When the barman came back and announced the price I asked him, as usual, to repeat it. However, Peter, who was standing on my left, told me what it was. It was at moments like this when I would be reminded that I had a hearing problem – Peter had heard him clearly enough, but I hadn't. With that and my failing eyesight I was destined for a stressful life.

We chatted at the bar for a while as people came to talk to us on a regular basis. He knew a lot of people too and I would first try and guess who they were then ask Peter to see if I had guessed right. Many people sounded similar and some of their features were similar too, but most of the time I could guess correctly before hearing their voices.

A young lady approached with a great big smile on her face. She looked similar to Samantha with curly brown hair but she was a little taller. She also had much thinner lips than those kissable lips of Samantha. It was Maria, and I had guessed it was her before she started talking to me. We had an interesting conversation before she left with her blond friend.

About three months previously, we had dated. She was my girlfriend for about two months. We met at my local Martial Arts class. She also went roller-skating and while I was out one night clubbing she was very brave and asked me out straight. She was the first girl that I had sex with and again it was my fault that we split up. So far I haven't got a good track record.

The first girl who I remember going out with was called Chelsea. I was about eighteen years old and well overdue! We met at the Sports Centre in Rugby where she used to come and watch us train with another friend. I took a liking to her friend even though I did have secret feelings for her too. Her friend ended up going out with a friend of mine and that lasted for years. After a while Chelsea began to act shy around me but as usual, being a typical man, I couldn't read the signs. I had feelings for Chelsea but I didn't think that she liked me more than as a friend so I concentrated on training (how thick am I).

Then one day at the Sports Centre Chelsea's friend said to me; "I think Chelsea wants to see you. She wants to tell you something."

Chelsea eventually emerged from the ladies toilets.

"Your friend said that you wanted to tell me something, is that true?" I asked her.

"How embarrassing! Um, yes I do, but I don't know how to say it."

"Why not just start and see what happens."

"Can we go and sit on the seats to watch the swimming?"

We went and sat and had a bit of privacy.

"So what did you want to say, what's happened?" I asked.
"Well, I don't know how to say this, so please don't laugh."
I sat in anticipation.
"Here goes," she said. "I had a dream and it involved you. We kissed and… well I liked it and… this is too embarrassing!"
"You had a dream about me? Well I feel really special," I answered happily.

I reached over and kissed her on her lips and we became an item after that. One day I took her to my home at 128 Murray Road and we went into my room. We kissed and touched and enjoyed each other's company. She had long dark hair, a slim figure and a beautiful smile. She lay down on my bed and I caressed her body. Slowly I moved my hand down to her legs where she was wearing a pair of tight jeans. Then slowly, I undid her zip and put my hand inside. It felt great and I began to get horny so I then opened the buttons on her blouse and felt around. Then just as I was about to go further she said; "I'm not ready for that. Another time maybe?"

I was ready! I was waiting! I was horny, but I also respected her too much so I agreed and we didn't go any further. We met up a few days later and she was looking beautiful. Her long glossy hair and irresistible smile was upon me.

"Do you think that I should cut my hair?" she asked.
I looked once more at her hair and it was stunning.
"No, I like long hair and it looks beautiful on you. It really suits you and I think that short hair will make you look ugly!"

I was young and foolish and I didn't know that words could hurt so much. I wasn't very good at expressing my feelings and she didn't take it too well. Over the next few days we didn't see much of each other. Then one day I saw her, only I wasn't sure that it *was* her. She had cut her beautiful long hair short. She looked fine but I have to admit that I preferred her with longer hair! I stopped and asked her something.

"Are you avoiding me?"
"You told me that I would look ugly with short hair and you offended me," she replied.
"Oh, I'm sorry Chelsea. Maybe I used the wrong words; I didn't mean to upset you. It does suit you having short hair."
"It's too late, I'm too hurt."

She walked off and out of my life. It had only lasted two weeks but we remained friends forever. I was no good at chasing women. When I look back I suppose I could have swept her off her feet with flowers and chocolates and all that, but I was young and knew that there were plenty more fish in the sea. My actions were wrong but it's too late now.

The second girl who I dated was Sarah. I was nineteen years old and we met at roller-skating. My friend Johnny was already dating her sister. Sarah was about five years older than me and I was about to find out that she was much more experienced and too hot to handle. We had arranged to meet at the fireworks display on 5th November. While we were admiring the display her sister asked me to meet Sarah behind the outdoor swimming pool, so I went. She was waiting for me. She almost jumped on me. We kissed and cuddled and it felt very intense. As we kissed I began to feel that she wanted more. She was taking over and began to devour me. I was still horny and wanted more but not there, not with hundreds of people close by, supposing someone saw us? I was outdone by an older and more experienced woman. I wanted her but not there, but she wanted me now. She wanted to take the risk of being caught. I looked at her blond hair; it was quite long, just past her shoulders and her lips were quite big and tasty. I gazed at her and imagined but I couldn't bring myself to take the risk. She was disappointed; I could hear it in her voice. This was a woman who liked to get her own way and didn't like being turned down. All my years of training prepared me to beat other men but here I was being beaten by a woman. I was scared of her; maybe she would hurt me! I imagined making love to her and then her turning to me to do it again. She was too much for me, out of my league and I had to admit defeat. We eventually returned to the others and stood holding hands as we watched the end of the firework display.

We arranged to meet at the next skating session. She didn't live in Rugby so found it hard to come and visit. Occasionally she asked to meet me during the evenings but I, like an idiot, put my sports first and was unable to work around my training program. I must have embarrassed her because I didn't even take her phone number. We met up a few times but somehow never got the chance to finish off what we (she) had started. I'm not sure how it happened but somehow we returned to being friends. The kissing and cuddling soon stopped and then a few months later she never returned to Rugby. My friend Johnny had also split up with Sarah's sister and they were never seen again. I blew it, another relationship down the drain. Obviously I left a lasting impression on her!

The third girl was Samantha, who I've already mentioned. We also met at roller-skating and she was a few years younger than me. Her friend Hanna was seeing my friend Peter and we were all friends! It was a group thing but then I blew that relationship too. I concentrated on training too much (again!) and never gave her the attention she deserved. She soon got fed up of being treated as second best and one day when I had a lot on my mind (probably training!) she asked if we should split, I said yes and that was that. Another relationship came to a sudden end. I never blamed any of my disastrous relationships on the women. It was entirely my fault and I'm man enough to admit it. You would have thought that I would have learned from my mistakes, but I was about to do it again!

The fourth person that I dated was Maria. She used to train at my local Martial Arts class and we slowly got to know each other better. We saw each other at our skating club and organised to meet later. We were in a club chatting for ages, getting to know each other more intimately. Then I offered to walk her home.

"Do you like me?" she asked.

"Yes, you're lovely," I answered.

"Would you like to see me?"

"Yes I would."

She kissed me and so started another relationship. We got on well but I was devoted to my training (yes I am stupid!). I thought that this relationship would have lasted because of my love for training. She trained too and we always had something to talk about but I did ignore her, slightly, when we were training. She smoked and that put me off a little. I don't smoke and didn't really want to be with someone who did. I tried it once, when I was fourteen. We were on the way to school and a friend was smoking. He asked me to try it and I did, but I hated the smell and have been against smoking ever since. She was thoughtful enough not to smoke around me but I felt awful. She deserved better than boring me who didn't smoke.

We arranged to meet for some privacy. It felt good and the time was right so we began our quest for sex. We kissed and cuddled lots and I enjoyed it. Cuddling made me feel special, wanted and loved. Without cuddles I think that I would go mad. She lay down and I touched and had a good long-lasting play. She moaned and I played! Then we swapped places and she played and I moaned! Then we swapped places again and we ended up making love. For a few weeks afterwards I walked around with a permanent smile on my face but then, like an idiot, I went back to concentrating on my Martial Arts. She wanted more attention and I wasn't giving it to her so one day she asked me if we should split and I said, "Yeah, maybe for a while." A while became permanent and yet another relationship went to waste. But I had my eyes on someone else!

We had finished our beers and my friends wanted to go to another pub. On the way out I went to the toilet to make space in my bladder for more beer! I made my way through the crowd and found the toilets. The door had an obvious picture of a man on it and underneath it was written 'Gentlemen'. After I had finished I washed my hands and went to rejoin my friends. We made our way out and into the other pub, where I tripped on a step that appeared from nowhere but I didn't feel too embarrassed because other people were doing the same so I just looked like another drunk person. We approached the bar and waited to be served. I observed my surroundings to see if I could recognise anyone. There were a few blurred images of people who looked familiar. Asking my friends for assistance in confirming some, I learned that I was correct in most cases. It was getting quite easy to determine people's identity from the blurred images I saw. Most people dressed in similar fashion, wearing dark clothing, mostly black. As we stood there, a group of young ladies came over to talk to us. They were dressed in black too. Their clothing was plain looking and hairstyles similar. I knew them well and worked out who some of them were before they spoke. Once the others began to speak I recognised their voices.

We chatted and flirted for a while as we drank our beer. Although I struggled to hear them clearly, I was able to hold a conversation. Most of the time I managed to position myself on the far right of the group so that everyone was on my left, but sometimes they moved around and ended up on my wrong side. Then one of them pointed at the way a young man was dancing. They all looked at him and began to laugh and make additional comments. I looked but I couldn't see what they were all seeing. As I looked over I saw a few shadows but could not determine that they were even human. There were no details or facial features to build on, yet the others were commenting as if everything was perfectly visible. They commented on his clothes and the colour of them and about his face, but through my eyes there was nothing.

"There's nothing there but a shadow moving sporadically. How can they see the colour of his clothes and the style? Are my eyes that bad?"

After commenting several times that I couldn't see what they were all laughing at I began to humour them.

"I might as well laugh like I can see that guy," I thought. "I bet no one even notices that I can't actually see him."

I joined in and began to laugh and comment as if I could see. I didn't want to be left out every time we had a conversation about other people. After a while I would have been left there, all alone, waiting for them to finish humouring themselves. It does get lonely sometimes, so I mostly end up pretending to see.

This kind of conversation went on throughout the night and I had to continue to pretend to be able to see. There were lots of shadows that were commented on, lots of remarks about people's choice of colour even though through my eyes most of them were wearing black and looked fine. It frustrated me not being able to see the red dress, or the yellow shirt that seemed to stand out so much to the others. I also felt uncomfortable not being able to hear clearly and having to ask others to repeat what they had said. I enjoyed the night but it was frustrating.

The lights came on to signify the end of the evening; the pub was about to close. As I stood there beside my friends including the group of people who had joined us during the evening, I was surprised to see that the black clothing that they were wearing magically became colourful as the lights became brighter. Plain black dresses became beautiful red with sparkly bits that reflected the lights. Their tops became revealing. Black tops became almost see through or had pretty little patterns on. Skirts and shoes changed colour before my very eyes. The white shirts also changed into different shades with their own unique patterns. Rings, necklaces and earrings appeared almost from nowhere. Similar hairstyles became more detailed revealing length, style and colour. Trousers gained pinstripes and black became blue and red and grey and brown. How wonderful it felt to be able to see again.

"This is what others see? I'm so jealous! If only they knew how beautiful they all look. If they lost their eyesight and then regained it they might be more grateful and appreciate having the ability to see rather than commenting on every little blemish. If only they knew how lucky they all are."

We continued to talk as we finished our drinks. Some of them were still commenting on people's choice of clothing. I looked at some people who they were referring to. Although through my eyes they were still not clear, I could see their dress code and some facial features.

"Is this what they could all see in the dark? How could they see colour and other people's faces so clearly? Do they see this brightly in the dark? If so, just how dark *are* my eyes? Now I understand why I can't see red in poorly lit areas. Now I know why so many people think that I'm colour blind!"

Then I became emotional.

"Why me? Why can't I be like them, see like them and hear like them? It's so frustrating not being able to see or hear well. My eyes are useless, I feel incompetent."

As we made our way outside more and more people began to reveal themselves. I was able to identify some of them by guessing who they were from their blurred features and others I had to wait until I heard their voices. We all crowded outside and chatted. I had a headache from thinking too hard (I was drunk). It took a lot of concentration to constantly work out who people were or trying to hear what they were saying, either that or I was very drunk and it was the beginning of a hangover! After a while we went to get some food. A take-away was a regular treat after nightclubbing. I got a doner kebab and chips and we made our way home.

CHAPTER 9
THE ART OF WINNING

Many weeks had passed and I had trained and worked hard for my black belt exam. After waking up bright and early I sat there in my room for about half an hour, meditating. With all that was happening in my life I had to somehow put it to one side while I concentrated on passing this exam. I had to empty my mind, not think of my failing eyesight, not worry about the blurred world I saw or about my hearing problem. It was a lot to ask for because my disabilities affected my every move.

After a while I got dressed in a tracksuit and went into the garden to warm up. John had shown me how to use a nunchaku so I started with that. Spinning them in my hands and around my body always warmed me up fast. Then I stretched, kicked and went through as many techniques as I could manage on my own. Then I stood there and imagined myself in fighting situations and practised my counter attacks in my head. I was getting nervous again and my mind began to wander.

I remembered about two years ago I was attacked by someone with a knife. It happened as I walked through a park with my brother. A friend of ours had upset this person and he was out looking for him. He knew that my brother was a close friend of this person and so wanted to harm my brother. As we walked I heard him shout something to us. He was with a friend and as they walked towards us we stopped. He shouted something else and my brother answered and in an instant he produced a knife and ran towards us. There was no time to think and I went into autopilot mode. As he came towards us I turned sideways so that if the knife made contact it would hit my arm. Just as he came into hitting distance, I shoved my brother to the side out of range and kicked this guy straight in his groin with a side kick. It was with my left leg, which was my fastest at performing this technique. It made contact and he flew backwards falling to the ground and the knife flew from his hand. Before I could do any more my brother had jumped on top of him to finish him off. I looked at his friend and told him to stay back or he would get hurt too. He listened and my brother sorted out his friend. It was a scary moment that was over within seconds.

Another memory was being given the nickname 'Superman' by some Martial Arts friends in Germany. It was given to me because of how easy I made press-ups look.

About two years ago our Martial Arts club was invited to Germany to fight – Rugby twinned with a club in a town called Ruesselsheim. It was my first time on a ship out of England. We travelled to Dover by coach. I was a little scared of travelling so I never closed my eyes. When I was ten years old, I had been involved in a car accident and ever since then I have always kept my eyes open, just in case.

The coach drove onto the ferry and we had a four-hour journey to France. Most people slept, but not me. We had already been travelling for ten hours and I was very tired but somehow I kept my eyes open. We drove through France and stopped in Belgium. This took several more hours and I was still awake. After about an hour or two we continued our journey to Germany. By the time we arrived in Ruesselsheim we had been travelling for eighteen hours and I had not slept at all. A very warm welcome awaited us with amazing entertainments and food and some nice German beer. I stayed at the instructor's house with a fellow student who also went on to take his black belt exam with me. We got in the instructor's BMW and travelled along the autobahn. He went a little fast and although I was quite excited, I was also wary of the fact that the autobahn has no speed limit! We arrived at his home and were spoiled rotten for the four days that we stayed.

Whether we won or lost the competition was not that important although I did win my fight! I was amazed by their hospitality and warm welcome; it was like we were old friends. There was so much food on display to eat for free that we couldn't finish it. It was my first trip abroad and I loved it and eventually I did get some sleep!

They took us on a train journey and we were comparing techniques. One of them got down on the floor and proceeded to perform press-ups on one hand. My group urged me to do something even better so I got down on the floor and did the same as the German fellow, first performing one-hand press-ups then switching from my right to left and back to my right again. Then I performed some press-ups on my fingers on both hands. Slowly I took off one finger from the floor to perform press-ups on four fingers, then three, then one finger and a thumb and then just my thumbs. After a short while I went back to performing press-ups on one hand and ended up with only two fingers and a thumb touching the floor. They congratulated me enthusiastically and named me Superman. Although I enjoyed the recognition I knew that I was not the best because my friend John, who I trained regularly with in the gym, could perform it using one thumb.

My mind drifted once more and I remembered a previous fight. It had happened about a year before on the way back from a youth club. There were two of us walking home and as we passed a group of young lads one of them called out to us. We turned and they proceeded to call us names. I asked them not to be so rude because they didn't even know us, but they persisted so I asked the one with the biggest mouth to apologise or he would be sorry, but he took no notice of what I said. I still contemplated whether to walk on because, well, I wasn't exactly scared. I had a few years of Martial Arts behind me and my confidence had grown. He walked up closer to me and I warned him but he was too cocky. He went to punch me but within a split second I had moved and punched him in the face. I then grabbed him by the throat with my right hand and swept him to the ground, holding his throat tight. I could have squeezed at any time. My friend warned the others to stay away and they did. One of them ran off and we later found out that he had called an ambulance. I sat on the guy on the floor and squeezed his throat slightly tighter.

"If I wanted, I could kill you at any time," I told him angrily.

As I shook him, hitting his head on the ground a few times and listening to him gasping for air, an ambulance turned up. My friend told me to stop as the ambulance pulled up near us. I let go of his throat and got to my feet. He was still lying there but I was sure I hadn't strangled him. As I stood there I watched the ambulance men carry him off and whisk him away, then we quickly left the scene of the crime.

After reliving these few memories I went back inside to have a wash and eat breakfast. My sister had ironed my Martial Arts suit so I didn't have that to worry about. I had tried ironing and although it looked pressed to me, it apparently didn't to other people. She said that she didn't want me going out looking like a tramp so she offered to iron it for me. My sister did most of my ironing. I wasn't lazy, I was just crap! But now I know the real reason. My deteriorating eyesight made it extremely difficult to see the creases so when I ironed something and thought that all the creases were gone, I was wrong (well that's my excuse).

My sister lived a few doors up the road from my mother's with her son Dyonn. My mother lived with my youngest brother Percy and me; all the rest had now grown up and left. My sister used to come every day to my mother's house to visit, eat or help out (or dump Dyonn). My mother was becoming increasingly ill. She was diabetic and suffered from high blood pressure, was struggling to walk, had kidney problems and her eyesight was also deteriorating from her diabetes. She used to go to church every week but as her illness got worse she found it harder and harder to get there. I used to go to church on a regular basis as well, but I was slowly losing interest as my sight was getting worse. I was doing what most people do and blamed the easiest person for my problems. God doesn't answer face to face so most of us can't even see that he is helping us all the time. It took me years to realise this but I now know that he *is* helping me.

After having my breakfast I was asked to help with the housework. I hated tidying up, it was tedious, boring and I wasn't very good at it because I seemed to be quite clumsy, dropping things or breaking glasses every now and then. It had to be done by my brother and I because my mother was struggling with that too. She was in considerable pain from her illnesses and took loads of tablets. Our house had three bedrooms so I had a bedroom to myself. I'd started off in the smallest room – it was *really* small, but as my mother had difficulties getting upstairs, we moved her bed into the living room downstairs and I moved into her bigger room.

My room was kept quite tidy, but at this stage of my life I wasn't that bothered about mess. We could both cook. Percy is younger than me yet he taught me to cook (how embarrassing). I could cook rice and chicken, Jamaican style. My mother had encouraged all of us to learn to cook just in case we ended up on our own, without a partner to help. I hated fish and was a fussy eater. Once my brother cooked fish and asked me to try it. I told him that I was too scared of getting the bones lodged in my throat and some time later he managed to get a small bone lodged in *his* throat. He coughed and choked but it wouldn't move. I tried to help him by patting his back, but still nothing. This went on for a few minutes and now that I look back on it we really should have called an ambulance but he insisted that he would be all right. He put his fingers down his throat and began to vomit and after a while it dislodged itself and came out. I still don't trust fish unless I know that it hasn't got any bones. My eldest sister makes fish sometimes and she'll go through my portion several times looking for any small bones that she might have missed. If she doesn't go through this vigorous ritual every time she cooks fish for me, I won't eat it.

It was now Sunday afternoon and time to go to my exam. I packed my bag carefully so as not to crease my perfectly ironed suit and walked to the Sports Centre. It was a fifteen-minute walk and I enjoyed both the exercise and the independence of being able to walk peacefully on my own. I arrived early and had enough time to relax in the changing room. There was a lot of pressure for me to pass. If I passed, I wanted to open my own class and teach, but first I had to overcome my nerves. I changed and went up to the training hall. There were one or two people already there but that was it. In the next few minutes about thirty people would be taking their different exams – there would be five of us taking our black belt exams. I practised and practised as more and more people began to arrive. This time I wouldn't be helping anyone apart from myself. I had already failed an exam about two years ago and there was no way I wanted to fail this one. Over the years I had helped quite a few people including two of the people who were going for their black belts today. I even missed exams to help them but it would make me so proud to see them pass.

More and more people entered and someone had brought a table and three chairs. All five of us had arrived and were working hard. Then we all stopped to bow as my instructor had entered the room with *his* instructor. We bowed as a courtesy to other black belts. Bowing was like congratulating others on their achievement in finishing their studying, completing their three year course, gaining their degree. My instructor was a third degree black belt and his instructor was a fifth degree black belt. He was one of the highest in England, learning Taekwondo from the army in Korea. He taught some of the best Taekwondo teachers around today, from leaders of the WTF Olympic

Taekwondo organisation to the ITF governing body. At some stage in my life I have fought against most of them. It was an honour to learn from him and it would prove to be a bigger honour to receive my black belt from him. We became more nervous and practised harder. Then we saw my instructor opening a very large and heavy bag. It was full of bricks and as they lay on the ground I began to chop the wall with my hand. For months I'd been performing this act, trying to toughen up my hand for this moment. After repeating everything needed I resolved to relax and tried to meditate again.

The third examiner entered the hall, we bowed and it was time for our exam to start. We lined up and I was at the front of the class. I remembered just a few years ago when I had been a beginner and had to stand at the back. As time went on I slowly moved towards the front of the class. Now there I was, hours away from being put in position one. Our instructor asked one of us to lead the warm-up and we exercised for about ten minutes. We then all sat down in a line with our backs against the wall and waited our turn. He started examining some beginners first so we had about half an hour to rest. Then he sent all five of us out to practise for fifteen minutes before he called us back in to begin our assessment.

He told us to stand up and perform a series of kicks. This went on for a few minutes and I was already feeling tired but I was no longer nervous. Once I got started I took advantage of the adrenaline rush. We then had to perform lots of press-ups on our knuckles. It had to be just our two big knuckles but I found that quite easy. The press-ups finished, our instructor asked us to do some sit-ups. We were then asked to perform some more kicks and then show some hand techniques.

After that we put on some boxing gloves and showed some boxing, hitting some focus mitts. By that time I was really tired but the instructors still asked us to do more. They were seeing how much stamina we had. We then had to perform a few katas, which are standard set moves used in most Martial Arts styles. Being so tired, I lost concentration and went wrong when performing a kata.

"I don't believe I've just gone wrong," I thought to myself. "I've done that kata hundreds of times and knew it off by heart, how could I go wrong?"

After a few more minutes of intense work we were asked to sit down. Then we were called up a few at a time, asked to find a partner and perform some more set moves and then some self-defence. As I sat there watching the others performing well I slowly began to worry about my mistake.

"I hope I don't fail because of that silly mistake. I only hesitated for a split second, maybe they didn't see."

It was my turn again to perform and I put as much effort as I could into each and every technique. After I had shown my self-defence moves I had to show some more self-defence, but this time against a knife. I looked at the knife and imagined that I was in a real-life situation.

After my knife defence was over, I felt that I had performed well. We went through a few more techniques then were asked to hold our legs out in a side kick position. Over the past few months I had done this many times but as I held my leg up I lost my balance and began to wobble slightly. I was not happy with my performance and now began to really worry. We were then asked to stretch on the floor. I got down and went into front splits, I could do that but when I turned to perform side splits I was not quite there. We then answered some questions that the examiners asked and were told to get ready to fight.

I sat there watching the others fight and tried to plan my actions and work out a strategy. The chief examiner then asked me to take up my fighting position. With my hand and feet pads already on, I rose to my feet, bowed to them and took up my position. The chief instructor asked to see me and I began to worry.

"What have I done, what did I do wrong?" I muttered to myself.

When I got to his table I bowed to show my respect.

"Can you fight without your glasses on?" he asked.

"Yes sir."

"Remove them and give them to me."

"Sir."

As I removed them my world became really blurred. It was hard enough seeing and fighting with my glasses on, but here I was at probably the most important time of my Martial Arts career, about to fight without my glasses on. It was something that I had anticipated and was used to. I've entered many competitions and have always fought without glasses, but now I was fighting for a black belt and I would have found it easier with my glasses on. After I gave him my glasses I bowed and returned to my place.

My opponent was chosen and we bowed to each other to start the fight. We began and they watched closely. Through my eyes he looked really blurred, out of focus, and it looked worse than usual. I could still see his hands and feet; it was his features that were missing or more out of focus, like his eyes. We were taught to look into people's eyes because you can usually tell what they are thinking or what their next move will be, but now I couldn't see my opponent's eyes. I was back to guessing and as we fought I quickly learned his style. He kicked and I blocked then he came in hard with his arms. I stood there as we exchanged a few punches. Although it was a semi-contact fight, being of large build we both hit quite hard whilst still showing some control. As he backed off under the pressure I kicked him to his head with a left turning kick. It made contact and he backed off again. We fought on and I started hopping on my right foot and executing some side kicks with my left; as my left leg touched him I quickly executed a side kick to his face but he blocked it. I repeated the same technique to lead him into another counter. Instead of trying to kick him to his head with a left leg side kick, I quickly turned and executed a back kick with my right leg into his chest and it made contact. I continued to control the fight and after another minute or so the fight was over. Our chief instructor asked me to fight a few more times before I was asked to stop.

After the five of us, the black belt candidates, had all completed our warm-up fights we were matched against each other. This would prove difficult because they were pretty much equal to me in skill and size. We fought and constantly tried to control the fight, but each of us knew what the others would do. We all knew how each other fought so I changed my fighting style. I decided to copy a black belt student who I admired; he was excellent and his techniques confused the others when I used them. A few more minutes had gone by and I was now very tired. We were down to the last fight. We had to fight against two people – you needed eyes in the back of your head for this and I didn't even have eyes that worked in the front of mine!

We started the fight and the two blurred figures came towards me. It was hard enough fighting one blurred person, with two I had to think extra fast. When they came towards me, I moved. Then they tried to surround me with one in front and the other to my rear but I moved into a position that kept them both in front. One of them was more aggressive than the other so I tried to keep him away from me. We kicked and punched and moved around a great deal. Then I sensed that the aggressive fighter was getting frustrated. This was exactly what I was waiting for and as he rushed in I caught him with a side kick to his ribs using my left foot and he went down. Then I quickly finished off the other person by punching a few times to get him to cover his face then I lifted my right foot high above him and dropped it back down on his shoulder executing an axe kick and the fight was over. I was ecstatic. I had fought two people without being able to see them clearly and won! Some students called me 'thunder-foot' because I was able to use both my legs almost equally. Although it turned out well, it had happened by accident. About two years previously I had been warming up with a fellow student and as I stood with my back against the wall I put my right leg into his hand for him to stretch me into front splits. He pushed my leg up fast to touch the wall, knowing that this movement was normally fine for me, but on this occasion I hadn't warmed up properly and the result was that I pulled my hamstring at the back of my right leg and it was injured for months. Before that moment my right leg had always been much better than my left, but now it was damaged. Being so dedicated to training, I refused to rest and trained my left leg instead, so that's how I became good at using my left foot as well as my right.

The fighting rounds finished, it was now time for the final event, which was breaking. We took our hand and feet pads off and waited for our names to be called. We had to take it in turns to perform the same breaking techniques and I was third. The first technique was the side kick; we had to break two wooden boards. The two people before me had broken it first time so I had to match their standard. Two people held the boards and I tested them with my hand to make sure they were secure, but they moved quite easily.

"Hold tighter please," I asked.

As I pushed them again the boards still moved. I wasn't happy.

"Still not tight enough."

I tested the strength of the boards yet again and they still moved slightly.

"That isn't solid enough and I'm not sure they'll be able to hold on when I kick. Maybe it's me. The others broke them so I'm just going to have to go for it," I thought as I lined up to get ready to kick.

After going through all the rigorous motions, I kicked the boards. As my leg hit they moved and I felt the boards go back. I had missed on my first attempt.

"That's it, I've failed. I can't believe I missed my easiest kick," I muttered in disappointment.

"Would you like another try?" the chief instructor asked.

"Yes sir."

A few seconds later I was preparing to hit again.

"Come on guys, hold this tight because I'm going to kick it real hard," I advised.

With an almighty thump, I hit the boards with more aggression than usual. My foot smashed through them. The two men still weren't holding tight enough and one of the boards flew out of their hands and hit one of them in the face. I felt a little sorry for him, but it was his fault. He was hurt and bleeding and was taken away and replaced with someone else.

I was really worried about failing. I'd made a few mistakes and was no longer sure that I'd pass my exam. I tried even harder than ever and I succeeded in breaking all the other boards first time. We'd reached the test of the last board before having to break the brick. Some of the others had missed a few boards so none of us were sure of passing any more. In this final board test we had to jump over someone and then break a board with a flying side kick. The first competitor broke it first time, the next took two attempts and then it was my turn. After setting up the board and moving the person that I was going to jump over into the right position I walked over to where I would be starting my run. The board was blurred and so was the person bending forward.

"That board looks more blurred than usual," I thought to myself. "I'm just going to run and guess where to jump from then I'll have a split second to focus on the board. Let's go for it."

First I did a test run and counted my steps. As I got close to the person bending forwards I looked at the board; it wasn't clear but I could see it. I wasn't allowed to try and kick the board on my test run so I simply ran towards it and stopped. I returned to my starting position and was told to begin.

I prepared myself for a few seconds as I concentrated my attention on the challenge. "It's about eight steps before you have to jump off your right leg, are you ready?" I mumbled to myself.

My run started and I picked up speed fast. As I got closer to the board it became more visible but first I had to jump this person who I struggled to see clearly. My eight steps were up and it was time to jump, so I leapt off the floor and jumped high. Everywhere went completely quiet for the second that I was in the air and it felt like forever. It was as if I was travelling through the air in slow motion and I had extra time to focus and then kick the board. Over the person I flew and on towards the board. My left knee was bent and ready to power my leg into the board.

"Not yet... now!" I shouted to myself.

Thrusting my left leg out straight, I executed a flying side kick. It hit the board and I kept my leg straight until I was sure that the board had broken. As I landed on my feet between the board and the person bending down, I peered eagerly at the board.

"It's broken! I did it!" I screamed to myself.

I sat back down and watched the other people who were about to attempt the same technique.

The final part of breaking was upon us; we were asked to set up and break a brick. The first person broke it on their second attempt and the following candidate failed to break it. I was now under a great deal of pressure.

I knelt down and set up the bricks, whilst my mind raced with a mixture of excitement and trepidation. "I *have* to do this. I can earn extra marks that might make up for the mistakes that I've made. If I don't break it on my first attempt, it's really going to hurt my hand, no... I have to go for it – give it everything I've got."

The area was a little dusty from the last break, but my bricks were now set up. I went through the motions as I continued to concentrate and focussed all my energies on the task in hand. I took my time; my right arm went up and then back down to touch the brick, then I repeated this action again. When I thought that I was ready I paused with my hand placed against the brick. I took a few deep breaths and… changed my mind. I decided that I wasn't comfortable enough yet and went through the preparations once more. After another few seconds I paused with my hand placed firmly on the brick. This time I felt good, comfortable and confident. I was about to hit this brick as hard as I could so that it would break and not hurt my hand. If I missed, then all the energy I used would be reflected and could be enough to break my hand. After about three more seconds I let out an almighty shout then lifted my hand fast and high. As my hand hit the brick I bellowed once more. There was a rumble of noise as my hand made contact with the brick and as I looked through my steamed up glasses I noticed that several more pieces of brick had appeared. This was the final challenge, probably the hardest of them all, and I had broken the brick first time. There were many people watching and they all began to clap their hands. As I smiled I looked up at the three examiners and they were smiling too. I was almost overwhelmed with emotion but I knew that it wasn't all over yet. The final two candidates had their attempts and then we had to wait while the examiners decided who had passed. After I rose to my feet I bowed to my instructors and rejoined my fellow students.

After everyone had finished we all sat in silence for about a minute. The examiners were talking between themselves, contemplating our results. Only five results would be announced today – those of the black belt candidates, and I was one of them. The chief instructor asked us all to stand and get into our rows, as we would do at the start of a class. We stood there while the examiners continued with their deliberations.

"I've failed; I can't believe it, I've failed," I thought to myself in a panic.

The next minute seemed to take forever. They were still discussing and I became increasingly worried.

"Did they see me lose my balance? Do they know that I'm deaf in one ear and that's why I find it harder to stand using one leg (excuses, excuses!). Do they know how hard I've worked to resolve this problem of mine? Has my instructor told them how difficult this has been with my limited sight? Surely I can't fail again."

They were ready to read out the results and the examiners rose to their feet. They all looked very serious as the chief examiner began to speak.

"Here are the five results."

He paused, almost as if to increase our tension.

"Paul… you have… passed. Congratulations. Please come and receive your new belt."

The crowd went wild and clapped with happiness as Paul made his way to our chief instructor.

"He deserved that, he performed really well and hardly made any mistakes," I thought to myself.

He shook their hands and bowed to each of them, then took his new black belt and returned to his place.

"Anthony… you have passed. Congratulations."

The crown began to clap once more and I did too but my nerves were in shreds. I was shaking and almost having a heart attack. I was really scared now because I knew that it was my result next. I was always third.

"I performed as well as Anthony, please don't fail me," I cried to myself.

I was almost collapsing under the pressure. Part of me knew that I had performed well but because I made a few mistakes I couldn't be sure that I had passed and I began to doubt my performance.

"Vendon!"

There was a pause as I held my breath.

"Congratulations, you have passed."

A big smile came to my face as the crowd went wild once more. I bowed towards the examiners before approaching them. First I bowed and shook the hand of our visiting examiner from Northampton, then I shook the hand of my instructor and bowed to him too.

"Thank you for your help sir," I whispered to him.

Slowly I made my way to my chief instructor and looked him in the eye. He looked like he was proud of me too. He smiled as he shook my hand with his right hand and passed me my black belt with his left. We bowed to each other as he congratulated me once more.

"Well done."

"Thank you sir."

As I turned I saw everyone looking at me and clapping their hands and I smiled with gratitude. The years of hard work had finally paid off and now here I was, standing with the highest prize in my hand, my black belt. It was an emotional moment where I, a big tough man, became tearful.

I had achieved my goal of qualifying for my black belt. Just like many others, I'd had moments when I'd felt like quitting because the level was too hard. Two years ago I failed an exam and contemplated quitting but I persisted to the end. As I took off my old red belt and replaced it with my new black belt I noticed that my belt had my name inscribed on one side. It was beautiful and I was proud to wear it. Then another thought came to me. It was of my second goal, to become an instructor.

The very next day I designed a poster to advertise my new class. My advertisement was placed in the local newspaper and the opening day came fast. I arrived at the training hall early and waited for any new students who had seen the advert. Slowly people began to enter and the hall became full.

A few minutes later I started the class and asked everyone to line up in rows. I counted sixty people, so many at my first class. As I stood there peering at the crowd I concentrated on the people on the back row and thought, "Just a few years ago I stood there, I stood at the back. I worked my way to the front and now here I stand as an examiner, an instructor, a teacher of my own class with my own students. In a few years someone from the back row will be standing here with me."

CHAPTER 10
A VISION OF MY FUTURE

Nearly two years later I was still teaching Martial Arts. I had one class and many students of all ages. The youngest was just five years old and I taught both men and women. Some of those who had come to my first lesson were no longer with me, but that was to be expected and others constantly joined to replace their numbers. When I first took up Taekwondo there were thirty or more students at a higher level than me and that didn't include the black belts, but over the five years that it took me to achieve the black belt level, less than ten of us managed to gain their black belts. I always considered achieving my black belt to be similar to completing a three-year college course (so it took me five). Many people drop out and only a few go on to take the final exam. That's why we give so much respect to other black belts and I lasted five years doing the same thing and being tempted to quit on the way.

Now I was teaching for myself, passing on my knowledge to others, hoping to help others achieve their black belts too. Several of my students were progressing well and were only a year or so away from becoming black belts themselves. These students needed more guidance, and I watched their every move to help them improve. Standing close, I would observe them and correct their small mistakes, fine tuning them for their final exam. Sometimes when they were slightly too far away I would miss an incorrect technique so most of the time I made sure that I stayed quite close to them so my lack of eyesight wouldn't affect my judgement.

I had already joined my instructors by sitting on the examiners board, behind the table and marking others taking their exams. It felt great to be sitting there and to finally find out what they discussed behind the table but it also opened my eyes to another problem.

"Look at him on the left," my instructor said one time.

"He's great isn't he?" I replied.

"Yes, he's outstanding at kicking and puts a great deal of effort into each technique."

"He does, I'm impressed."

We continued to observe other candidates and then my instructor saw a mistake.

"That boy in the middle has his thumb inside his fist when he punches; did you see? He does it all the time. I'll have to correct him."

What I saw through my eyes was slightly different; I couldn't see such detail. I could see his fist but not his fingers or thumb, they appeared too small through my eyes and I couldn't see them clearly.

"How can he see so clearly? I would normally be able to see his fingers and thumb when I stand closer, but sitting here behind this examiners table, he is a little too far away from me."

Although this only happened a few times when sitting behind the table, it slowly began to get on my nerves. There were also other times when I was constantly reminded of my impairment. At the beginning of a Martial Arts exam I would be given an information sheet by my instructor to fill in. I had to look at it very closely to be able to read the questions and filling the form in was another problem. With my failing eyesight I was struggling to see to write. Reading what I'd written was another complication and as the months went by these problems became increasingly arduous. I found a way of coping by memorising the questions on the forms, then I was able to write my marks and comments in the correct places as though I could see what I was doing. It was slowly becoming even harder to see and I knew that I would have to put some changes in place.

The time came for me to attend my next eye appointment and things were not looking good. I had already noticed that things that I had been able to see a few months before were now much less visible. I didn't know to what extent my sight had changed, nor by how much it had deteriorated. Remembering what had happened on my previous visit to the Eye Hospital, I went prepared for bad news and took a friend along with me this time to guide me back home safely.

We caught an earlier train and arrived at the hospital with time to spare. As I stood at the reception desk waiting to be served I began to feel distinctly nervous; I didn't really know what to expect and that was scary. We were told where to sit and the long stressful wait began.

"Will they be undertaking the same tests? Has my eyesight got worse or am I just imagining it? Will they be putting those awful eye drops in again? Have they found out more about my condition?"

The memories began to resurface. I was feeling stressed and depressed and I hadn't even been in for my appointment yet.

There were a lot of people waiting to be seen by the doctor and most of them were elderly citizens.

"I shouldn't be here. I'm so young, too young to be partially sighted. I've even had to bring someone along to help me get back home afterwards and now I feel completely hopeless. I can't do anything for myself."

Half an hour passed before I was finally called in for my first test.

"Can you cover your left eye and read that board please?"

The moment had finally come for me to find out how much my eyes had deteriorated or whether they had miraculously cured themselves! I proceeded to read the big letter that was all on its own. Then I read the first line and felt somewhat relieved, I struggled with the second line and when I tried to decipher the third, I couldn't.

"I could read that line last time," I thought desperately. "I had to strain my eyes, but I did it. Now I can't read any of it, not one letter."

It was obvious that my right eye was worse than it had been and I became slightly tearful, but I knew that my left eye had yet to be tested.

"Can you cover your right eye now please and read from the board with your left?"

"Here we go," I thought to myself, "maybe my left is the same or better than my right."

I did as I was instructed and covered my right eye. The large letter wasn't looking too clear and I began to have a bad feeling. As I struggled to read the first line I knew that there was no hope of me reading the second. I sat there despondently hoping that my eye would slowly get better and become clearer but I waited in vain. So I proceeded to guess the letters on the second line. I tried everything because I wasn't ready to accept the obvious. After making a dismal attempt I returned to my friend who was still sitting in the waiting room.

"I knew there was something wrong, I felt it," I thought to myself.

The next half an hour wait seemed interminable; it was as if someone had stopped time. I sat and had plenty of time to become sorry for myself.

"What's happening to me? Why does this have to happen to me? How bad are my eyes going to get? Can't they just stay the same so that I can readjust my life to cope?"

My eyes were getting worse and there was nothing I could do about it. My left eye was worse than my right and continuing to deteriorate at it's own pace.

"Maybe there's a cure," I thought as I was called in for my second test.

I followed the doctor and entered his room. He removed my glasses and put a patch on my left eye so that I couldn't see through it. As I sat on the chair I put my chin on the chin rest and peered at the white satellite dish that represented my field of vision. I remembered the test; they were about to shine a small light that looked like a torch and move it around the dish to see where I could and couldn't see it. The parts where I couldn't see were my blind spots. They had drawn up a graph with the results of my last test and would compare this to the new graph they would draw today. This would determine where the deteriorations were taking place. I had to press a button every time I saw the light. I remembered playing it like a game last time, but this time it felt like I was responding less, which set alarm bells ringing in my head.

My emotions began to trouble me and I felt that there was something seriously wrong. The doctor asked me to put the patch on my other eye and we began the same tests again.

"Can you see the light yet?"

I looked hard but there was no light.

"Where's the light? It must be there somewhere, but I can't see it. My eyes *can't* be this bad," I thought to myself.

"No I can't see the light," I answered nervously.

After a few more seconds the light appeared. It was like magic. A normal sighted person would see the light all the time. They would be able to see it at any part of the satellite but here I was struggling to see it at all. The doctor first brought the light from the top, in the middle, and then slowly moved it down until it ended up in the centre. I saw the light just before it got to the centre. That meant that most of the top of my eye was covered by blind spots. If someone threw a ball up and I tried to keep looking straight, the ball would suddenly disappear as it entered my blind spots.

The button wasn't getting much use with my left eye. He then took the light back to the top of the satellite dish, moved it slightly to the left or right and then proceeded to make his way towards the centre again. He performed this movement from the side and from the bottom going up towards the centre. I could feel which parts of my eye had blind spots and it was an awful feeling.

"Are you pressing the button whenever you see the light?"

"I am. I can't see the light very often."

He continued to mark his sheet.

Watching carefully I noticed that I could see the light earlier from my left.

"Does this mean that I can see more clearly from the left?" I wondered.

After a few more minutes he moved the light around in my blind spots and although I could hear him moving his light around, I couldn't see it. Then I heard him joining all the dots together and shading in the parts where I couldn't see.

I put my glasses on and waited for him to complete his sketch.

"How bad is it?" I asked.

"It's quite good."

"Then why did you ask me if I was pressing the button?"

"There was quite a large area where you couldn't see and I was just checking."

"Has it changed much from the last time?"

"Your left eye is showing a significant increase in areas where you have no vision."

"Is it a lot?"

"The professor will go into more detail."

He led me back out to the waiting room. My body felt weak. I was drained and not looking forward to anything else. I wanted to go home and cry. Thoughts rushed through my mind and I felt like someone had just died. The fight to go on had almost disappeared. It was too much for me to accept so early on in my life. I felt tearful but there were too many people around for me to get hysterical. I didn't say much to my friend, no, I didn't want to talk about slowly losing my eyesight. I sat and looked at my surroundings, waiting for my next test, hoping that it wouldn't be much worse.

After ten minutes I was called into another room. I sat with my chin on another chin rest and a doctor asked me to remove my glasses. He then moved a blue lens on the machine closer to my eye, first my left then my right. The lens was so close that it actually touched my eyes. To prevent me from blinking he held my eyelid open with his fingers. After writing a few things down he looked at the back of my eyes with a special light called an ophthalmoscope.

"I need to put some eye drops in to dilate your eyes."

"Do you have to?" I pleaded.

"Yes, it's the only way we can get a good look at the back of your eyes."

I really hated having this done. These were the eye drops that had made me see people as ghosts and that was scary. Though very reluctant, I let him put the drops into my eyes and then he sent me back out for another twenty minutes to let them take effect. I sat and watched as the world slowly disappeared before my very eyes. The lights gradually became brighter and more distorted as my eyes started to dilate. As this happened they began to hurt more and more and I struggled to keep them open. The leaflets on the shelves looked like someone had poured water all over the words and they were starting to smudge. The magazines on the table had disappeared and the details on the photos were distorted as if they were melting. Someone appeared to have rubbed the letter off the large sign that said 'Desk A'. The person sitting opposite suddenly had one-tone clothes and she looked like she was wearing a mask over her face. Everything around me looked as if it had been thrown into a giant blender and mixed together until nothing was recognisable. My world was changing and I had to sit there until the transformation was complete. The group of people walking past were so blurred that they didn't appear to possess any limbs. They all looked like ghosts. It felt really uncomfortable looking at the ghostly figures before me, they began to scare me so I closed my eyes and thought, "The ghosts are back so the transformation must be complete."

My friend could tell that I wasn't feeling well. Maybe it was the tears dripping from my eyes that made it obvious. He went to the cafeteria and brought back a sandwich for me.

"Look at the world through my eyes," I thought, "it doesn't even look real, ghostly figures everywhere. Not even the person next to me looks real. I'm really going to need help getting home."

It was my turn to see the doctor and I entered the room once more. I opened my eyes and peered around. The view was horrifying. The doors blended in with the walls, which had no obvious corners. Empty chairs looked like spilt paint. The view before me looked like a canvas that had been splattered with different coloured paint by a one-year-old. It was a mess and they expected me to make sense of it all. This time I had to link arms and be led into the room. The doctor looked at my eyes with a brilliantly bright light and it hurt. He held my eyelids open once more and told me to look straight ahead. My eyes kept trying to close but he wouldn't let them. Sometimes I looked away because of the sheer pain that the light was causing me. It felt like a massive torch being held against my eye or as if I was looking straight at the dazzling sun. My eyes were dilated and it made things appear larger.

"There's quite a lot of scarring here. Your disc is dark," he said as he continued his examination.

When he had finished he wrote down a few notes and asked me some questions.

"Have you noticed any pain in your eyes?"

"Yes, they seem to hurt quite a bit on a daily basis."

"The pressure in your eyes is a little high so I'll prescribe some eye drops to it bring down."

"What's causing the pressure?" I asked.

"You also have a condition called glaucoma."

"Oh great, I have RP and glaucoma?"

"Yes, but the eye drops will help to reduce the pressure."

"So what's next?"

"There's no need to do any more tests. We already know you have night blindness so you just have to see the professor for the results of your tests."

"Thanks, but I think that I already know my results."

After a few more minutes he led me out to wait to be seen.

It took about twenty minutes before I was called in and it was a long and depressing wait. I had plenty of time to sit and think.

"Glaucoma *and* RP? What… I knew something was wrong but I never expected another eye disorder. How much am I supposed to take before I crack? I've gone from being a clumsy short-sighted little boy to a complete misfit. Most people have enhanced hearing when they have poor vision but oh no, not me. I can't hear *or* see and now glaucoma? I give up, I can't take any more."

I felt like I was going to have a nervous breakdown. The tears streamed down my face before I entered the professor's room.

He read through my notes as I sat in silence. Then came his verdict.

"How do you feel?"

"I came here with short sight and now I have RP and glaucoma. It's humiliating; I'm young. Why am I suffering so much? What's happening to me? I don't even know if I'll be able to see when I wake up in the morning. It's not exactly a bright future to look forward to. I feel useless. I'm probably going to need help and assistance for the rest of my life. I'm an independent person. How am I supposed to live with this?"

"I know it must be hard for you to accept what's happening. Tell me more about your family."

"My parents haven't said much so you'll have to tell me more about RP and if there's any cure yet."

"From what we have seen in your eyes, you have one of three RP strains. It appears that you have a strain that runs in the male line of your family. We need to find out whether it comes from your father's or your mother's side, but this type lies dormant in females."

"Are you sure? Two of my sisters are short-sighted, isn't it possible that they have it too?"

"We'll have to test all of your brothers and sisters to make sure. Can you persuade them to make an appointment?"

"I don't think they'll be too happy but I'll try."

"Your results show a gradual deterioration of both eyes, but it's more pronounced in your left. Your field of vision is showing more blind spots but you still have your central vision."

Still struggling to hold off my emotions I squeezed out some more questions.

"What about my night blindness, you didn't test for it, why?"

"You're already suffering from night blindness and it will gradually get worse as your eyes deteriorate further. There's no need to test for that any more, the previous results were conclusive."

"So my nights will get darker?"

"Yes, you could say that, and the colours will slowly fade away."

"Is there any cure?"

"Not yet. Our eyes are complicated. Maybe in about ten years we will have a cure. RP is quite new and we don't know much about it."

"Is there anything I can do about my short sight?"

"Yes, go to your opticians and they should be able to give you stronger strength glasses."

I prepared myself for the biggest question, the one that scared me more than anything.

"Am I going blind?" The word seemed to echo around my head as I uttered it.

"We're not sure. You might never completely lose your eyesight or you could wake up tomorrow and be blind, we just don't know. Are either of your parents blind?"

"No, but my mother is losing her sight due to diabetes."

"Then it's possible that you won't go blind. We need to test your family to find out more. It's possible that your genes have mutated."

"What about being deaf in one ear?"

"That's why we need to test you. We're not sure which strain you have because you shouldn't be going deaf. Are you sure you didn't damage your ears? Or maybe it happened after an infection?"

"I'm deaf in one ear and my brother who suddenly went blind is experiencing problems with *his* hearing."

"This is very strange."

"It's too much for me."

"I recommend that you seek a councillor. They will help you to cope with your condition."

As I wiped my weepy eyes I muttered, "I'm fine."

He booked a further appointment for the following year and I left.

My helper was waiting patiently. He had been waiting for over three hours, but he was very understanding and hadn't complained once. He led me outside where I was met by that blinding light. I trembled helplessly as he slowly walked me to the train station. I felt old and frail. There were many ghostly figures; everywhere I looked I saw one. They had no faces as if their features had been eaten away. Their white clothing blended in with the yellow, cream and other light colours and the black, blue, red and grey were jumbled so that it looked as if they were wearing either light clothes or dark clothes, but no shades in between. As we walked along I saw cars that looked like solid blocks, windows without window frames, bikes without wheels and doors without handles. Notice boards and leaflets appeared to have lines drawn all over them without any visible words.

The light was still hurting my eyes and I resorted to looking down and occasionally closed my eyes as we walked. Steps had disappeared and I had to be told when to lift up my foot and be guided to step up when I reached a pavement. When we arrived at the train station I was amazed at the amount of ghostly figures. They were all rushing around and paying no attention to others. Occasionally they would collide with me and just rush away as though nothing had happened. It made me feel invisible. We sat on the train and I had to close my eyes because I felt disorientated. I couldn't work out who was closer to me and which people were further away. My sense of depth was affected. We spoke a few words on the journey home but not many. I sat on the right so that I could hear more clearly, but the noise of the train made it difficult so most of the time I sat in silence.

We arrived in Rugby and I opened my eyes again. Everywhere appeared even more blurred. It was probably because I had slightly forgotten how blurred my vision had become. We stood at the door and I waited for someone else to press the button to open it. The button had disappeared and if I had been on my own I wouldn't have been able to get out. I was then told when to step down and when to take a big step over the gap between the train and the platform. We then made our way out of the station. I was terrified as I struggled to avoid colliding with other people. We walked slowly and carefully towards my home.

"I feel completely useless," I thought to myself. "I have to be told when to step, where to step, mind the post, mind the people, mind the child and the small dog and mind the kerb. I'm hopeless and having to ask for help feels so degrading."

That evening I sat around and did little to help my mother. It was an uncomfortable feeling to see the world like this. I didn't feel able to do *anything*. I sat with my eyes closed in front of the television and just listened to the sounds. In my head I tried to put pictures to the sounds that I was hearing. When my family spoke to me I responded but I remained almost motionless. I couldn't see any point in looking at someone who appeared as a ghostly figure. They told me that my pupils were still dilated and my eyes were bloodshot. Feeling tired and drained I went to bed early and cried as I relived the events of the day.

"There's no cure? How am I going to face this? It's too much to cope with. I felt so useless having to be helped around. How will I be able to tell my boss at work? She'll probably want to be rid of me and then I'll struggle to get another job. What a tough life ahead and… I could wake up blind any day."

The thought of waking up and opening my eyes and not being sure whether they were open because I would be blind, scared me.

The next day I was woken by my alarm. I didn't know what to expect so I opened my eyes slowly and was immensely relieved to see light.

"Yes, I can see!" I thought cheerfully.

I opened my eyes wide but everywhere still looked blurred.

"Oh yeah, don't forget your glasses."

After feeling around for my glasses I placed them on my face but was presented with another challenge.

"Are they broken?" I thought frantically.

The room appeared to be just as blurred with my glasses on as off so I took them off again and replaced them once more but was horrified to see that there was no real difference.

"I don't believe this, my eyes must still be dilated. How will I be able to work?"

Sitting back down on my bed I contemplated the situation. I wasn't used to this view and decided to ask for an extra day off. Leaving my room was difficult. There was no door handle to be seen so I stopped and concentrated on where it *should* be. Groping around with my hand I located the handle and walked out of my room. Then

I navigated to where I knew the stairs were, but I wasn't quite sure exactly where they began. If I overstepped then I would fall down the stairs so I walked slowly, creeping forwards with my hands out in front so that I could break my fall if I accidentally tripped. One of my feet was at the top step and hung over it slightly. Now that I knew where the first step was I made my way carefully downstairs. I wasn't sure how many steps there were so I counted them as I descended. When I got to ten I slowed right down preparing for the last step. I held onto the banister as I crept down. When one of my feet was unable to go any lower I knew that I had reached the bottom step and committed the number to my memory.

"There are thirteen steps so I'll remember that for next time."

I stopped to think of where our telephone was kept. It was in the living room on the window ledge so I slowly made my way in. It was hard enough finding the door, now I had to find the phone in this distorted room. I walked a few steps before hitting the settee with my leg.

"I guess I should know where the settee is. I must remember that."

On my next step I heard a cracking noise like I was breaking something.

"That must be a little toy. I hope that I haven't broken it."

Shuffling my foot out of its way I proceeded to take a few more steps before hitting my knee on something sharp.

"Ouch! That really hurt. Must be the coffee table," I decided.

I rubbed my knee and crept on. When I looked over to where the telephone used to be I saw a hazy mass of different shaped outlines but no phone. One of those shapes was a telephone but as hard as I tried, I was unable to determine which one. So I resorted to touch and felt around until I came across what felt like a telephone. I straightened it out and picked up the receiver and then replaced it once more.

"Where have the buttons gone?" I thought to myself.

Now I had to work out where the keys were. If it had just the numbers zero to nine then it would have been easy but this telephone had additional buttons.

"I think the zero is on the last line and second from the left."

Working my way along I found the zero. Then I slowly typed in my work number that I knew off by heart and… it was the wrong number!

"No; there's a line of additional buttons on the left so that means the zero would be the third one across from the left."

I tried again and was successful.

My boss was very understanding and agreed that I could take another day off as sick leave. I struggled to put the receiver back on the holder then turned, thought for a few moments to get my bearings and then made my way carefully across the room to the television. Then I had to remember where the button was; I put my hand out and searched slowly until I came across it. I switched it on and found somewhere to sit. The picture on the screen was too distorted and I began to try to work out what was being shown. When people stood still they blended into the background. I only knew that there were people there from the sound of their voices and from the movements on the screen. I sat right in front of the television to see if being closer helped. Although things became slightly clearer, they were still not clear enough to make me want to watch these outlines moving around. The background was so distorted that it all looked the same – it was hopeless. Then I decided to change the channel, but I couldn't find the remote. I hunted around for a while, dropping a few things, but not breaking anything (well, that's what I told my mum), but I still wasn't able to find it.

After a few minutes of trying to decipher the picture I returned to my place on the sofa. The screen appeared so distorted that it was straining my eyes to look at, so I closed my eyes and listened. It was easy to work out what was going on with the news because most of it was verbal information. When a show came on I imagined pictures in my head of what was happening. It was like reading a book. An hour or so had passed and I was still in front of the television. The programme wasn't very interesting and I was unable to change the channel. As I opened my eyes I noticed that objects were a fraction clearer. Looking around at the distorted room depressed me so I rose to my feet and started to make my way to the door. Suddenly I stopped as I vividly remembered that there was a coffee table around somewhere, so I slowed down, as I didn't want to bash into it again. There was no door handle in sight so I felt around until my hand was upon it. I slowly made my way to the kitchen and observed the multitude of distorted images.

"How am I supposed to make breakfast?"

The sight I saw was horrific. All the cups had disappeared. The cutlery, the plates, pots and pans all looked the same.

"Where do I start?" I thought.

I went over to the sink and felt around to see what I could recognise.

"This feels like a knife and that a spoon. I need this."

Then I rummaged some more.

"Whoops, I nearly broke a glass. Lucky I was moving my hand so slowly."

Everywhere I explored I tried to remember what was there.

"This feels like a cup and another one and this is a bowl. I need that too."

Slowly I made my way over to where the table would be if I could see more clearly. I placed the bowl down cautiously sliding it into place and trying not to knock anything off the table. It looked like a pile of mess and I didn't know what anything was. After placing my spoon in the bowl I turned and approached the cupboard where the breakfast cereal would be, not forgetting where I had placed the bowl. The boxes of cereal all looked the same so I picked each one up and brought it close to my face to see if I could recognise anything. The 'W' on the Weetabix box stood out slightly and it was also a thinner box.

"This is the Weetabix so that bigger box must be the Corn Flakes."

It was all a guess. I wasn't sure but I had to eat something. I took the box of, hopefully, Corn Flakes over to where my bowl was and tipped it gently. The sound I heard indicated that my guess had been correct, but it sounded as if there were Corn Flakes spilling on the table as well as into the bowl, but I couldn't see. After I had finished pouring some in I returned the box to the cupboard.

Then I walked over to the fridge to get the milk. Once again everything looked the same and I picked up a few items before finding the right bottle.

"How am I going to pour the milk into my bowl without spilling it?"

An idea came to me.

"I know, I'll hold the bowl with my left hand so I know exactly where it is and pour until I think that I've got enough milk. Then I'll put one of my fingers into the bowl to feel how much milk is actually there and pour more if I need to."

So that's what I did. My finger was wet but I had successfully poured milk into a bowl without being able to see it.

Then I squashed the Corn Flakes into the milk trying to wet them all. I like my Corn Flakes soggy (real soggy!) and I decided to go and brush my teeth while they soaked up the milk (yum, yum!).

Walking slowly, I managed to find the stairs.

"How many steps were there again? Was it twelve or thirteen?"

I began to walk upstairs and counted my steps as I went. When I got to ten I slowed down and stepped even more carefully as I proceeded to get to the top. As I turned to head towards the bathroom my hands struck the door. I felt for the handle and entered. As I stood by the sink I saw many outlines that appeared to be similar. I felt a few and found several toothbrushes but I was unable to see which was mine. A few seconds passed as I tried desperately to remember where I had left it but was still unsure, so I washed my face with water and returned to my room where I lay waiting for my breakfast to go soggy.

"I can't even have breakfast properly. I might as well close my eyes because I appear to be doing most things from memory or touch. How am I going to brush my teeth? Do I have to ask for help again? It's like I can't do anything for myself. If I could see I would be able to find my toothbrush and toothpaste and the television remote. Now I have to go back down and find the sugar. I feel so useless."

As I lay there I heard my brother rummaging around. After a while I also heard my mother.

"How can I help my mother in this state? My brother's going to work so he can't."

Ten minutes later I heard the front door. It was one of my sisters coming to help my mother.

"Saved by my sister," I thought as I made my way out of my room.

Although I found it difficult to say, I asked my sister to find my toothbrush and toothpaste. Putting the toothpaste on the toothbrush was another challenge. Somehow I managed it, maybe too much toothpaste and not all of it on the toothbrush but I managed it.

I went downstairs remembering the amount of steps and entered the kitchen. I asked my sister to find the sugar and I carefully put some on my soggy but tasty breakfast!

"I feel like an invalid," I thought to myself. "I'm so independent and find it difficult to ask for help. I might as well go back to my room because I'm no use to anyone."

When I'd finished my breakfast I apologised to my family and went back to my room. I lay there with my eyes closed.

"I'm no use to anyone," I repeated to myself. "I may as well stay in my room. Maybe this is why so many blind people become reclusive and stay in their homes."

Occasionally I opened my eyes to see the world slowly reappearing. After about three hours my eyes were no longer dilated and my sight was restored to normal! It was a scary view of my future, not being able to have clearer sight. It was amazing the amount of complications it caused me. Not being able to find my toothbrush, toothpaste, find items in cupboards and not being able to watch television. It opened my eyes and made me think.

"I could wake up any day and see like that permanently. How scary. I'm going to have to find ways to get around because I'm not going to ask for help all day every day for the rest of my life. I would prefer to stay here in my room and become a recluse. I'll have to find ways of putting a label to some of the outlines I see. I need to be more organised so that I can find things. It's time to make some serious changes to my life."

CHAPTER 11
GIVING UP THE GHOST

It was April 1989. My mother's ailments were getting progressively worse and I had little time to think about my own problems. She had already been in hospital for breathing problems and was experiencing them again and she was also suffering from several other afflictions. Arthritis in her hips, that gave her pain when she walked, a kidney failure, and heart and lung disorders that made it hard for her to breathe. Her diabetes had now made her blind, and she had high blood pressure. She had also been in hospital for an operation on her eyes; they had performed laser surgery on both eyes to relieve some distress that had been caused by her diabetes. She now wore special glasses that had lenses in the centre because they had removed the lenses from her eyes. She never spoke much about her family so I always wondered if the problems with her eyes had anything to do with RP, but she was being treated by the hospital so surely they would have diagnosed her. She always blamed the problems with her eyes on her diabetes and that is something I will have to accept.

She needed constant care, which we provided, and we did all the normal household chores. After tidying up reluctantly, I would make her a cup of tea and ask what she wanted me to buy at the shop. My sister would then take over the nursing duties. We were all very worried about her and did our best to care for her. She had been sick for over fifteen years; it began soon after she gave birth to her last child, Percy. He was a difficult baby and must have put her body under too much strain. Then again after having eleven children, I think most women's bodies would be strained.

One morning I walked to the town centre to do some shopping. My mother had given me a list and I also had a few things to do in town for myself. I went to the bank first and then I was going to look for a present for my mother, as it was her birthday in two weeks time. When I arrived at the bank there was a queue for the cashiers. I had used this bank for a few years and was used to where things were. The queue slowly got smaller until finally it was my turn to be served. The person behind me in the queue had to tell me which cashier's desk to go to; there were numbers above each of their windows and they flashed when the cashier was ready to serve the next customer. I used to be able to see the numbers quite clearly but now they looked out of focus. As I walked towards the number it became clearer and I was able to read it. I handed in a few cheques that I wanted to pay into my account. I was able to fill in the credit slip to say how much I was paying in. After being served I went to look for a present for my mother.

There were a few steps leading up to the door of the shop I wanted to go in. Going up them never gave me much trouble; the light would shine off parts of the steps and there would be a slight shadow where the light was unable to reach. Although this sounds trivial, it would become important in my later life.

My mother sometimes complained that she was cold so I had decided to buy her some warm clothing. I could see most of the garments clearly enough, but some were displayed in darker parts of the shop and I had difficulty making out the colours and styles. My main problem was reading the price tags. The print was very small and the poor light in parts of the shop made it worse. I didn't mind asking one of the assistants once or twice, but I needed help to read nearly all of them. So instead of bothering them all the time I picked up each item I was interested in and held it close to my face so that I could read it. Sometimes I also had to angle the price tag towards the light to gain brightness. This generally proved successful, but when I still couldn't see a label properly I put the garment back and hunted for something else. Unable to decide on a piece of clothing I set on my way to a shoe shop.

On the way out I tripped down the steps and nearly fell. I had forgotten about the steps, but more important, they were now invisible! Most steps are of one colour and to a normal sighted person this causes no real problems, but to someone with poor vision it becomes hazardous. The edges of steps are almost non-existent and our depth of vision is poor so we can't see that the ground is getting lower. When the light shines onto a horizontal step it appears to be on one level so without clear markings on the edge of them it looks as if there is no step. This caused me problems and they would get worse!

After composing myself I walked along to the next shop to look at shoes. Finding shoes wasn't too hard, but I had trouble reading price tags again. Another problem was being able to read the different sizes. Each shoe had a clear label inside stating the size, that is, it would be clear to normal sighted people but to me it was like trying to read the distorted line on the optician's board. By bringing the shoe very close to my face I could read most of the sizes, but one had a very dark sole and I couldn't make it out so I resorted to asking for help.

I found one of the assistants. "Excuse me, but what size is this shoe?"

"It's written on the label inside the shoe," the lady replied.

"I…"

I paused while I decided on my choice of words.

"Should I say that I'm partially sighted? No, that's too embarrassing, I can't. They probably wouldn't believe me anyway," I thought to myself.

"I have poor eyesight and am struggling to see it," I said instead.

The shop assistant looked without picking up the shoe and was able to read it for me.

Although I looked at a lot of shoes, each pair that I studied was either not quite what I was looking for or was too expensive so I went into several different shops and encountered the same problem in each one. Eventually I made a decision and went to purchase the chosen shoes. My money was a little difficult to decipher so I held it closer to be able to see it, then I paid for the shoes and left the shop.

As I walked through the town centre I passed the clock tower. I looked up and took note of the time. There was still enough time for me to look in one more shop so I went to one that sold watches. As I got close to the door I became confused. It was a glass door and I couldn't work out whether it was already open or not. I couldn't see a handle, which made me think the door must have been open, so I tried to walk in and bumped my head on the door. It was closed!

"This door is a plain sheet of glass! How is someone with low vision supposed to see it? If they had posters or something stuck on it that would help, but clear glass confused me into thinking that the door was open."

I rubbed my head and felt around until I found the handle and entered the shop.

"I hope no one saw me. How embarrassing! Hitting my head by bumping into a glass door. My eyesight is affecting my judgement even more these days."

The watches in the shop were all behind glass but I could hardly tell. From where I was standing it was a little difficult to see the details of each watch so I asked to see one or two of them, but then decided to leave the shop rather than embarrass myself asking for assistance regularly. As I walked along to the grocery store I looked through shop windows and peered at the signs but most were just out of my focus range and I would have had to be much closer to be able to see clearly. A few things went through my mind.

"I keep on denying it but my eyesight is getting worse. I'm struggling with glass doors where sometimes I'm not sure whether they're open or closed. Those watches were hard to see and I would feel hopeless asking them to bring out all the ones that I was interested in. It felt humiliating to ask the shop assistant to read the labels on those shoes. The numbers on the cashiers' desks at the bank are almost impossible to read until I'm right up close. I even struggled a little seeing what was written on those cheques and as for steps… I'm really starting to have problems."

I continued to wonder how much worse things could get as I entered the grocery shop.

Finding what I needed was becoming increasingly difficult. I'd ask for assistance a few times but on most occasions I would manage on my own. I was already trying to remember where items were in certain shops and I would try to do most of my shopping in those stores. In the grocery shop I walked to where the sugar should be and checked it was still there, then I picked one of the bags up and held it close to my eyes to be able to read the label. There were different kinds of sugar and I didn't want to purchase the wrong one. Sometimes I had to take my glasses off to read the small prices and labels, it was strange but it worked for me. I had to pick most things up to read them whereas most people would take a quick glance and then walk on.

I couldn't see through the glass fridges to find out what products were inside so I ended up opening most of them. Then I would take something out like chicken and assume that the fridge was full of chicken and nothing else. This was guessing of course because sometimes there would be several different products in the same fridge and, having realised that, I would end up going through each fridge several times. If someone had been watching me they would assume that I was buying a mass of shopping from the amount of items that I picked up. I would take a quick look then put the item back, then pick something else up, read it and put that back too. It was a slow process but it worked. It was frustrating not being able to read things like labels or prices and I also felt useless having to ask several times for assistance when I couldn't find things I needed. I really despised the organised shops that would change the positions of their products around. It's annoying to a normal sighted person but it's like the end of the world to someone with poor eyesight. It would be like walking into a shop with no labels on anything. These were the times that I would ask for assistance the most.

"Excuse me, but I can't find the tins of tomatoes."

"They're over there on the second shelf down," the girl said as she pointed me in the right direction.

"I've looked but I can't see them; can you find them for me please?"

She led me to the correct part of the shop, stood with me next to them and pointed once more.

"Thank you... thank you."

I wanted to say something else but it just wouldn't come out. I tried, I really did, but I wasn't ready. I was going to say that I needed to know which were the tins of whole plum tomatoes and which were the chopped tomatoes and that I needed assistance with reading the labels, but it wouldn't come out because I would have had to explain that I was partially sighted. I had been doing well, informing most of my friends of my disabilities but I felt uncomfortable opening up to strangers. It was just about bearable to ask where something was, but to ask them to show me and read the label for me felt degrading. One statement just meant that I couldn't find where the products were stored, but the other meant that I couldn't see or read them. That was the one I couldn't deal with yet. I hadn't got a blind person's stick because in theory I wasn't that bad, but actually that's what I really needed.

On the way home I noticed that people's features were slightly more blurred than before. I could still see their eyes, nose and mouth but in slightly less detail. Many people also told me that I was now confusing colours more regularly. I would sometimes see yellow as white and red as grey but not just at night, it was also happening during the day now. Crossing the road was becoming a definite pain. Sometimes I wouldn't see bicycles and motorbikes and I would hesitate to cross the roads. On several occasion I had near misses, but had only once been hit by a cyclist. My hand and my leg were cut although nothing too serious, but I did feel sorry for the cyclist seeing me step out right in front of him.

When I got back home I put the shopping away and began to make my mother some food. She loved chicken and rice and that's what I made for her. As I passed her the plate she struggled so much to hold it, her hands were constantly shaking from her illnesses. Everyone was getting really worried about her but she was more concerned about my father. He hadn't visited for two weeks now and she said that she had a bad feeling. Most of the time we ignored her superstitions but this time she scared us. At one time my father used to come and visit everyday, but slowly, as he became more senile, his visits became more infrequent. Every day became every two days and then every few days, but two weeks without seeing him was the longest. Throughout the day she voiced her concerns for him, first telling my brother Percy and then my sister June after she finished work. We couldn't take it any more and agreed to go and see him. So I went with Percy and June to find out if he was all right.

The house looked quiet and almost spooky. My brother knocked at the door, but there was no answer.

"Maybe he's gone out," I said.

"He hardly ever goes out these days," Percy replied as he proceeded to knock a few more times.

Then he crouched down and called through the letterbox but to no avail. Now we were worried. We looked up at his bedroom window as he would often be there looking out, but he wasn't there. After a few more minutes of vigorous knocking, we decided to go around to the rear of the house and try the back door. We walked through the alleyway and entered the garden, which was overgrown and badly in need of some work. My father had said that he would attend to it and stubbornly wouldn't let us help, but obviously he had not. We knocked several times before giving up.

We stood and wondered what to do. My mother suspected that something was seriously wrong with my dad and wouldn't be satisfied unless we had seen or spoken to him. She was very superstitious and many years ago she had saved my elder brother and sister from a fatal accident. They had been invited to a party in London where hundreds of teenagers were gathering. People were going from all over the country to attend this party. My mother awoke that morning and told them that she'd had a terrifying dream that there was going to be a serious accident at this party where several people would be injured. It took many hours for her to persuade them not to go, but living with my mother for years with her constant vivid dreams that sometimes came true finally did it. Many others from Rugby went to the party and the next day on the television news came the breaking story that would change our perception of our mother's dreams. The house where the party took place had mysteriously burnt down and many people had died including a brave young man from Rugby. My brother and sister could have been in that fire where many people had jumped to their death, but they had been saved by a mere dream. Since that incident we had grown to trust my mother and felt that we had to stay until my father was found safe.

We were tempted to wait until he returned but we soon decided to break in and make sure that he wasn't inside. Somehow we were able to force open a window and my brother climbed in and opened the back door for us. We crept in slowly calling my father at the same time, but there was no reply. We checked all the rooms downstairs and then we thought that we heard a noise upstairs like something heavy had dropped. My heart was beating very fast and for some reason I became scared and chills took over my body as we raced up the stairs. We slowly opened his bedroom door still calling him and there by the window, on the floor, lay my father. We rushed over to him to see if he was still breathing. His eyes were open and he looked as if he was trying to say something. We all panicked and didn't know what to do. He was alive but needed immediate hospital treatment. We were hysterical and rushed around frantically looking for the phone. When we found it we discovered that it was disconnected so my sister and I rushed outside to ask some passing pedestrians. Someone had a phone and we called for an ambulance.

Within minutes the ambulance arrived and we rushed back upstairs to help Percy. They said that our father had suffered a stroke and would need hospital treatment. Within another few minutes he was gone and we rushed back home to inform my mother. On hearing the news she broke down and cried saying that she knew something was seriously wrong. We tried to calm her down and suggested we all go to the hospital to see him, but she refused saying that she was too upset. So we left her and rushed to the hospital. After a while he was brought out of the emergency room and put on a ward where we could visit him. He lay very still with his eyes open swallowing his saliva vigorously. I was scared and very upset. It wasn't time to lose my father; he was the fit and healthy one. My mother had been sick for years and still going strong, it couldn't be time to lose my father.

The next few days were stressful and depressing. My father was still in hospital and had not improved and my mother was still refusing to visit him. She had another dream and saw that he was just waiting for her to visit before he finally give up the ghost. We didn't know what to do. I was very emotional and thought that she would turn out to be right again so we waited... and waited.

Sometimes we sat around quietly thinking to ourselves and other times we argued, trying to come up with a unified solution. While we were quiet, I had time to relive some memories about my father. He used to drive us to school in his van, which had about twelve seats. It was like a day out because there were so many of us. Sometimes he would drive us to Birmingham to buy some Jamaican food and he always complained about me not liking very many of the traditional dishes. Sometimes they had to cook separate food for me.

We were always so excited to see him. Once we had a car accident on the way to collect him from work. My eldest brother was driving with my mother, my sister Carline and me – Daddy's son! We were in the fast lane and a car suddenly pulled out in front of us. My brother slammed on the brakes and the car skidded because the road was wet. He lost control and we veered off the road and into a ditch. The car rolled a few times during the episode. I somehow held tight and didn't get thrown around the car but my mother and sister did. I woke up to see my mother with broken glass all over her and my sister was still unconscious. We were all taken to the hospital and found out that my sister had seriously damaged her neck. She had to wear a neck brace for months. It was a miracle that I suffered no injuries, but ever since then I've been scared of driving fast and still get flashbacks today.

My father sometimes played his guitar and always made me laugh because he wasn't very good. Sometimes he would take out his false teeth and chase us around the house. He used to attend church regularly and read his Bible every day. He told us about some Bible study competitions that he took part in and said that his team always won when he was present because he answered most of the questions.

Nine days had passed and still no sign of improvement. He had suffered a stroke and had a brain haemorrhage. There were many discussions about him. Some agreed with our mother not to visit and to keep him going with the hope of improvement and others wanted him out of his pain and misery. We gathered together and finally persuaded our mother to visit him one day. At the hospital she bravely held back her tears and stroked his hand. We were all there watching and waiting but nothing happened. After a while we all went home to comfort my mother. She was still adamant that something was going to happen. That evening, that same evening, we received a phone call from the hospital. My father had passed away. Just a few hours after my mother had finally visited he left our world.

"I told you he was just waiting for me to visit," my mother cried.

She cried hysterically for hours. I couldn't take it any longer and left to visit a friend called Paula. After I told her what had happened I broke down and cried in her arms. I had never cried that way before nor have I since. He was the first person in our family to pass away and it was a total shock. He had been a healthy man and nobody had expected him to die. He was just sixty-three years old and had to take early redundancy a few years earlier. Things hadn't gone quite according to his plans and he got into financial difficulty. Three of us helped him out for two years and clubbed together to pay his mortgage. It didn't leave me with much money to spend but he was my dad and more important than any amount of money. I'm sure he was heartbroken from having to depend on us and it probably caused him extra stress. A year or so went by without him redecorating and

I know he wasn't happy with the temporary split of our family, but I guess his pride got in the way of finding other solutions.

Just three days before my mother's birthday, on the 4th May 1989 after nine days of fighting, my father finally left this world.

CHAPTER 12
HAVING TO ADAPT TO COPE

After the sudden loss of my dear father, the next few years were hard. I found it was difficult not to keep thinking about him and whether there could have been anything more that I could have done. Finding my father there, lying on the floor dying, haunts me. If I hear his name, it brings back memories. He was very devout and every time I hear about people reading the Bible, I remember that he used to read it every day and used to give us money for doing the same. I even remember receiving money for being able to recite the names of all sixty-six books off by heart. We were brought up in the church but slowly I drifted away and didn't continue where my parents left off. The world is full of challenges and I felt that I had suffered as much as I could take, so my faith floundered. I found it easy to blame my mishaps on God. It took a long time, but eventually I would realise that it was God who kept me going.

That first year was extremely depressing for me. Some nights I lay in bed crying to myself. His sudden death had made me realise that anyone could go at anytime. I wanted to spend as much time with my mother as possible, knowing that her life could soon come to an end and I wanted her to enjoy what time she had left as much as possible. Sometimes we would have disagreements but I always looked for ways to make up, even when I thought that I was in the right. I was scared of losing my mother so I tried my best not to have arguments. It was an emotional year that ended with some great news. On the 7th October 1989 my first child was born. Her name is Michaela Wright and she is beautiful. She needed a great deal of attention but she's worth it.

My mother was moving house to a bungalow; she was hardly walking at all and was mostly confined to a wheelchair. There was no room for me in the bungalow so I bought my first house. It had three bedrooms and the bathroom was downstairs, but it needed a great deal of improvement. When we first moved in it was infested with cockroaches. I was scared of them but I still had to remove them from around Michaela. I called an exterminator and was rid of them forever.

I visited my mother every day. My younger brother Percy had moved in with her and my sister Angela cared for her daily. She was frail and needed assistance in most situations and was now registered as disabled and had acquired a car for mobility. My brother drove her wherever she wanted to go and she would then get around with the aid of her wheelchair. We could all tell that she was still suffering from the loss of her husband and we were doing everything possible to keep her happy. Her health was deteriorating rapidly and we were afraid that we would soon lose her too. We began to take her to places that she had always wanted to visit or see. I took her to her first visit to the cinema; she really enjoyed it although she couldn't really see the screen clearly, but she was grateful. I also took her to a reptile exhibition and she touched a snake for the first time. She was ecstatic and spoke of it many times. She was happy to achieve her lifetime goals but every Christmas she would say that it would be her last. We were always grateful to see her in the New Year but would become increasingly worried about her close to the next Christmas. We were on edge with my mother's poor health for a long time.

My vision was also deteriorating more rapidly. Some mornings I would open my eyes and thank God that I was still able to see something, then moan about the challenges I had to endure for the rest of the day. My faith was put to the test and every few months I would notice a slight difference in my vision. I realised that it was time for me to learn to adapt and find ways of coping with what I could and couldn't see. It meant adjusting my lifestyle and also giving up some things that I cherished so much.

The first sport to suffer was roller-skating. It was something I loved doing and was a good way of getting away from the stresses of life. It made me laugh, smile and kept me happy. That was until my last skating session.

My problems started as soon as they switched off the lights in the skating hall. There were lights from the disco, but they weren't bright enough for me to see proficiently.

"It looks a little darker than usual in here today," I thought. "That corner over there was the only really dark area before, but it all appears to be dark now."

As I skated around weaving and dodging through the other skaters I kept nearly colliding with people who seemed to appear in front of me from nowhere. Their features and outlines that I already found difficult to see were even more blurred. Sometimes I would be skating happily along through what seemed like an open space and the next second I would be on the floor after bumping straight into someone. Other times I would be skating past a group of people and crash into someone because the group was bigger than I could see. This happened too many times and I was beginning to hurt people, but I was also hurting inside from not being able to see enough. I was becoming a hazard to others and it was making me feel depressed. Many thoughts buzzed around my mind.

"I know that my vision is getting worse but I can't give up roller-skating. Can't my eyes just stop deteriorating so that I can get on with my life? It's my life and I enjoy skating so much."

Peter and Adam were there and sometimes I skated with them, but most of the time I was unable to find them or unable to keep up with them due to the amount of collisions I was experiencing. On many occasions I just stood there looking for them.

"Where are they? I can usually identify them from their outlines but everyone looks so faint that I can hardly tell the difference between male and female. It's like looking at a load of ghosts."

All I could see were moving shadows, mostly grey, some darker than others but none of them were clear. There was no difference between their faces and their bodies, they were just shadows. There were some little kids there and I didn't want to skate into them so I skated very carefully. I had reduced my speed and stopped doing stunts like skating backwards but I was still experiencing problems.

My skating partner was there as usual and she came up to me. "You were standing on your own near me for ages. Why didn't you come over?"

"I didn't see you," I answered.

It was apparent that she had forgotten about my poor vision and was expecting me to recognise her in the dark. She genuinely had forgotten and I felt uncomfortable having to remind her. When she had approached me she hadn't said her name so I had to struggle listening to her with only one good ear to work out who she was. I had to do this with most people and although I told them to say who they were, most of them didn't. It began to bother me a lot and I had to think of a solution before it depressed me further.

"Reminding people all the time is really upsetting me," I thought. "I need to find a way of knowing who they were without having to keep asking them. I don't want to lose their friendship, so what can I do?"

We skated around and I continued to ponder.

"If I can't hear someone who I've told several times to stand on the other side of me, then I'll just guess what they're talking about and if I get the subject wrong... too bad. If people can't be bothered to take someone's disability into consideration, then why should I care about their feelings? If they can be ignorant... then so can I."

I was still skating with my friend Sally and thinking of other ways to adapt and cope with the problems my sight and hearing loss were causing.

"If people complain about having to repeat what they've said then I'll pretend to be listening but not make much conversation with them. I'm deaf in one ear and can't help having to ask people to repeat themselves, so if they lose their patience with me... too bad! I didn't ask to be deaf and I wouldn't wish it on anyone so why should I make all the effort? Others have to learn to compromise too."

I could feel my attitude towards others changing. My personality was slowly being reshaped. Life had treated me unfairly for long enough and now I was getting a little frustrated and slightly angry.

"If people who I've known for a long time start talking to me without telling me who they are, I'll talk to them but I won't be that interested in what they're saying. If they know that I can't see very well, the least they can do is to show me some consideration."

The anger inside me grew as time went on. Slowly I could feel my character changing. I didn't seek to change my personality or alter the way I was on purpose; it just felt like it was the only thing I could do to prevent full-blown depression setting in. My fight had already started to deal with the many difficulties I was experiencing: hearing loss, glaucoma and... well, I had not realised it, but also going blind.

Skating was finished and I returned home. There was no hanging on the back of trucks that day; I skated home safely on the pavement.

The next day I went out for a solo skate. I skated behind my father's home, where I often went to be alone. I was trying to see how fast I could focus on objects because I still loved skating too much to give it up. After a while I decided to try and jump over something. Usually I could jump, skate fast and skate backwards proficiently, but I was struggling slightly and wanted to practise until I overcame my disadvantage. I was determined to practise until I became adept again. I jumped a few times and it felt fine but I needed to know if I could still jump over an object and if I still knew where to take off from the ground. It was becoming hard to focus, but I was determined to overcome it. There were two car tyres lying around in the alleyway so I placed them in the middle touching each other so I wouldn't have that far to jump! As I skated to my position for my run up I paused for a minute.

"Come on; you can do it. You can't give up yet," I coaxed myself. "There must be ways to modify how I skate so that I can carry on safely."

The tyres looked so far away from me and so out of focus. They looked like two blurred blobs in the distance. They looked nothing like tyres.

"I'll just skate towards them fast and as they come into focus I'll have to make a quick decision about where to take off from. I'm used to this; I can do it. Just think fast."

I decided to go for it and started skating towards the tyres. The alleyway was quite smooth so I was able to pick up speed well. As I approached the tyres they began to come into focus. The closer I skated, the more detailed they became. I was almost ready to jump when I felt one of my skates hit a small stone. It was too late to stop so I jumped and flew through the air over the tyres. It became apparent that I had left the ground a split second too early because of the stone and not being able to see clearly enough to know the exact point of my take off. I had guessed as usual, but this time I had guessed wrong and was about to pay for it.

It felt a fraction too early as I started floating down. As I got lower the tyres were still underneath me.

"I'm going to hit them," I thought hysterically.

I started to panic as I brought my knees up higher trying not to hit the last tyre, but as I got closer I felt my skate wheels clip the edge of the tyre. It held on to my wheels and I began to topple. As I felt myself falling I straightened out my hands to break my fall. I was still travelling quite fast and as my hands hit the ground I continued to slide on my knees until I eventually ground to a halt.

I lay there for a few seconds and felt a tingling sensation in the palms of my hands. As I turned them to have a closer look, I saw blood gushing from both hands. There were also little stones lodged into my skin. I was hurt and needed to get home to wash the blood off. I sat up and checked my knees, which were beginning to feel rather painful. A weird sensation came over me as I pulled up my tracksuit to reveal my knees. They too were cut badly and I had scratches on my shins. Now in more pain from knowing the extent of my injuries I rushed off as fast as I was able to get cleaned up.

As I bathed my wounds I contemplated what to do about the future of my roller-skating.

"Maybe it's time to quit. I may love skating but I'll probably incur many more injuries. I checked the path and it appeared clear but because of my impaired vision I was unable to see the stone. Others would have seen it clearly."

My knees were a mess and I was in pain and I began to get angry.

"Why do I have to give up? Why are my eyes failing? It was so dark in the skating hall it almost scared me. What am I going to do, stand on the sidelines and watch others enjoying themselves? Oh no; I wont even be able to do that will I because I can't see enough."

Trying to decide what to do was frustrating me. I'd been skating for ten years and really enjoyed it.

I continued the battle with myself.

"Maybe I'm better off quitting now while things are still quite good. I've had my fun and now it's time to grow up. Maybe it's better this way. At least other people can skate safely without me being a hazard. Now I won't cause any more accidents."

It was a tough decision to make, but I knew deep down that it was the right one – I quit roller-skating that day. It was hard giving up something that I had grown to love so dearly. I was tempted to continue, I could perhaps skate slower, but that would have made me feel useless and it was also too much of a risk for others. Innocent people would probably get injured from me colliding with them or skating over their fingers. I could always tell people that I was getting too old for skating, at least then I wouldn't feel so hopeless. I changed my mind a few times but I followed it through and finally gave up roller-skating. There were no more Saturday morning skating sessions for me, no more weaving, dodging and laughing, no more holding hands with Sally or skating fast, no more taking risks hanging on the back of trucks and no more jumping over ridiculous objects. It was all over and I had to find other ways of bringing me some pleasure. Although I felt very sad and emotional at the loss of one of my main sports, I still had my Martial Arts to keep me going. From then on I put even more effort into achieving great things.

After making the decision to give up roller-skating I had more time to concentrate on Martial Arts. With my increasing problems of marking grading exams I set out to pass my second-degree black belt and gained the ability to make changes to exams.

So I opened up another class. At the next exam I brought out some new student record forms. The writing was bigger and the names of techniques were abbreviated to fit onto one form. With these changes marking became easier and I started looking forward to marking exams again. Another way I coped with my impaired vision at a grading was by asking the students to perform the techniques closer to the examiners' table. My new system was working and I was now ready to sit with a group of instructors and using my marking system, promote my first students to the black belt level. There were three of them and I sat there watching them perform techniques that I had taught them. They looked fantastic, the way they jumped, kicked and fought each other. They even succeeded in breaking a brick thanks to my instruction. It was like looking at myself being duplicated.

At the end of their exam they lined up in their rows awaiting our decision. The instructors discussed their decision with me and I agreed with their criticism. At last I heard what the examiners discussed when assessing black belts. All three of my students passed and I was ecstatic. It made me so proud watching them receive their black belts from my instructor's hand. Two of my black belts went on to open classes of their own and the duplication process started all over again. I also continued to adapt my teaching methods and produced some outstanding students.

During classes I was now walking closer to the students when they were performing techniques so that I could see well. I was getting used to where to stand to be able to see what they were doing. When my students were performing set routines I would only have a few up at the same time so that I could get closer. It took longer to tutor everyone but I was able to see when they were making mistakes. It would have been great to be able to stand at the front of a class and see the people at the back clearly but that was just a fantasy. I had to adjust my teachings to be able to continue. Some insurance companies refused to cover me because they felt that I wouldn't be able to teach proficiently and safely but I persisted and found other insurers who accepted my policy.

I had made several changes to my training too. I used to love fighting everyone, big and small. Sometimes when I was fighting someone, I would find it difficult to see smaller students so I moved them further away to avoid accidents. Slowing down my techniques was another change I had to make. Sometimes I would see people at the last second fighting near me and I would stop, thinking that I was about to collide with them. When I was demonstrating techniques I would ask all the students to stand slightly further away from me so that there was no way that I would accidentally kick them. When I kicked pads that were held in someone's hand I would occasionally hit their fingers because I could hardly see the pad, so I adjusted and kicked the pads slower or sometimes aimed to miss it so that my feet were nowhere near their fingers.

I also hosted a few competitions in Rugby. I designed leaflets in large print, before shrinking them to normal size once I was satisfied with the designs. Each competitor had to have their name written on a sheet of paper. Most competition organisers would write down the names as each student arrived in their own handwriting. Since I was having trouble reading handwriting I tried my best to know in advance who would be entering the competition and type their names onto a spreadsheet and print it off. I made sure that a minimal amount of information would need to be handwritten. Sometimes I would leave others in charge but at other times it would be left to me. I also did a great deal of judging. There would be four of us sitting around the edge of the fighting mat, but eventually I had to stop that because the fighters became too blurred. One minute they would be close to me and I could see who was scoring points, but the next they would be in the far corner, away from me and too far for me to be able to mark points effectively. I never gave up, I adapted. When I could no longer see clearly I became a referee. This is the person who stands and moves around with the fighters. That way I was much closer and able to see them fight.

For years I continued to enter Martial Arts competitions. Although I was often tempted to quit competing, my students were more likely to enter if I led the way. I was amazed that I won most of my fights; my opponents were of high standard and all black belts like myself. I had to fight without my glasses, which put me at a greater disadvantage. It must have been my experience with being able to judge what techniques people were about to execute that helped me win. Someone with my low vision shouldn't have been winning regularly.

My vision was still deteriorating and it was becoming increasingly difficult to see without my glasses on. It used to take me a split second to focus, but that split second slowly got longer. The people I fought were powerful and fast and if I couldn't focus quickly enough I could be knocked out. I was taking some hazardous risks and wanted to quit, just like when I had quit roller-skating but my students wouldn't let me. They were wonderful students but they had no idea how difficult it was all becoming.

One of the competitions that I remember being in was a team competition. I had been training with one of my instructors in a small town called Hinckley, a twenty-minute drive from Rugby. Once a week I would travel with a fellow black belt and train there. Many of the black belts who trained there went on to become champions. We were both selected to fight in the team. Although I was good I still thought that with my poor eyesight they should have chosen someone who could see their opponent clearly but they believed in my ability even though I didn't. After winning a few fights, our team made it to the semi-finals. We were against a team with some really fast black belt fighters. I had won my fight and we were competing as a team and were level on points at the end of the final fight. The rule was to put our best fighters to battle against each other and the winner would progress their team into the finals. Surprisingly I was selected to fight for our team. As I looked around at the mass of people watching, I couldn't help wondering at the situation.

"Here I am preparing to fight for a team full of great fighters. I bet it would surprise a great deal of people if they found out that I was registered as partially sighted. Telling them would be like showing someone that you're tired, they would take advantage of the situation. I'll keep it a secret."

The team members were all watching closely. It was a very intense moment where the whole future of my team was put on my shoulders. If any of my competitors found out about my disability, they would use it to their advantage and fight me with more confidence. I had to keep it a secret and was now prepared to fight my team into the finals.

The fight started and he came out fast. I struggled to see his hands because they were too blurred but I could still see his legs. I countered with a few shots but he was fast and avoided most of them. We fought on and I tried to catch him with some spinning kicks but only made contact a few times. He was a nifty fighter and I had to think fast. I needed a strategy to beat him. He was their best fighter and it proved to be a difficult fight but eventually I worked out how to beat him. He was fast and I was more powerful. After he kicked he was fast enough to dodge my technique so I decided to kick at the same time as he did. Although his techniques were touching me a split second before mine hit him, I was hitting him harder and began to hurt him. He backed off to try and recover but I kept the pressure on for the rest of the fight. I never gave him enough time to recover and went on to win the fight for my team. Then I sat with my team members and waited for the finals.

"I'm so glad that hardly anyone knows that I'm struggling to see," I thought to myself.

I was so proud of myself. There I was, a partially sighted fighter who felt that he was no longer efficient enough to be fighting black belts of this high standard but somehow managing to win. Now I knew why my students wanted me to continue. They saw me as a great leader and fighter so I had to lead.

We were in the finals and I was exhausted. We were against a team with three British champions. I had observed them fight closely and was impressed with their standard. They were going to be a tough team to beat. Our first fight was already on the way and our team member was suffering from some good techniques that were landing and bringing him down to the ground. We had lost the first fight and so far we hadn't fought against any of their champions.

The second fight started and this time it was against one of their champions. Our man performed well but the champion slowly took over the fight. Early on our team member was hit to the ground and he flicked back to his feet, which impressed everyone. He gave the fight his best shot, even knocking the champion to the ground but the end result was now two losses.

Our third fighter was my fellow black belt from Rugby. He too was against a champion and fought well. Somehow in the second round he was able to work out the champion's style and went on to win. I was ecstatic. Although he was a fellow black belt, I had vigorously trained him to that level, giving up some of my spare time to assist him. He has gone on to become a fifth Dan black belt with many classes. He's an outstanding fighter who I'm very proud of.

The score was two wins to them and one to us. We needed to win the last two fights but we were against their biggest fighters. There was another champion and a fifth Dan instructor. Both of them were much bigger than me (that's my excuse). I was the next fighter and I was against their tallest and best champion and I was still tired from my last fight! The battle began and we caught each other with a few impressive kicks. He was taller than me and fought from a longer distance. When I wore my glasses I was able to cope with this well, but on this occasion I was fighting without my glasses and he looked slightly too blurred. This caused a problem because I had to wait for him to move slightly closer to me to see and figure out what he was about to do. That split second cost me and he caught me with a few shots. He was also great at using both his legs and it was like fighting against myself. Towards the end of the first round I changed my style of fighting and caught him with a few jump kicks, which levelled the points.

The second round started and I moved in closer so that he would struggle to use his long legs. As we traded some punches I became aware that he was just as powerful as me and we slogged away at each other. He backed off and made some noises, which indicated that he was tired, but as I moved in to prevent him from regaining his energy he caught me with a side kick to my stomach and I went down. It was perfect timing and he caught me off balance but I wasn't hurt. He had obviously seen me pressure my last fighter when he was tired and had set me up. I was as tough as him and was ready for more. I got to my feet quickly and the fight continued. I was beginning to tire and he started to pressure me more. We almost traded point for point and I wasn't able to gain the upper hand. The fight was over and I had lost – the fitter fighter won. It was quite scary fighting against someone so fast and powerful, but it was even scarier not being able to see him clearly.

The score was three to them and one to us. We lost the last fight but we had already lost as a result of my fight. At the end of the event we went up to receive our second place trophies and it was the biggest trophy I ever won, standing at one metre high.

One year later, in another competition, I met the same champion again. This time it was an individual championship and he was the defending champion. We both battled our way through the competition, beating everyone in our path, but we knew we would have to meet at some stage of the competition. It turned out to be in the semi-finals and everyone crowded around to watch us. We were in the heavyweight section of the black belts, the most feared category because of the size and power of the candidates. Our fight was well on the way and we kept up with each other. He was faster this time but I still managed to hit him with a few kicks. I began to tire under pressure and he started to come in after I had executed a kick. I spun around fast with a jump kick towards his head missing by a whisker. As he moved in for a counter I kicked again catching him in his stomach. He staggered, but didn't quite go down. I moved in and we exchanged some punches. The final whistle blew and it was a draw.

He had worn me out and I wasn't looking forward to the next section. Somehow I had managed to draw with a champion.

"A draw?" I thought to myself. "I drew with a champion? Someone who would probably kick my ass if he knew that I couldn't see well."

My success was short lived and we had to fight for another thirty seconds to determine the winner. We began once more, kicking and punching but both missing our targets. Time went on and I began to wish that I was a little fitter. He was definitely fitter than me and it began to show as my stamina grew thin. He came in with his hands and we hit each other hard gaining points both ways. Then almost out of nowhere he delivered a kick to my stomach knocking me off balance and gaining a point. I never saw the kick. All I saw was a blurred image that was too distorted to work out. As I was trying, the kick hit and it was too late.

The whistle announced the end and he had beaten me by one point, but I was overjoyed with my performance. Only I knew how little I really could see. Entering competitions was my new thrill. It made up for the loss of my roller-skating. It made me feel like I was still worthy of something. I had lost to the champion and I was happy. He went on to win the finals. Afterwards he came over to see me and congratulated me for being such a worthy opponent and we became friends. A few months later he even came to teach a few of my classes and I felt honoured.

CHAPTER 13
THE THICKENING FOG

My adjustments were complete and for a while I enjoyed my new lifestyle. My teaching was going well as a result of the changes that I had made. Once again I was able to see my students clearer by standing nearer to them when they were performing techniques. With my new grading exam forms I was able to mark more effectively. Whenever I went to the gym I would now ask my friend to change the weights for me. It made me feel uncomfortable but it had to be done. The biggest change that I had to get used to was asking other people to read my letters. Most letters were fine but when they had to read some of my more private letters, I was embarrassed. They even asked questions about some of the letters they were reading and they found out whether I had money in my bank account. I felt useless having to ask and having to share my secrets. It was like my independence had been taken away from me. I had adjusted to the way people looked through my eyes and being able to guess who the distorted faces belonged to.

Then one morning I woke up and noticed a difference. I got ready for work and went to catch the bus. Everywhere looked misty but it wasn't that cold.

"That's strange," I thought, "maybe my glasses are dirty."

Replacing my glasses after cleaning them made no difference so I tried once more. Everywhere still looked misty. It was a strange feeling that baffled me.

It was like fog. It wasn't thick but it was definitely visible and affecting my vision. Windows looked grey and were no longer completely transparent. The doors of houses, bricks, walls and gates seemed to have a cloudy finish to them. People's faces were slightly hazy. It felt like someone had turned down the contrast on a television so that all the colours were starting to blend in with each other. Cars began to blend in with the road as well. Something was wrong!

"It must be foggy. I've cleaned my glasses so I know it's not that."

As I walked past a lamp post it became more visible from the side. It was as though I could see more clearly from out of the sides of my eyes. From the front, the lamp post almost blended in with the sky and the pavement, everything had a grey haze to it. As I passed the lamp post it appeared to stand out more from the pavement and the other surroundings. It baffled me and I began to worry. My eyes darted around as if they were confused with where to look. Sometimes I would be looking straight on then found myself focussing on objects to the side of me. I kept switching from my left eye to my right and sometimes I could see double. I discovered that when I closed one eye I could see more clearly. When I looked at a passing car it seemed as if there were two vehicles very close to each other and when I tilted my head or closed one eye, it would become one car again. This began to scare me and I didn't know where to look.

"What's happening now? Why is that lamp post more visible from the side and why is everything slightly grey like fog? *Is* it foggy? Maybe I'm still half asleep but then why have I got double vision some of the time? I'll clean my eyes with water when I get to work."

By this time I had arrived at my bus stop. It's only a two-minute walk from my house, literally around the corner and there are no roads to cross. As I stood there for a second I observed the mist. A friend was also waiting at the bus stop.

"Good morning!"

"Morning and how are you?" he asked.

"I'm fine thanks but it's a little foggy today."

"Is it? It seems clear to me. It's cloudy but not foggy," he replied.

"Well it looks slightly foggy to me but my glasses probably need cleaning," I said jokingly.

I knew that my glasses were clean but until I found out what was happening, I thought that it was the easiest thing to blame while I tried to figure it out. While we waited for the bus I continued to wonder why I was seeing fog.

"Now I know that it isn't my glasses and I know that it's not really foggy. It must be my eyes. Maybe I still have some sleep in them and it's affecting my vision. I will definitely clean my face at work."

That was the only conclusion I could arrive at to explain the foggy vision I was experiencing.

Then I noticed that objects appeared slightly more blurred and slightly darker than usual. My surroundings looked slightly more distorted. It did occur to me that my eyes might have become worse but there was no reason for me to see fog.

A bus was coming so I looked out for the number. My friend told me that it was our bus. When I asked how he knew he said that he could read the number. The bus was too far away for me and I was surprised that he could really see that far. It wasn't until the bus stopped that I was able to read the number and I noticed that it was very large. I paid for my ticket and found a seat. As the bus moved off I peered through the window, which also appeared to be misty. It wasn't thick mist but enough to impair my vision further. Then I began to blink quite vigorously to see if I could clear some of the sleep. When I looked through the window once more I noticed a slight difference. It had cleared up some of the fog a bit and everywhere seemed a little less hazy.

"It's working," I thought to myself. "If it *is* sleep then blinking a few times is obviously removing it. At least I can see a little clearer again."

However, everywhere slowly became just as foggy as it had been before I had blinked rapidly. I was beginning to worry even more. After blinking a few more times the mist appeared to lift slightly, but then returned again. This time I narrowed my eyes slightly and frowned. This helped me to see more clearly and lasted a little longer but I thought that I would look a little ridiculous squinting all the time so I only did it occasionally.

The bus had arrived at my work and I made my way in. After putting my bag down in my room, I switched all the computers on and went to wipe my eyes in the washroom. I washed away the sleep from my eyes and replaced my glasses. Although the difference was very slight, it had helped but everything still seemed a little foggy.

"Now I know that it's not real fog because it's still slightly foggy in here," I thought to myself. "But there can't be any sleep in my eyes because I've just washed them."

Then I went to look at my reflection in the mirror.

"Where have my glasses gone and why does my face look grey? If my eyes are worse, then why the fog?"

I returned to my duties.

I then discovered that my keyboard was very difficult to read. Sometimes I would have to remove my glasses to be able to see the letters. I experienced the same problems with reading words on the computer screen.

"It's my eyes isn't it? They've become worse. I can't believe this. It's my job as a computer technician to type and read screens. If I can no longer do this how will I cope? Everything appears to be more distorted."

It frustrated me as I tried to focus. Sometimes when I typed I would press the wrong key because of not physically being able to see it. As this problem persisted I began to feel angry.

"Why does this have to happen to me? I have to work. There must be a way to deal with this. Everywhere is so misty."

Over the past year I had learned to cope with my visual impairment, I had adjusted my life to cope with the changes to my eyesight. I was writing less frequently, reading with books much closer to my face, I'd had to give up roller-skating and had changed my teaching methods. Now it appeared that my sight had decided to deteriorate further which would require even more changes.

"I used to read words on the computer screen in font size 14, which is already quite large. Maybe I should increase the size again."

After adjusting the size of the text on the screen to 16 point, I was able to read once more. The only problem with this was that not all the text could be enlarged so I still had to remove my glasses sometimes to be able to read. Removing my glasses seemed to help me to focus on closer objects.

"How am I going to deal with not being able to see the keyboard well? I need to learn to touch type so that I know where all the keys are."

These adjustments helped me to perform my job efficiently but there were more changes to come.

As I went downstairs I noticed that it had become more difficult to judge where the steps started so now I had to walk around much slower and more cautiously. Some parts of the building were much darker than others and would give me a great deal of trouble. To cope

I walked slower, held on to the sides and tried to remember where all the steps were. Sometimes I had to carry computers and would worry about missing a step on the stairs and dropping one. It was fine to cope with on my own because nobody could see how much I struggled on stairs. If I had to walk with someone else I would pretend to be looking around at my surroundings but really I was looking for where the steps began. I told my boss about the problems that I was experiencing and she helped as much as she could. She assigned me two prefects who helped with some of the jobs that I was struggling with.

I was in the process of entering all the books in the school library onto a database. Along with other tasks, I had to read a barcode on each book, but this was no longer possible with my glasses on so I had to take them off to read the tiny figures. I also had to read the barcodes of new computers and with the increased amount of times I had to take my glasses off, I was adding to the strain of my eyes and this would often leave them in severe pain.

Nobody knew how much I was frustrated by not being able to do my job as well as I used to. Slowly my independence was being taken away from me and I had to put my trust in other people's hands. Sometimes I would help out in classes and be overwhelmed with rage, yet somehow I would continue to smile as though I had no problems. Sometimes my every thought would be about my disability and I would continually try to fight the thoughts and erase them from my head. Hatred and anger were ripe in my mind. I would often become angry from not being able to perform well and would sometimes get aggressive towards others for not understanding after I had told them about my problems. Being aggressive was my way of coping, an outlet for my frustrations. I didn't mean to be like that, I just had to or I could see myself becoming more and more depressed. My mind was full of thoughts that hurt to think about and I desperately needed to find ways of stopping them from taking over my head and my life.

When helping during classes I experienced some more problems.

"Could you help me please?"

"What's the problem?" I asked.

"I was trying to delete something but I've deleted the wrong section; can you see where it's gone?"

As I looked at the computer screen from where I was standing I could no longer read the text so couldn't see where the cursor was. In these situations I would sometimes ask the pupil to stand to the side while I corrected it for them. There were many different problems involving text that I found hard to see. Sometimes I would have to use my computer to find their work but I preferred them not to see me struggling to see my screen but sometimes it couldn't be helped and I would almost feel incompetent. Then I would feel sorry for myself and the thoughts would continue to bombard my mind.

Another problem that I experienced was with colours. Many students would draw objects in different colours then want to move some of them. Sometimes they couldn't get the program to do what they wanted and they would ask me for help.

"Could you help me move the yellow circle inside the red one please? It doesn't seem to want to move for me."

"Where is your yellow circle?" I asked.

The pupil pointed to what looked like a blank section of the screen.

"There's nothing there," I answered.

"It's just there on my screen."

Yellow appeared white to me and it didn't matter how hard I looked it stayed invisible. More thoughts clouded my mind.

"My eyes really have become worse. Where is the yellow circle? Why can't I see it? I'm not colour blind. How much worse are they going to get? Why can't I see the keyboard? Why do I have to suffer so much? Why do I have to write in bigger text and why can't I see barcodes? How am I supposed to walk safely without seeing steps? Why can't the suffering stop?"

The thoughts continued until something else interrupted them.

"I have another appointment in a few weeks and I'll find out how much worse they've become then."

Colour caused a major problem for me at work all the time. I would struggle one way or another several times a day. Every time I encountered a new difficulty it would add to my anger and would sometimes prevent me from finding solutions. I wasn't ready to give up though and I found out more about how each program worked, then I memorised the shortcut keys. The next time someone asked for help I asked them to click on the section that I couldn't see, then

I used the shortcut keys to move it, asking the pupil which direction to go in and when to stop. Most of the time I couldn't see what I was moving, but successfully performed the tasks many times.

Computer cables also became a challenge because I could no longer see where to plug wires in, but after memorising where everything connected, I was able to rewire a whole room full of computers, printers and control boxes literally by touch alone. I would place a finger behind the computer and run it along the back. After feeling where all the sockets were I would then guide the cables in. Being able to turn the computer around wouldn't help much because everything appeared blurred. My lack of clear vision was causing problems throughout my working day and although I really enjoyed my job I was sometimes grateful to reach the end of my working day.

One day on the way home I went to see my mother as usual; my sisters were there and it was obvious that they weren't feeling too happy. Three of them had been to the Birmingham Eye Hospital for tests; my brothers were still reluctant to go as they were worried about the possibility of receiving bad news and I didn't blame them. It's a crushing blow to be told that you may go blind and that it could happen at any time. They were not prepared to accept the possibility and so avoided going. They wanted to enjoy their lives as much as possible by acting as though nothing was wrong with their eyes.

However, my sisters were curious. Angela, Carline and June had gone along to be tested and had their results. Jennifer had some problems and was short-sighted. I felt that she should have gone too but she was reluctant like my brothers and didn't want to know, she wanted to carry on with her life. All three of my sisters who had been to the hospital were suffering the after effects of the eye drops that had been used to dilate their eyes. Two of my sisters were blessed, it had been confirmed that they didn't have RP, but their relief and joy was overpowered by the fact that Angela had been diagnosed with the condition. She was very upset. She had gone to her appointment thinking that she was just short-sighted but had wanted the doctors to examine her eyes in the hope that it would provide them with more knowledge that might help my brother and me.

Some of her words rang bells in my memory – they were the same words that I had used not so long ago. She had known that she was just short-sighted, but deep down she had also known that something else wasn't quite right. When she was younger her eyesight had been so good that she had taken some driving lessons. She is ten years older than me and has experienced the changes much later on in her life than I did. Angela was very distraught from the news and felt like her life was over. After watching our brother suddenly become blind she knew the dangers that may be upon her at any time. She now had the same worries as me, like waking up one day but in her eyes it would still be dark, still dark forever.

At my next appointment I was already expecting bad news. It wasn't clear to me how much my eyes had deteriorated further but it was obvious that there had been a change.

"Please let my eyes be the same. They don't have to be worse. Please let me be able to read the same amount of lines down this chart. Please, I've suffered enough."

In my mind I was hoping for the best, pleading with myself and asking God to help me. I knew something would be wrong but it didn't have to be significant.

The first test was over and my result was already clear. My right eye had gone from reading two lines down, to just one and was now seeing what my left had a year ago. It was frustrating to hear and to know, but there was nothing I could do about it.

"I don't believe this. Why does it have to get worse? It doesn't, it can remain stable, why does it have to deteriorate so much? A year ago I thought that my left eye was really blurred compared to my right, but now that one is going exactly the same way."

My left eye had gone from reading just one line to a dismal amount that wasn't worth seeing. The first time I had my eyes tested at the Eye Hospital I thought that the solitary big letter was huge and pathetically easy to read, so big that anyone should be able to read it with their glasses on, yet that was all I could now see with my left eye. That was all I could read and even then it wasn't very clear. It looked distorted. It was vaguely ridiculous to think about and I had trouble accepting it. I was only a few years into my tests and was just about able to read the top letter, but it was only just legible. The letter was slightly out of focus and I was able to determine it by guessing.

"How bad are my eyes? Can't they just stay the same now? How much worse are they going to become? At this rate what will I be able to read next year? My left eye is so distorted that sometimes I don't even bother to use it. Most of the time I just use my right but if that's going to become as blurred as my left, how am I going to cope?"

The thoughts worried and distressed me as I fought to keep them out of my mind.

"How many times am I going to have to readjust to cope with my ever decreasing eyesight? I'm only just getting used to how things are at the moment, have I got to adjust my lifestyle again? I've already given up roller-skating, which I loved. What else am I going to have to give up? What other activity is going to suffer because of the deterioration of my eyesight? Maybe I should just give everything up now and become a drunken recluse."

"No you can't give up," another voice in my head said, "you're strong and you'll learn to cope." The fight in my mind slowly escalated.

"What's the point, who cares about being strong? This is too much for anyone to take."

"You can do it. You're brave. Show other people that you can cope with anything."

"Who cares what other people think? I can't take this any more. First my hobbies suffered, now it's affecting my job. I might as well be a depressed wreck."

"Don't give up! There are lots of people out there who are worse off than you. Your brother is coping and what about those poor people in wheelchairs, would you prefer that? Not being able to walk again?"

The anger and frustration built up as I continued to fight off the arguing thoughts.

The next test was the satellite dish to determine my field of vision. My patience was wearing thin as I progressed through to the end. The parts of my eyes on which I had blind spots were growing rapidly. They were beginning to take over my eyes and were also affecting my central vision, which is why I was appearing to see some objects better from out of the sides of my eyes. The doctor asked several times if I was pressing the button whenever I saw the light. The more he asked the clearer it became that my eyesight was failing and the angrier I became.

"I can't believe that I have so many blind spots. I can hardly see the light, it just keeps disappearing and this doctor is getting on my nerves thinking that I should be able to see it more often. I would love to be able to see it all the time then I wouldn't be here. It's obvious what's going on in my eyes and it's killing me not being able to do anything about it."

Upset but not tearful from the news I thought some more.

"It's like seeing a small cloud in your eyes and it's slowly getting bigger but there's nothing you can do but watch as it finally takes over your eyes. There are parts of the cloud that have small gaps but eventually it will become whole and take over the entire view. At least the cloud hasn't completely taken over yet, I've still got some vision at the centre of my eyes, but for how long?"

The next doctor tested the pressure of my eyes and looked into the back of them with his ophthalmoscope. He put the wonderful eye drops in. This was always the highlight of my appointment because my eyesight was already grossly distorted, but with the addition of the eye drops things became even more blurred. Objects that were already difficult to see would either vanish or become even more confusing to look at. The only slight benefit of being dilated was the way the contrast of objects brightened up. Suddenly an item would come back to life as its true colours became more apparent. Dull black clothing would spring to life and reveal its true blue colour or white would become yellow or greys turned red. It was a benefit, yes, but only slight because it would also brighten the rays of the sun, which would become brilliant and blinding and painful to see.

It was during the twenty-minute wait for my eyes to become fully dilated that I experienced my most confusing emotions. I felt sorry for myself as I thought of the problems that I had to endure and then felt humiliated at the thought of having to ask people to assist me for the rest of my life. Frustration overcame me as I battled to find ways of dealing with what was happening and was so angry at being treated this way. A tear came to the corner of my eye, but it wouldn't fall. It was trapped by the anger lingering inside. The thoughts continued to confuse me. I sat in silence beside my friend who had come along to help me on the journey home. He was not aware of the terrible fight that I was experiencing within my head.

"What's the meaning of life? To see how much stress we can take? To see how many challenges it takes to push us over the edge? I don't know how much more I'm supposed to take."

I became emotional but still no tears appeared. Thoughts and feelings rushed around inside until I felt like I was going to explode. I wanted desperately to cry but my tear ducts seemed to be empty. The death of my father had used them all up and my personality had changed. My emotions from dealing with the loss had drained me of my tears and now I was in desperate need of some. It would have made me feel much better to have a good cry but I was unable to. Maybe it was not my father but the anger and the bitterness that had taken over me from dealing with the sad moments of my life. It was the only way I knew how to cope. I wasn't scared of anyone. My Martial Arts training had taught me to face anyone, but not how to face the thought of going blind.

After the test the doctor said that there was more pressure in my eyes and that I had to give up the heavy weight training that I had continued to do.

"So there it is," I thought. "There's the next activity that I love to do that I'm going to have to give up. All these years of building myself up just to be knocked back down again, surely I'm not going to become a recluse? That's not my future… is it?"

"It could be worse."

The fight in my head started once more.

"This is bad enough thanks. Am I supposed to sit here and just take it?"

"There's nothing you can do about it so accept it."

"It's not that easy to accept. My independence has been taken away from me and I'm a very independent person. I'll feel embarrassed to have to keep asking others for assistance and it's not going to be just for one or two things; no, I will eventually have to ask for help for everything."

"There's got to be a cure out there, surely."

"Why is this happening to me?"

The anger and rage took over me once more.

The doctor referred me to the professor for the rest of my diagnosis and as usual the professor took a few moments while he studied my results.

"Your eyes appear to have deteriorated even further. Your left eye is still considerably worse than your right. The tests show that your left eye is almost unable to read from the board and slowing down when reacting to movement. Both your eyes are showing signs of tunnel vision."

All I could do was sit there and listen to someone pronouncing my sentence. One after another he stated my problems as he continued to rip my life to shreds.

"Can I look into your eyes and see your discs again?"

"Help yourself. It won't make any difference to me."

"I understand how you feel, but it will help you in the long run. It will help us to know more about RP and speed up the process of finding a cure. Most doctors don't even know what it looks like so would be fascinated to look into your eyes."

He took a good look into my eyes and then wrote down a few notes.

"The pressure in your eyes is a little high. Have you got a strenuous job?"

"No. I work with computers but I do lift up heavy weights at the gym."

"The pressure from lifting heavy weights will put more strain on your eyes. I would recommend that you stop. It doesn't mean that you can't lift weights, just keep them light."

"What's the point of going to the gym?" I thought to myself as the professor rambled on.

"The discs in your eyes are showing more signs of damage. Are you having many more problems getting around?"

It was my turn to talk and I unloaded some of my thoughts onto him.

"My whole life has changed. It's like it's no longer in my hands. I just have to accept whatever happens. I've had to give up roller-skating because it's done mostly in poor light and I'm really struggling in the dark at the moment. Everything also looks more distorted so that's affecting my job and general lifestyle."

"In what way?" he asked.

"Well I can no longer read barcodes. The text on the computer screen has to be bigger. I work with software companies that design their installation sequence in small text. Sometimes I have to take my glasses off to read it and my face is literally touching the screen. The keyboard is nearly impossible to read. If I didn't know where the keys were I probably wouldn't be able to continue my job."

"You're experiencing quite a few problems then?"

"That's nothing. It's affecting me throughout the day, every day now. I'm struggling to find my toothbrush. Most of my clothes look the same colour and sometimes I put my shirts on inside out because of my lack of sight. I can no longer see myself in the mirror; I look like I'm wearing a mask. When I shave I can't see my hairs, I just guess. Now I can't see dirt and keep worrying that things are dirty. I'm struggling walking around. Sometimes I bump into things and I'm terrified when crossing the road. I have to ask for help when I'm in a shop because I can hardly see or read labels. I have to guess people's names because I can't see them clearly. Now I've just found out that not only am I struggling with colour at night but also during the day."

"Is there anything else?" he asked.

"I wake up every morning not knowing whether I'll be able to see. Everywhere looks so distorted that my sight is cloudy. I can hardly read a book any more and it makes me feel so jealous seeing other people reading. My writing is getting worse and I struggle writing cheques and using cashpoint machines. It's not worth me watching television these days because the picture is so distorted that it hurts my eyes to look at it. Sometimes I have to ask other people to read my letters. Do you realise how humiliated that makes me feel?"

"I wish I could do more to help. We've had your sister's results and I have to admit that we're confused. She wasn't supposed to have RP. She should have been a carrier. We will need blood tests. Oh, and we're moving to new premises, so we'll send you the details."

"My sister wasn't supposed to have RP and we're not supposed to have hearing difficulties? What's going on?"

I became angry and confused. Here I was with a specialist who had performed numerous tests and was still unsure of the nature of my disabilities.

"Let's wait for the results of the blood tests, and then we'll know. Have your parents said any more about their family history?"

"My mother said that nobody suffered blindness and my father passed away recently, and there was so much that I wanted to ask him."

"I'm sorry to hear that. Have you seen a counsellor yet?"

"I'm fine. I don't need one. I just need a new pair of eyes."

"Have any blind associations been in touch yet?"

"No; why?"

"They'll provide you with some help with getting around. I'll contact them again."

The conversation came to an end and I made my way home with my friend. When I arrived home I was met by a wonder of colours. My kitchen was painted yellow and I had always thought that it was off-white. With my eyes being dilated, they let in more light, which had increased the intensity of colours.

"Wow!" I said. "That's a bright yellow. This is amazing. I can see yellow."

It was a brilliant yellow that stood out so clearly from the white. The other colours in my house stood out more too.

"So this is what people see. There's colour everywhere and it's so beautiful. Other people are blessed to be able to see this all the time."

Although it was hurting my eyes, I stared at everything, wishing that I could always see colour like this, wishing that the colours wouldn't fade away and wishing that I could see more clearly.

CHAPTER 14
MY GROWING OBSESSION

By lightening the weights I was able to carry on working out at the gym. The doctor had warned me to stop exerting myself with heavy weights because it was putting a terrible strain on my fragile eyes. It felt different to train so light. Whenever I felt like I was beginning to strain myself, I would stop. After years of pushing my body to the limit, lifting lighter weights was like a walk in the park! It took a while to get used to it and others questioned me regularly, trying to encourage me to train harder but I refused for the sake of my health. I wasn't ready to lose my eyesight over a few weights or to impress my friends. Maybe if they had been going through the same medical problems, they might have had more sympathy.

My new training program included lots of walking and jogging on the treadmill, sit-ups on a lower incline and lifting much lighter weights. When I did lift a heavier weight I would only be able to lift it about six times before having to stop due to exhaustion. Eventually the weights I chose to exercise with were so light that I could sometimes lift them twenty times and still have energy to lift more. It became therapeutic. Somehow I found myself going to the gym to relax and find peace away from my stressful life. Sometimes I would walk and feel so relaxed that I would think of solutions to some of my daily problems.

It was while I was walking on a treadmill one day that I thought about taking up yet another Martial Art to keep me busy. Since I was experiencing so many problems seeing long distances, I decided to take up a Kung-Fu style called Wing-Chun. It involves mostly hand techniques and you're much closer to your opponent. It was the same style that my friend John was doing at a new class that had opened in Rugby.

Another reason for taking up Wing-Chun was because I had recently visited my doctor due to pains in my hips. He diagnosed me as having arthritis. The more I kicked the more pain I experienced. This was very annoying since Taekwondo was mostly kicking. Maybe I had also pushed my hips too hard because I could do the front splits and almost the side splits too. It hurt my hips and was also hurting my knees. With the deterioration of my eyesight, it seemed that I had trained too hard to take my mind off my problems.

Wing-Chun was fun and totally different from Taekwondo. It involved lots of close contact techniques. After a year of studying Wing-Chun my instructor entered me into my first competition. I had already paid to enter but on the day of the event I would have preferred it if I could have got my money back or just not have gone. My daughter had been fretful and restless during the previous night and I hadn't had much sleep. Somehow my instructor persuaded me to fight; he said that I couldn't get a refund so I may as well fight anyway.

The competition started with some outstanding demonstrations. One of them was a small Chinese master who put a bottle in someone's hands and asked them to hold it tight. He then jumped and somehow brought both his legs in at the same time to meet the bottle. His legs were almost horizontal as he hit it. The bottle broke from the pressure of both his legs trying to meet in the middle and he must have hit it hard to break it (well I thought that it was spectacular!).

The competition got under way and somehow, still half asleep, I was able to reach the finals. It must have been my previous knowledge of competitive fighting that helped me because I was really struggling to see. I always fought without my glasses now and this time everyone looked incredibly distorted. It was like fighting in thick fog. Their faces were completely out of focus, they looked like they were wearing masks and I couldn't see their eyes, mouths or noses any more. Their arms and legs blended in with their bodies so much that most of the time I couldn't tell that they had executed a technique. Every time the distorted image appeared to move I went into autopilot and reacted accordingly. For the first time in a competition, I was wary of my opponent. I was no longer sure whether I should fight in the finals since I had another battle going on in my head.

"How did I manage to get to the finals? It's so difficult to see people. I'm a bit worried about their vanishing limbs. It's too difficult fighting against someone you can hardly see."

"You have years of experience, you can beat him," I argued to myself.

"It's not just him, it's life. I don't think that I can carry on with coping under this pressure."

"Let's just win the finals and see."

"It's not important to me any more. I know that I can fight but I shouldn't need to prove it all the time."

"What about your students and your instructor?"

"What about me? Isn't that more important? My eyes seem to be deteriorating faster these days and I should put all my effort into coping. I'm so terrified of going blind."

"It might not happen, just go and fight."

"It's happening… and you know it."

I found myself arguing in my head, with myself, and it was very stressful. Although it was always my voice that I heard, there was definitely a conflict starting. Part of me wanted to carry on and never give up on anything else in my life, but another part of me was more emotional and understanding and knew that I had a tougher fight to contend with ahead of me dealing with the changes that had to happen in my life to cope with going blind. I didn't even like saying the word. It scared me more than any fight that I'd ever had. Somehow I convinced myself to decide after I finished the finals.

My final fight got under way and it was very demanding trying to fight someone who I knew was as good as me, yet I couldn't see what he was doing. It was hard but I found it harder to fight what was going on in my head. While we were fighting my mind kept wandering away from the fight and onto myself. Many thoughts coursed through my mind.

"What are you doing here? You can't even see him because your eyesight is getting worse. Everywhere looks more blurred and distorted. You can't even see the judges or the referee. I'm sorry but you can't see. Your opponent looks like he has no arms or legs. Admit it; it's too much for you and you can't continue. What's the point? You've got nothing to prove."

At the same time I was trying to finish the final fight. The thoughts kept racing around my head and I became confused about what to do.

"You've got nothing to prove any more. You need to concentrate on coping with the constant deterioration of your eyesight. The fog will soon thicken so you need to be concentrating on other parts of your life. You don't need this any more. You don't need to be here. Just stop the fight and confess that you can't see enough to fight on."

I'd been fighting my whole life and I wasn't ready to quit, I didn't want to lose another sport that I'd grown to love and become passionate about. I tried so desperately to stop the thoughts but they persisted and took over my mind. There was no space left to think about how to fight my opponent and I began to lose. In my mind I tried desperately to shut myself up but the arguments grew.

"Stop the fight."

"No! I'm not ready to quit."

I kept talking to myself but somehow I was able to continue to fight at the same time. There were two fights going on now, and it seemed like I was losing both, and as the voices argued in my head and I became more confused, I was hit by my opponent.

"You never even saw that kick, did you?"

"I can still do it. I'm going to finish this fight."

"Where are his arms? You can only see them when you're right next to him. It's too dangerous and you'll get hurt."

"I'm used to this pressure and I'm used to guessing so I'm not giving up, but why do my eyes have to be so blurred? It's scary."

"You're tired too. Maybe it was a sign when your daughter made you stay up all night. You shouldn't have come."

"It's not time to give up yet."

The thoughts in my mind lasted the entire length of the fight. I'm not sure how I survived without getting hurt. I was concentrating on the fight in my head more than the physical fight out there. The thoughts were driving me mental and I was glad to hear the final whistle. I had lost the fight but I didn't care. My frustration grew as I became closer to deciding the future of my competitive fighting.

"You lost see, but you're not hurt. Quit while you're ahead."

"What will I do if I quit? What will my students say? They all rely on me to pave the way forward. I'm their leader and encourage them to enter competitions. I can't quit on them."

By this time I was sitting on my own. It would only be a few minutes before my instructor would find me and by then I was hoping to have my final decision. I was shaking with rage because I knew that I should give up but I couldn't accept it. Confused thoughts raced through my mind. The anger was building up inside and I was losing control.

"I don't know what to do."

"Yes you do, just quit. If you enter any more competitions you might actually get hurt. You can't see, so face the facts."

"But I'll feel useless and like a failure. Fighting is all I know."

"Do you realise how dangerous it could be if you decide to enter more? You're good but there's no need to fight blindfolded, you've got nothing else to prove. People admire you for fighting for so long with poor vision and they would understand if you had to give up. You have a bigger fight on your hands now. Your eyesight isn't getting any better and you need to concentrate on learning to cope."

"Why do I have to give up on so many things that I enjoy? Why? WHY?"

My anger grew even more.

"I've given up roller-skating, I've had to give up heavy weights and now I have to give up competition fighting? I hate my eyes and hate not being able to see."

"Yes! This is the perfect time to give up. You can't see. You couldn't even see when he was executing some techniques. Do you realise how dangerous that is? You can still fight during your classes with your glasses on."

"Why is this happening to me? Why can't I see?"

My instructor was approaching and I knew that he would want to discuss my fight. It was time to make a decision.

"Good fight. You still came second so you'll go home with a trophy. Better luck next time."

I paused while I thought of what to say.

"There won't be a next time. I couldn't even see when he was executing a technique. My eyesight is really bad and… it's getting worse. It's a miracle that I didn't get hurt. It was so difficult to see any of my opponents. I'm crazy even being here. Everything and everyone is so blurred and foggy, what I see is ridiculous. People look so distorted that if they never moved I wouldn't be able to tell that they were human. When I turned my back to execute a reverse technique, and lost sight of my opponent, it took me several seconds to readjust and focus on them again. Do you realise how dangerous that is?"

"I'm sorry, I didn't realise that your eyesight was that bad."

"I'm sorry too, but I can't do this any more and you'll never know how much this decision is going to hurt me, but… I have to give up. There'll be no more competitive fighting for me."

The decision made, I collected my last trophy and returned home, bitterly disappointed and upset.

Within a few weeks my eyesight was worse than ever and I experienced more problems. It was after another difficult night when I hadn't been able to sleep, I was up, wandering around the house, agitated with thoughts about my eyesight.

"Where did I put my glasses last night? They're usually here on my table."

There was no point looking because without my glasses I couldn't see to find them anyway. So I felt around with my hand until it touched what felt like my glasses.

"Ah-ha, here they are."

I placed them on my face.

"I really must remember to put them in the same place every night!"

Then I went to have a shower. When I was ready to use the shower gel, I noticed that it wasn't to be seen. I didn't have my glasses on so that didn't help the situation. After a while of searching around with my hands and trying to remember the texture of the shower gel, a thought went through my mind.

"It would be much easier if everything was always in the same place, that way I wouldn't have to search around like an invalid or constantly ask for help!"

After getting out of the shower, (after I was clean!) I put my glasses on and went to brush my teeth, but now my toothbrush had disappeared too.

"Where's my toothbrush?" I thought to myself. "It must be here somewhere. There are two over there, I wonder which is mine."

It was difficult to tell which one was mine so I decided to keep my toothbrush separate in future so that I could always find it. Then as soon as I had found a solution, my next problem popped up.

"Now where's the toothpaste gone?"

My search started as I moved my hand slowly across the shelf where the toothpaste is usually kept.

"It's not here. I don't believe it. I'm going to have to ask for help."

I had to ask for the toothpaste and it was given to me.

"That would have been easier to find if it had been left in the same place too!"

Slowly but surely I became more organised.

After I had finished brushing my teeth I prepared myself for a shave. The shaving foam was in a bottle that looked (and felt) like the air freshener and various hair products. Somehow I was able to find it.

"Maybe I should put this to one side too so that I always know where it is and don't get it confused with another bottle."

I found my razor and looked into the mirror to see where to shave. My face looked like it was hiding behind a mask. I was unable to see any facial hair.

"How can I shave? I don't know where to shave! I know, I'll keep running my other hand across my face to feel where the hairs are and to feel when my face is smooth so I'll know when I've removed them."

When I'd finished I returned to my room to get dressed. There were no socks left in my drawer so I went to the wash basket. Lots of socks there, but which two made a matching pair? Most of my socks looked pretty much the same but were slightly different, so I had to ask for help again. Then I got dressed. I managed to put my tie on, but I couldn't see whether it was straight or whether I looked tidy enough for work. The distorted image I saw of myself wasn't clear enough. I asked for help and went to make some breakfast.

I needed a bowl, but struggled to find one.

"Why can't they leave the bowls in the same place? Now I'll have to search for one."

When I eventually found a bowl, I went to get a spoon and then poured my cereal into the bowl. After finding the sugar and the milk I started to eat my breakfast (after leaving it to get soggy!). Many thoughts went through my mind as I ate.

"How long will it be before I get on other people's nerves asking for help all the time? If things aren't left in the same place it causes me serious problems. Instead of asking others I'll become more organised and that way I don't need to rely on them so much. I'd need to do it all for myself if no one else was here."

My breakfast was finished and I went to catch my bus to work.

After work I returned home. As I walked into the living room I felt something hard underneath my shoe. Bending down, I retrieved a piece of Lego, one of my daughter's toys. It had been innocently left on the floor, it's easily done and I didn't want to break anything.

"Rather than risk breaking some toys that I can't see, I'll enter the room more carefully and whatever is in my way I'll pick up!"

I slid my feet carefully, trying not to step on anything. Then I bent down to scoop up some toys and put them in the correct place.

While I was closer to the floor I saw a few pieces of paper, they were only small.

"They weren't there when I was standing up. I couldn't see any bits on the carpet. I wonder what else is down there?"

Kneeling down I was able to see the floor more clearly and saw a few pieces of dirt so I removed them and went to wash my hands.

"My hands feel slightly sticky but I can't see anything on them. I'll wash them until I think that they're clean."

When my hands were clean and I went to dry them but I couldn't find the tea towel and there was nobody there to help me.

"I'll have to put the tea towel in the same place so whenever I need it I can use it!"

I fancied a cup of tea so I went to the cupboard and took out a cup. Then I reached for the tea bags, but couldn't find the box so I rummaged around for a while with my hands. Eventually I found it and went to put a tea bag in my cup. Not being able to see clearly I bent forwards to get my head closer to what I was doing, but I'd forgotten about the cupboard door and banged my head as I straightened up.

"Ow! That hurt," I said to myself, rubbing my head. "Who left the door open? Oh, it was me! I must remember to shut the doors straight after I've finished in a cupboard."

I looked up at the cupboard door and it looked so distorted that it blended into the background. Only by looking really carefully was I able to tell that it was open.

"I seem to be using my hands an awful lot these days. My eyes must be getting worse because sometimes I feel like I'm using my hands more than my eyes to see."

Instead of looking for things using my sight I was now starting to feel around with my hands to find them.

Then I went to find the sugar. In the morning I'd put it back in the cupboard where I'd found it, but it was no longer there – someone else had used it and not put it back. It only took me a few seconds to lay my hands on it and after taking what I needed I put it back in the cupboard in its usual place. Then I went over to get the water that I had previously boiled in the kettle, but while I was pouring it in the cup I heard noises that told me it was spilling out of the cup. As I looked down to take a closer look I saw that there was too much water in the cup and it had spilt on the work surface. I quickly fetched the dishcloth and wiped it up. Somehow I knocked into something that I didn't see.

"What was that? It sounded like a glass."

As my vision deteriorated, glasses became almost invisible. Unless there was something dark in it, it was like there *was* no glass. It made me feel useless not being able to see the glass and not being able to clean it up. It smashed on the work surface and I became slightly angry as I tried to clear it away.

"Stupid me; why couldn't I see that? Why are glasses invisible to me now? I'll have to be more careful in the future and leave glasses in the corner beside the wall. I can't seem to see anything these days. I'm so clumsy, so useless."

It was obvious that I would have to use my hands to feel where the pieces of glass were. So I slowly moved my hand across the worktop, picking up the broken pieces as my fingers touched them. Luckily there weren't too many pieces but I did get worried a few times as I touched the sharp bits. Using my hand in this way was very dangerous and could have resulted in a nasty cut, but it was the only way that I could do it. It didn't matter how hard I looked, I just couldn't see the glass. After cleaning it up I took my cup of tea into the living room and drank it while watching the television.

My head was throbbing from the bump on the cupboard. Although accidents happen, it made me feel even more hopeless, not being able to see clearly enough to know that the cupboard door was open.

"This is ridiculous. I know that I need to learn to cope with the changes to my eyesight but it appears that I have to change my whole life. It seems like I have to be aware of everything around me and organise things more so that I have less accidents and can find things when I need them."

Every time I walked on something or became aware of something on the floor, I couldn't stop myself picking it up. Then I had to wash my hands each time. If there was something on the kitchen worktop that shouldn't have been there, I would clear it away so that I wouldn't knock it over. Gradually I was finding myself tidying up more and washing my hands more and it was causing me distress.

The next day I experienced similar problems and broke yet another glass. I became even tidier and tried to keep the worktop clear of obstacles. As I went to watch television I bumped my leg on a chair. It was out of place and I hadn't seen it. My shin was cut and I nursed it before sitting down to watch the television.

The programme became boring so I decided to switch channels.

"Where's the remote disappeared to?"

I looked around but couldn't see it.

"It must be here somewhere."

After taking another look around I started using my hands again, shuffling them around the settee. My hand knocked into something.

"Ah, this feels like the remote, but I just looked there and couldn't see anything. God my eyes are getting worse."

The fight in my head began again as I tried to convince myself that I could cope.

"This is too much for me now. *Everything* needs to be replaced exactly where it's kept or I can't find it. I feel ridiculous shuffling around with my hands all the time. How can my eyes suddenly get so bad? I don't want to lose my eyesight."

"That's something you're going to have to accept."

"Why? Why me? It's so difficult and I feel so frustrated when I can't find something."

"That's why you need to rely on others and trust them."

"It's not easy to change your life in an instant without feeling something. I can't rely on others. They won't be here every time I need their help."

My head got warm from the confusing thoughts rushing through my mind. I became frustrated, nervous, anxious and then angry.

"You're going to have to learn to let go and trust others. You can't find things by yourself. If someone moves something that you've put in a particular place, you have to ask them anyway. Just face it, you are hopeless."

"I can't give up! I *can* be organised. I'm not relying on others, it's too much for them running around after me. I can do it myself."

I became hysterical. It felt like I was going out of my mind. The conflicting thoughts drained my energy and the more I thought the angrier I became. The anger was aimed at myself for not being able to perform daily tasks as efficiently as others could or as easily as I used to be able to.

When I switched channels a few times I noticed that I was struggling more than usual to see the screen. The picture looked even more distorted and out of focus. Nothing looked real on the screen. It was like watching cartoons of people moving around and it made me wonder if it was time to buy a larger television so that the screen would be easier to see. I could always sit closer to it, but I'd literally be on top of the television before it became clear.

"Look around. Everything is blurred. New glasses won't help, this is as clear as I will ever see. This is scary. People are starting to look like ghosts again but this time my eyes aren't dilated from the eye drops. I hate seeing people as ghosts; I want to see them as people again. Why can't I see?"

A few more weeks passed and my problems escalated. It was a daily contest that I had no option but to take part in. Occasionally when I was making food for myself I would reach into the fridge to get the butter or something and would be unable to find what I needed. Sometimes I would search for ages without success. My eyesight was so poor that most things looked the same; blurred! I found that I needed to ask for help more regularly, and the frustration was almost unbearable if there was no one there. How could I finish making my meal when I couldn't find the ingredients that I needed?

Small trivial things began to get to me and made me feel like a failure. If I couldn't find my own nail clippers that I had put away safely because someone else had used them, I would become upset and angry. Doing things that were second nature to most people had become insurmountable obstacles for me. Sometimes I would be searching cupboards for food items that I knew were there somewhere because I had put them in a certain part of the cupboard so that I would be able to find them for myself, but someone had moved them, so I was lost. I would get upset and angry again – I hated what I was turning into but I couldn't help it. My new personality was the direct result of my failing eyesight.

My obsessions grew as my eyesight deteriorated. Even my personal hobbies were affected. My music tapes are now labelled clearly and kept in a particular order. Sometimes I wouldn't be able to see the label of the tape that I wanted but I would know how many tapes from the left it should be. It then made me more upset when other people disturbed my routine and caused me to centre on my inability to see. While I was then searching for a tape that I had organised proficiently I would be wishing that I could see clearer. This would then upset me again and I would eventually become bitter.

I was terrified of going blind and worried constantly how it would affect all aspects of my life and what other changes I would have to make. I wasn't sure how long I could go on with my job before the problems became too much for my employer to cope with. After a long time of debating on a change of jobs I enrolled at my local college on a teaching course. They recognised that I had a propensity for computers and if I was unable to have hands-on experience with them, I could revert to teaching computer skills. The course involved lots of reading and studying and somehow I was able to cope. I would read with the book close to my face or read without my glasses but I would read. I even went to my opticians and purchased a pair of contact lenses. They sometimes helped me to see more clearly but I seemed to be able to read a little better without them.

Once while I was wearing my contact lenses I decided to do some gardening. The lawn was slightly overgrown so I took out the mower and started to cut the grass. I had a little routine when mowing the lawn. It was very difficult to see the cable so I would cut the grass in straight lines and keep lifting the cable as I drew closer to it. It started to rain, but only lightly so I pledged to finish mowing the lawn. I was congratulating myself on being able to see the cable a little clearer with my lenses in when suddenly I heard the lawnmower struggling.

"This must be long grass," I thought to myself.

Then something told me to let go so I did and the lawnmower switched off. When I took a closer look I saw that I had cut through the cable. It was severed and it was raining and I had no circuit breaker. I could have been killed that day. Just by coincidence, I heard on the news later that a woman had died from cutting through her lawnmower cable. The next day I purchased a circuit breaker so that I would avoid any more accidents like that. From that day I always thought that God had another plan for me and it wasn't my time to go.

CHAPTER 15
LIVING WITH MY DISABILITY

At long last help was on the way. In 1993 I received a phone call from an association to assist me with my disability. They were sending over an assistant to give me more information on how to cope with my visual impairment.

A young lady turned up at my house at the prearranged time. Her name was Rita and she worked for the Warwickshire Association for the Blind (WAB).

"Good morning, I'm Rita from WAB. How are you?"

"I'm fine thanks."

"We received information that you're in need of assistance. I need to know how much vision you have left and if you're working so that I'll know how we can help you."

It felt uncomfortable talking about it, but I was in for a surprise.

"Well as usual they're difficult questions to answer. Although I can see, my vision is so poor that I'm registered as partially sighted. I can see the picture on the television, but not in great detail. I've recently bought a television with a bigger screen and although it helps a great deal, I'm still struggling to see it clearly. Most of my friends know that I'm partially sighted but I still feel uncomfortable sharing it with others."

"Well, I want you to try and relax while you're telling me about your eyes and the problems that you've incurred. I know that it's difficult to open up and share your thoughts, but it will help. I must admit that… I'm registered blind!"

This came as a shock to me and I felt a weird sensation.

"How can she help me if she can't see?" I thought to myself.

She had come with a helper so I assumed that he would do her work.

"You're blind?"

"Yes," she said. "So I understand exactly how you feel. Now tell me more about your problems."

"I can't see the video below my television any more and my hi-fi is a dark blob to me so I have trouble using them both."

"That's because your eyesight is darker than you realise. Other people wouldn't have any problem seeing them."

"But I can see fine outside in the sun."

"Your eyes are trying to let in as much light as possible to help you see. Although it's bright enough outside to see more, others see even more."

She seemed to understand what I was trying to say and it soon made me feel comfortable enough to share some more thoughts.

"Most of the time I can cope with my dark eyesight but I really am struggling to cope with the ever increasing blurred vision. It's so blurred now and getting worse. In the evenings I suffer from night blindness too, and can hardly see anything. Colours fade from my sight and it's like living in a black and white world. I'm very independent but at night I rely on others quite a lot. I'm very hesitant in my steps and now I have to walk slower. It really gets on my nerves when others ask me to speed up – it's like they've forgotten that I struggle to see. They say they understand but they don't. They don't know what it feels like or they would be more compassionate."

"Do you work?"

"Yes, I'm a Computer Technician."

"That must be hard. How do you manage to see the screens?"

"Yes it's very difficult. I'm struggling much more now to see the screens than I used to and I don't know how much longer I can cope with the problems it's causing me with doing my job."

"We can help. I'll get someone to see what equipment you need to keep you in work."

"Thanks. That would be a great help."

I became more relaxed knowing that there were people out there who were willing to help me.

"Tell me more about your mobility problems."

"Well I'm used to having my independence and going out quite a lot but as my eyesight is deteriorating I don't feel like venturing out so much."

"What about walking?"

"Most of the time I walk on my own. I'm struggling to see lamp posts and other obstacles like wheelie bins and I bump into them, but most of the time it's at night. It's only happened a few times during the day because I avoid them at the last second but at night I don't see them at all. Sometimes I see things that aren't there and other times I don't see what is and bump into them. Most obstacles are so distorted that they're almost invisible. Then just as I'm about to collide into them they appear and I've got a split second to stop. Sometimes when I see shadows, I'll stop and try to work out whether it *is* a shadow or not. It's so confusing working out whether things are there or not. It can sometimes be as simple as a darker part of the pavement or a shadow from an object that I can't see or different patterns on the floor. It's very confusing and sometimes I wonder why I even bother to go out because it distresses me so much. It's very difficult to see and avoid people especially when they walk fast. Everyone looks blurred until they come closer to me and sometimes when people are in a hurry and I only see them at the last second, I'm startled and will stop suddenly. It's so scary. It's like one minute your path is clear and the next someone is about to crash into you. People appear from nowhere and can vanish just as quickly. They should slow down. Their faces are so blurred that I can only just see their eyes and mouths but not in detail. The colours of their eyes are no longer visible. Looking at them is like looking at a picture of someone that a child has drawn. Their clothes coloured in with a felt tip pen, no details just the outlines. I hate seeing people like this."

"What's your eye disorder called?"

"RP; I hate it. I hate what it's doing to me. They say that I might go blind and I don't know if I can cope and there's no cure. It's too much for someone to suffer from. It's not fair; life's not fair. I do admire you though, but I don't think that I could cope if I actually went blind. This is bad enough. Having to ask people to help you throughout the day, no, I couldn't cope if I went blind. I'm already finding it difficult to ask others to help. Sometimes they can't and I feel even worse and useless, not being able to do things for myself. No, I couldn't cope if my eyes got much worse."

"When you've got no choice you have to learn to cope or curl up in a small ball and disappear like many people do. It's your choice and you've got to be strong."

"It's a terrible disability to inflict on someone. The world we live in is a visual world. Without my sight I won't be able to do much without help."

"You're going to have to get used to that too."

"I never realised how much I depended on my eyes until now. Nearly everything involves sight. Seeing people, reading and writing, watching television, using a computer, finding things that have dropped, cooking, going shopping and crossing the road. There's too much to mention. I can't cope any longer, I hate it so much."

I became heated as I brushed my hands through my hair through sheer frustration.

"I don't want to be blind. Why is this happening to me? What have I done to deserve this? It really makes me angry when I can't do something simple that I would be able to do if I could see."

The anger and frustration built up as I shared my inner thoughts.

"Are you seeing a counsellor?"

"No; I don't need anyone, I'm fine."

"It's time to face what could happen. You will need to learn Braille and also learn how to get around using a white cane."

"Me! Using a white cane?"

It made me nervous. There was me, trying my hardest to cope with my visual impairment but I had never pictured myself using a white stick. I began to feel distressed and dizzy.

"Me!" I thought, "and a white stick? What's happening to me and when is this torture going to stop?"

"It's up to you. Would you like to learn how to use one? I can teach you."

I hesitated.

"Are my eyes going to get so bad that I have to use a white stick?" I asked.

"Probably; I do think that it's best if you learn, just in case."

"But they're long and... I might as well wear a t-shirt that says, 'I'm blind'. It's degrading; I can't, I can't!"

"You can carry it folded up until you feel comfortable using it."

I paused to think again.

"I don't know what to do," I thought. "I'd be too embarrassed to use one. How can I teach Martial Arts without people saying that I can't see what they're doing? And what about work? I don't know... but then it will help me in the long run. I don't know... I suppose there's no harm learning."

"What do you mean, that you will teach me? Can't I just have the stick?" I asked.

"No, there's a technique to using a white cane, I'll teach you."

"*You're* going to teach me? You're not going to ask someone else to teach me?"

"I can use one, I'm blind, remember?" she replied jokingly.

"Exactly; it would be like the blind… leading the blind. Now this I have to see!"

The thought of how Rita would be able to guide me when I could see more than she could fascinated me. We arranged to meet in a week and I eagerly awaited her return.

The week passed quickly and it was soon time for my lesson. Rita walked in with her helper and sat down. She took out my new toy – my white cane. It was folded up small, so she showed me how to unravel it and it became quite long and slim.

"Are you ready for your first lesson?"

"Yes, where are we going to practise walking?"

"We'll start on a road that's already familiar to you. I've taught a few other people there as well so I'm used to it."

She told me that it was Hillmorton Road, outside the Sports Centre that I used regularly and then we set out on our way.

Her driver drove us there. He never helped much; he just did the driving. She literally did everything herself. He stopped outside the park and we got out. She arranged to meet him back in the same place in an hour and we stood on the pavement as he drove off.

"Open your cane first," she instructed.

I unfolded it and the short sections interlocked with each other and my stick was straight and ready to be used. It was about five foot long and very slim.

"I'm ready," I said.

She linked my right arm and off we went. She began to talk to me and I had a little trouble hearing her. I wasn't going to say anything because I thought that she'd think that I was only fit for the bin, being deaf *and* partially sighted, but she sounded too muffled.

"I'm sorry if I didn't mention this, but I'm deaf in my right ear so I can hardly hear you on that side."

"That's fine, can you hear anything?"

"No; my right ear is totally deaf and so I usually have people on my left side. My left ear picks up what you're saying but it sounds muffled as if you were talking to me while I'm under the water in a swimming pool."

We stopped and she swapped sides.

"This makes a difference in the type of white cane that you need."

"In what way?" I asked curiously.

"White canes are for blind people, but if you also have a hearing deficiency then your cane will be white with red stripes."

"Wow! I didn't know that. I thought that all white canes were the same."

"No, they're not, we'll order you a new cane. Now let me show you how to use it."

We stood there for a moment while she opened her white cane too.

"Put your cane down to touch the pavement, now move it to your right. Then take a step closer to it with your right foot. Now move your cane to your left where you would walk with your left foot. Now take a step forward with your left foot."

"Like this?" I asked, having a go.

"No, try again like this," she demonstrated.

"That feels awkward, why can't I just hold the stick in front of me and walk?"

"Because your feet don't take the same path. Doing it that way you might still bump into things with your body. The way that I'm teaching you makes your cane search out the path of each of your feet just before you take a step."

"I'll try again then."

I followed her instructions and off we went, walking cautiously forward, both using our white canes.

We walked along, tapping our sticks on the pavement and then stepping forwards.

"Slow down, we're coming to the road. Right, stop here and we'll turn around and walk back," she said.

"This isn't as bad as I thought it would be."

"You get used to it."

"I'm not too keen on touching it on the floor though," I stated.

"Why?"

"Well, I'm always worried that I'm going to walk in dog muck and now I'm worried that my stick will touch some and… it's disgusting, we can't see well enough to see dog muck but selfish people still let their dogs do it and then leave it without cleaning it up. I hate it! I'm always worried that I've stepped in some and the more obsessive I'm becoming the more I can smell it."

"That's disgusting!" she answered laughingly.

"It is. It makes me really angry to know that normal sighted people can be so thoughtless. It's not just us; children can accidentally walk in it or people with wheelchairs can roll through it and then bring it into their homes. You're making my phobia worse thinking about it!"

"You started it," she answered with a laugh.

"I did, didn't I? Where am I going to put my stick when I get home? Nowhere hygienically clean like my kitchen work surface for sure, no, I'll keep it by my shoes."

She laughed at my obsession as we walked on.

"Let's take this path to the Sports Centre," she said.

"How did you know that was there, I thought that you couldn't see?"

"I've been here many times but most importantly, I try to memorise my surroundings wherever I go."

"You too? I thought that I was the only one who did that but now that I think about it, that's how most visually impaired people probably get around. It hurts me though."

"What do you mean?" she asked.

"Having to think of everything while I walk, it gives me a headache. It's usually after a hard day's thinking that my eyes hurt more too and it's really uncomfortable. The pressure is so great I have to take my glasses off and rub my eyes."

"Get used to it. You need to know when a lamp post is coming up before you get to it."

"It's too much to think about. Sometimes I feel like my head is going to explode. Everywhere I go I remember things that most people can just look and see when they need to. I know that there are two benches on the left of this path and at the end of the path it dips slightly before the opening in the fence on the left. It's almost unnecessary information but it stops me from walking into the locked gate that's straight ahead."

"You need to keep doing it, memorising everything because as your eyesight gets worse that's all you'll have to help you manoeuvre around objects."

"I will. You know, I often try to go out for a drink and I've found myself studying where the toilets are in each pub! It's so hard to read the signs on the doors these days. I've even directed drunken people to the toilet! I prefer to drink in the pubs where the toilets are easy to find. I've walked into a few ladies' toilets you know, accidentally of course! Most of the time I watch which door men go in and assume that's the men's toilets."

Just then I felt my foot slip.

"What was that?" I asked.

"What's wrong?" she replied.

"My foot just slid on something. Now I'll never know whether it was mud or dog muck. I can't see well enough to look at my shoes and... I feel sick."

"Here comes that gate. Let's stop and have a rest then we'll walk back."

We rested for a few minutes, exchanging thoughts. It was so soothing to find someone who really understood my thoughts. She had the same thoughts and feelings as me. She experienced troubled times and moments where she too felt useless. My confidence grew and we continued to chat.

"Sometimes I feel so useless and incompetent having to ask others for help all the time," I said. "People tell me that I should ask for help more often, but when I do, sometimes they're not able to help and then I feel incapable of doing things for myself. I feel like a burden to others and end up trying to do things for myself. Sometimes that's okay because if feels like I'm gaining some of my independence back. I hate going to parties where you have to help yourself to food. It all looks like merged clumps of blurred paint to me, and nothing's identifiable. Then I have to stand there with my plate while others tell me what's on the table. Most of the time, they then have to serve me. I feel like a baby, not being able to do things for myself."

"If you carry this white cane then people will understand," she advised.

"But I don't want to be labelled, I don't want to be partially sighted, I want to be normal again. I want to be able to do things for myself."

"How did you feel using the cane?"

"It was fun, a little embarrassing, especially when we were passing people. Imagine what they must be thinking seeing two people with white sticks walking together. A pair of misfits, that's what we probably looked like."

"Do you remember your surroundings from where we walked from?"

"Most of it, I think, why?" I asked innocently.

"We're going to walk back but this time I want you to wear these."

She produced a pair of sunglasses.

"Put these on."

My glasses were too big and I couldn't get the dark glasses over them.

"They won't fit."

"That's fine; take your glasses off first."

"But I can't see without my glasses."

"Exactly; you need to get used to this feeling just in case your eyesight gets any worse."

So I removed my glasses and put the dark ones on. They were special sunglasses, very dark, big and bulky and oddly shaped. They also had an added surprise.

"I can't see anything through these, nothing," I said desperately.

"Move them around until you can see through the little pinholes."

"Pinholes? Where?"

"There's a small hole in each lens that allows you to see through. It blocks out most of the light that can irritate your eyes. It also imitates what tunnel vision can end up looking like."

It made me feel very uncomfortable and disorientated. The view was so dark and so blurred it was as though I was looking through a tunnel and only seeing the faint light at the other end. There was someone approaching, I could hear them so I looked around, trying to line my eyes up with the pinholes and focus on the movement. I saw a vague line in the distance that slowly became wider. It grew as the person got closer but it never became clearer. It was so cloudy looking and so distorted that it looked like a very faint ghostly apparition. As the shape passed me I almost trembled. It was so uncomfortable and scary to see like this.

"No way would I come out of my house and walk around if I saw like this, no way," I thought to myself frantically.

I readjusted the dark glasses until I could see, (well, see something) and we walked on. I was nervous, this felt very different. I couldn't see the trees or the lamp posts or even the path. I was very wary of each step that I took. I walked much slower too. My white stick detected me veering off the path onto the grass so I straightened up. It was so hard to control my balance as I became disorientated. We continued to retrace our path cautiously.

"How do you feel with those glasses on?" Rita asked.

"Very uncomfortable, I can't see anything and with being deaf in one ear, I feel dizzy and keep feeling like I'm going to fall over. It's an awful feeling and I don't know where I am or how far it is until we reach the end of this path."

"This is where your memory comes into play, trust yourself."

"We're walking slower so my timing is out too. I would say that we're close now."

I carried on walking and using my stick like it would save my life. We slowed down as I prepared to hit the gate with my stick. After a few more moments the stick made contact and I searched around with it as I shuffled to my right to find the opening. It was awkward but somehow I managed it.

"I did it!" I shouted joyfully.

"Well done. Now let's walk to our left."

We set off and plodded slowly along. We were near the road this time and the sound of the cars frightened me. I could see thin blurred strips, which were presumably people and they moved in a jerky fashion. They were unsure of where to walk and dodged us at the last second. Then my stick hit something. It was a post that I had forgotten was there.

"That was scary. For a second or two I didn't know what it was and panicked," I said.

After manoeuvring around the post I continued to lead her forward staying in the middle of the pavement by guessing how far away the road was from my right.

"Slow down we're coming to a road again. Remember, we'll turn around and walk back again," she said.

"Why don't we keep walking and cross the road?"

"You're not ready, not with those dark glasses on anyway. We'll cross roads on another lesson."

"Another lesson! I have to do this again?" I cried out.

"Yes, next week I'll teach you techniques on how to walk up and down steps and then we'll cross roads the week after."

As we walked on my stick sunk down as it hit the road at the edge of the pavement. We stopped, turned and walked back.

"We'll walk back to the park gate and then rest while we wait for our lift back to your house."

Halfway along, I suddenly stopped as I remembered that there was a post around somewhere. I slowed down all the way past the post and to the gate. After we arrived at the gate she asked me to remove my dark glasses. Although my sight was still distorted, I felt relieved to be able to see more light.

"Did you enjoy your first lesson?" she asked.

"It was fun but at the same time I felt helpless, terrified and very vulnerable. I struggle to see anyway but that was different. I felt like people were watching me and I didn't like the attention the stick drew. I enjoyed it, but I didn't, does that make any sense?" I replied in confusion.

"Yes… I think," she replied as she laughed.

"I'm scared," I said.

"Scared of what?"

"I'm scared of going blind and seeing like that. People think that I'm strong and brave to have carried on going out but I don't know if I can do it if my eyesight deteriorates much further. I really am scared of going blind."

"It is scary but we learn to cope, we have to," Rita replied.

We spoke for a few more minutes before a car drew up in front of us and beeped its horn.

"That sounds like our lift," Rita said.

"Wouldn't it be funny if we got into the wrong car?" I said jokingly.

We laughed and nervously got into the car.

The next week seemed to pass quite quickly and we found ourselves at the Rugby College for my second white cane training session. We straightened out our canes and proceeded towards the entrance. This time I was lucky – she hadn't produced the dark glasses, though I would have been very reluctant to wear them anyway. We walked carefully towards the steps at the entrance and waited for our canes to hit the first step.

"There, did you feel the difference?" Rita asked.

"Yes, we've reached the steps," I answered.

"Use your cane to feel around and work out a picture in your mind of what's in front of you. Remember, don't rely on your eyes, memorise the feeling."

"Yes, it's definitely steps, I can feel them going up."

"Are there any railings beside the steps?"

"Yes, on the right," I answered.

"Remember that too; now let's move to the right so that you can use the railings to help you up the steps."

We made our way up the steps and into the college. She asked me to take her to the main stairs inside the building, so I led the way.

"We've arrived at the stairs, they're in front of us. Now what should we do?"

"When you walked into the building, up the outside steps, you used your eyes too much. Remember we're also practising in a way that will help you if you were to lose your eyesight completely."

"What do you want me to do this time? You haven't got those dark glasses again have you? I really would prefer it if I didn't have to wear them, they're so uncomfortable, and people know me here, it would make me feel humiliated."

"No, you don't have to wear them, but I want you to close your eyes and walk upstairs though."

"That's as bad as having the dark glasses on! Fine, I'll do it, but only because you forced me," I said jokingly.

"Some stairs don't have railings so I want you to try it with and without using the hand rails."

"I can't see so what do I do with my white cane?"

"Find the first step with your cane and then turn your wrist and hold your cane straight down so that it's vertical. As your cane hits a step, you should take a step so that the cane is always near your feet."

It was a scary experience. My eyes were closed and I felt very dizzy and off balance. I kept thinking that I was going to topple over backwards down the stairs.

My cane came to a smooth step and it confused me slightly.

"We've reached the top I think."

"Have we?" she replied. "You've used these stairs before, so are there any more steps?"

"Let me think. No, it levels off for a metre or two and then there are some more steps to the right before we reach the first floor."

I walked forwards until my cane reached the wall, then turned slightly to my right and felt for the next flight of stairs.

I heard a commotion. There were students coming downstairs.

"Stop and wait for them to pass, but try not to panic."

"How will I know if they've all passed?" I asked.

"Listen carefully."

"I'm deaf in one ear," I said sarcastically.

"Listen… carefully then."

I knew what she meant so I waited until I felt that it was clear to walk then I proceeded using the same technique that she'd taught me. We got to the first floor and I was safe.

"How did that feel?"

"Embarrassing! I must have looked so helpless and frail to those students. My eyes are open but they still haven't readjusted to the light so I still can't focus yet."

"Rest for a while and then we'll walk back down."

Thoughts began to invade my mind.

"That actually took ages. I didn't realise that we were walking so slowly. It scared me to walk any faster because I kept thinking that I would collide with someone who was in a hurry, or fall. I felt vulnerable. Now I'm even more worried about going down the stairs. It will be much easier to trip."

"Close your eyes again and find the first step," Rita's voice cut into my reverie.

I slid my cane on the smooth floor and walked slowly and cautiously towards the edge. My cane sank down a level indicating the first step.

"I've found the first step. What do I do this time?"

"Keep your cane there and slowly walk to it. Now take the first step and stand where your cane is. Then move your cane forward until it drops to the next step and walk onto that one. Take your time; remember you don't want to fall. Are your eyes still closed?"

"Yes, but this is scary. I feel as though I'm going to fall. I'm disorientated again and I don't know where we are."

"Visualise it in your head. Did you count how many steps there were on the way up?"

"No, you didn't ask me to," I replied.

"It helps to know how many there are before the last step."

"I can hear some people behind me."

"Let them pass and then continue when you're ready."

I could feel the people hesitating to pass us. Then one of them said hello to me as they passed. I know he was talking to me because he called me by my name.

"Who was that then?" Rita asked.

"I don't know. I've got a white cane and my eyes are closed and they still didn't have the decency to say their name. I get a lot of that from my friends, you know, and they know that I'm partially sighted – it makes me feel emotional."

"I get it too."

We finally made it back downstairs and I was allowed to open my eyes. Then we went up and down the stairs a few more times so that I could get used to the technique. My second lesson had finished and I awaited my final training.

The next week we started on Corporation Street, a busy street where the traffic travels a little faster. There was a small path in the centre of the road, and on either side there were two lanes of traffic. It was scary just standing there listening to the noise. Rita told me to close my eyes and walk along the pavement using my white cane. I felt a little more comfortable moving it from left to right to map out my path. Although Rita was on my left, I still found it difficult to hear her with the sound of the noisy traffic, but she was used to dealing with people who had more severe problems than mine and didn't seem to mind having to repeat what she said. Then my cane hit a signpost that appeared to be in the middle of the path and I found it quite difficult to manoeuvre around it.

"What's that in the middle of the pavement for? Couldn't they have put it somewhere else, rather than slap bang in the middle of the path? Don't they ever take pedestrians into consideration? Didn't they think about how difficult it would be for people with low vision to get around it?"

"There are many signposts like this," Rita said.

"Well I think that they're very thoughtless and inconsiderate! It's not even safe to walk on the paths round here. They should try it with a blindfold on. Maybe then they would realise how difficult it is and how ridiculously placed some of these posts are," I rambled.

"Slow down, we should be coming to a road soon."

"My cane has found the edge of the pavement. So what do we do now? My eyes are closed and I'm terrified."

"Wait until the noise of the traffic gets fainter, then cross slowly and carefully."

The traffic was on my right and I really struggled to tell when there were hardly any cars so… I admit that I cheated and had a quick peek through my eyes before crossing! Cars could turn left into the road that we were crossing and I was reluctant to take too many risks. I stepped down and walked until my cane reached the other kerb, then mounted the pavement.

"That was scary. It would have been better if there were traffic lights there or a crossing. It's very dangerous and I didn't feel safe."

"Trust me, I'll protect you," Rita said.

"Let me think about that," I answered sarcastically.

We walked on for a few more steps and then I bumped into another signpost.

"This is becoming seriously annoying!" I complained.

We walked on a little further.

"Stop!" Rita shouted suddenly.

"What's wrong?"

"Did you feel the texture of the pavement change?"

"No, why?"

"Walk forward and see if you can feel it now."

I took a few steps.

"Yes I feel it; it's like lots of small bumps under my feet."

"That means that we're approaching some traffic lights. All crossings should have bumps like that on the path. Remember that in future."

"It's in my memory bank, what's next?"

"Find the button on the traffic lights and then hold your hand underneath it."

"Hold my hand at the bottom of the whole box?"

"Yes, there should be a small ridged circle in the middle somewhere."

"Oh yes, I found it, what now?"

"Hold onto it until you feel it rotating. That will tell you when the traffic lights are on red and the cars have stopped to let you cross."

"That's very ingenious of someone. That person should design a better place for the signposts too!" I said.

"Some lights don't make a beeping sound when it's safe to cross, especially traffic lights that have a separate controller to get across the other side, so the circle rotates so that people with low vision know when it's time to cross."

The circle began to spin and I knew that it was time to cross but I was still very nervous of being run over by some maniac who couldn't be bothered to stop, and these traffic lights hadn't made a sound to indicate when it was safe, so I opened my eyes and took another peek to make extra sure that the traffic had stopped. Then we crossed slowly and felt for the traffic light box to get across the other side of the road. Once again I held my hand underneath the box until it began to rotate and yes, I took another peek at the traffic! We crossed and were safe.

"Shall we do that again?" she asked.

"Nope; I've got it perfect thanks; it's easy to understand," I answered cunningly.

"Were you scared then?"

"Yes, terrified. It's hard enough with my eyes open, no way am I doing that again with my eyes closed. If my eyes get that bad, then I'm calling a taxi to carry me over to the other side!" I said jokingly.

"You can't get a taxi to cross the road."

"I would! It's too dangerous walking. Blind people should get a lift in a car when they want to go out."

"It's not always convenient to others so they have to take a risk and walk."

"Now I know why so many blind people prefer to stay at home and become a recluse – it's safer. Walking is so scary, and cruel. How are they supposed to cope with their nerves? I would become a nervous wreck."

"Fine, I get the message. We'll walk through the town centre and get used to busy streets," she suggested.

"That sounds safer to me," I said with a smile.

This time I was allowed to keep my eyes open so I felt a little more comfortable. My confidence grew as I walked on and was able to see where I was going. There was a post in front of us that I saw at the last second before colliding with it so I moved to avoid it. The pavement around this area was very uneven and difficult to walk on without stumbling a few times. Every time I stumbled I became more embarrassed. I kept thinking that people must be watching and laughing at us as we struggled to walk with our white canes. We approached another road and stopped to make sure that there was no traffic. I listened carefully despite my hearing loss then I stepped down off the kerb and walked to the other side. We then walked on to into town.

It wasn't too busy but there were plenty of people around to avoid.

"Remember you have a white cane so you don't need to move out of people's way, unless they're in a wheelchair," Rita said.

My first target approached and walked around us. It felt fine. We walked on and soon came across a lady who didn't move. She panicked and froze on the spot, not knowing what to do. We judged that she was unsure and walked around her and she apologised. We walked on and came across two people who were talking and not paying much attention to their surroundings and one of them tripped over my cane, but just walked on. We walked further and most people moved out of our way but we had to walk around a few people who were standing in the middle of the pavement talking and seemingly unaware of our presence. A group of teenagers were messing around on the path and one of them dragged another to the side and out of our way. There were a few more incidents where people didn't move or were too busy rushing around that they collided with us. The more people who got in my way, the angrier I became. It was frustrating enough coping with poor eyesight but with the added problems of ignorant and thoughtless people, I felt too uncomfortable.

We walked around for a while then waited for our lift. While we were waiting we exchanged a few words.

"Did you enjoy your experience?" Rita asked.

"It was an experience all right and no I didn't enjoy it! Some people are so ignorant, the way they walk around without a care for other less fortunate people. It was humiliating when my cane got tangled in their feet and I found it difficult not to lose my temper and have a go at them. I was wondering who couldn't see, them or us and I wanted to hit them or shout at them, no I didn't like that. I feel much more confident without the white cane when I'm walking around town. Then I can pretend I'm clumsy. I'm very observant and actually move out of people's way even though I can't see them properly and sometimes I apologise to them even when it's not my fault. I felt very vulnerable and timid and like an easy target. I know that I can take care of myself but I still felt unsafe and like easy prey. This is going to be a hard one for me to get used to. Sorry, but I was definitely uncomfortable with that and I admire any blind person for using their white cane in town centres."

Her driver turned up and they returned me to my home. My lessons were over and I could get back to learning to cope at home. It took a while but I began to take the white cane out although I didn't open it. I was back to bumping and dodging people when I went out. Although I needed it, I wasn't confident enough to straighten the white cane to its full length.

CHAPTER 16
SUFFERING IN SILENCE

Within a few months, my obsession had escalated out of control. My eyesight was slowly getting worse and I was becoming terrified of what could happen. I didn't know what to expect and that made me extremely nervous. I couldn't accept that I might go blind; it was too much to cope with. Memories of eye appointments and words that the doctors had used haunted me. Then I would struggle to get back to reality and get the thoughts out of my mind. Throughout each day I would find myself reliving moments in my head and as my eyes deteriorated my personality changed. Then my conflict of thoughts grew as my sight worsened.

"What *is* going on? Everywhere looks so different. It looks cloudy everywhere and people are harder to see."

"Your eyes are much worse."

"They don't have to get any worse. It's so hard to see anything. When I'm indoors it's like night-time, so dark that everyone appears to have dark masks on their faces."

"You can't even tell the difference between white and black."

"If people don't talk I feel lost. When I walk into parties I have to wait for other people to acknowledge me first, I just can't see anyone and I can't take it any longer."

"Just enjoy your life and don't worry about other people's problems, sort out your own."

"Maybe I need to speak to a counsellor. I'm really struggling to keep smiling and pretending that everything is fine. I'm not coping any more."

"You don't need anyone, you don't need a counsellor, and they'll only put you on anti-depressants. You're not depressed, you're strong."

"Maybe I *am* depressed, I sure can't stop thinking about my sight problem and what it's doing to me. I worry about everything, like making sure I don't trip over something or making sure I don't knock something off the kitchen worktop. I get upset when someone moves things like my tapes or videos, or coffee or sugar. It's these simple things that are making me upset because I struggle to find them for myself. Why is this happening to me?"

"It is happening so learn to accept it."

My confidence in life slowly whittled away and I became more bitter and angry. As my eyes worsened so did my obsession.

My life was like a routine with most things organised in a way that aided my sight loss. I had to ask for help and assistance with certain things but I was still trying to hold onto what little independence I had left. Some days I'd wander around the house and see a small piece of paper on the floor, so I'd pick it up and then wash my hands wondering if there would come a time when I wouldn't be able to see things on the floor. The washing of my hands became far too frequent, an endless ritual, but I wasn't able to stop myself. There was no dirt to be seen but I knew that dirt and germs lurked somewhere and I wasn't happy about not having proficient sight to be able to see, so I would wash my hands until I felt that they were clean.

Since having my white cane lessons and using the cane to touch the ground, I'd become even more aware of dog muck. I was sure that it was everywhere because I smelt it in the air. So I put newspaper down by my front door and left my shoes there when I came in. No more walking inside with my shoes on just in case I had some dog muck on them. After touching my shoes with my hands to take them off my feet I would wash my hands. I never failed to wash my hands after using the toilet, but that also involved a ritual. I cleaned the toilet with a tissue or two or lifted up the seat using a tissue, always trying not to come into direct contact with the toilet. I also cleaned the handle before flushing. When I used toilets in a nightclub, I'd wash and dry my hands then I would wait for someone else to come in so that the door was open and I wouldn't have to touch the handle. Then I'd quickly make a dash for the open door and if I ever needed to touch it, I'd only touch the lower part of the door because nobody else would have touched that part. If on occasions I had to use the door handle, I would only use a finger so that one of my fingers would be dirty and not my whole hand. (Well some men don't wash their hands and that's disgusting!) Most of the time I would refrain from shaking men's hands, for the same reason and if I ever got food on the way home, I would wait until I got home and washed my hands before eating.

As time went on my obsessions grew. They even affected me when I was teaching Martial Arts. Sometimes I would pick up people's feet to help stretch them and could feel myself wanting to wash my hands afterwards. My sight was deteriorating and I could see it happening. People's faces were much more distorted and at only two metres away I could hardly see them. Their eyes were black and bold with no clear sign of the whites of their eyes. People with beautiful green eyes or bright blue eyes were no different and they too appeared black – it was as if people had empty eye sockets. It was getting a little scary to look at people over two metres away.

The voices in my head argued every time I had a problem seeing something or someone.

"Why can't I see that?"

"You know why you can't see it, your eyes are getting worse and you can't take it any longer."

"Yes I can, things could be worse."

"Worse than what? If your eyes get any worse you'll be blind."

"I'm not going blind, no, I refuse to accept that. Things will be fine."

"Haven't you noticed that people are beginning to look like ghosts again?"

"So what, I can cope. Nobody has to know what I see; I'll pretend I see people."

"It's like it was when you had the eye drops in your eyes to dilate them. You can't see any more than you could then."

"Yes I can. I see people fine close up."

"Who are you fooling? Look at them, they're blurred, distorted and look like they're standing in thick fog."

"Yes but there are worse things to think about. I can cope, I have to!"

The arguments escalated so much that my head hurt. I kept trying to keep myself busy so that I had little time to think negative thoughts but then I felt trapped because if I couldn't see something that someone was showing me, I would be plunged back to the frustrated arguments in my head.

"Why can't I see that photograph of my kid clearly and in detail?"

"Because someone's making you go blind."

"But why? Why me? Why does it have to happen to me? I don't want to go blind, I'm scared, so scared. I want to see again. Please God help me, help me to see again, you have the power, please," I sobbed in my head.

"Haven't you noticed that everywhere is darker especially at night? You are struggling more these days and you're bumping into more posts, just look at your shins, they're in bits with scars everywhere from previous collisions. You need more help getting around."

"No! I'm embarrassed to have to keep asking. It's so humiliating especially when people can't help after I've asked."

"Too much is happening to you at the moment and you can't cope. You just want to disappear."

"I *can* cope."

"What, you can cope with the dark, cloudy and distorted images?"

"I have to, what choice do I have? To stay indoors and never leave my house again? Give up work and teaching Martial Arts? I can't give up, not again. I'll have to try and use my cane – that will help."

"It won't help. It might solve one problem, but it will create some more. If you ask for more help and you have your stick, you might get around better but you'll feel degraded and become depressed, and you don't want to become depressed do you?"

"No! People seem to lose track of reality when they're depressed. No, I'll fight it."

"But if you use your stick you'll become emotional and that makes you feel weak."

"Yes it does. I'm confused; I don't know what to do."

"You've also noticed that part of people's faces appear to be missing."

"Yes, but only *I* know that. It's horrible. People look so scary from a distance or when they're in shaded areas. There's *got* to be a cure. My eyes can't do this to me. I almost can't bear to look at people."

Over the past few months I'd noticed that parts of people's faces were slowly disappearing. It must have been more blind spots that were becoming dominant. It began as only small sections, but like a virus, it was growing and there was nothing I could do to stop it. When I looked at someone, their face was horribly blurred and distorted. With the additional blind spots, parts of their faces appeared blank as though someone had rubbed out part of a picture. Part of one of their eyes would be missing and I would have to move my eyes around and look from an angle. This was how I adjusted to see people clearer, from out of the sides of my eyes. Another way was to close one eye and find out which one had the worst blind spots. Their faces were clearer if they were closer than two metres away from me. Sometimes I would go really close to someone just to be able to see them clearer. Close enough so that no parts of their face were missing. It would make me both happy and sad to see them this close – happy that I was able to see them reasonably clearly because I hardly ever got the chance, but sad because I was counting down the days that I had left to be able to see them at all, before I finally got tunnel vision and their faces disappeared forever. Some people like to sit in dim light because it makes them feel comfortable but it made me feel very uncomfortable talking to ghostly figures. I missed seeing my friends' faces; sometimes I even forgot what they looked like unless I got a chance to see them up close. I would have loved to be able to see a real smile again and not have to piece together a jigsaw puzzle of a smile. I'd started to admire other things too, like photographs, videos and films. Sometimes I tried so desperately to read books. It was now so difficult, but I suppose deep down inside I knew that one day I would never be able to read a book again.

I used to have conversations with people and my face would be turned away slightly and my eyes focussed somewhere else as if I wasn't looking at them or paying much attention to them, but that was the angle at which I could see them clearest. People asked me on numerous occasions to look at them when they spoke, that's what we were told when we were children – look at people when they speak to you, remember your manners! In my case it's selfish and inconsiderate to ask me to do this because I *was* looking at them when my face was to the side. When I looked straight at people they were darker and more parts were missing, and it made me feel useless when I saw their jigsaw image. It was very confusing and frustrating for me, but that's what I had to do. When I appear to be looking at you, I'm not, and when I appear not to be looking at you, I am!

Somehow, in the middle of all the problems and challenges that I was experiencing, my students persuaded me to take my 3rd Dan black belt. After experiencing difficulties, I had managed to pass before and then I'd vowed that I would never take another exam. My eyes were too blurred and it was taking me far too long to focus on people. It was also dangerous. Fighting against other black belts was similar to entering competitions. All it would have taken was for me not to see one kick and I could have been knocked out. Life wasn't being fair to me. If I could see more clearly I would have wanted to excel to the highest standard despite my arthritis. My techniques were proficient enough but my eyesight wasn't. Yet another dream had been taken away from me because of my lack of sight.

Life wasn't being fair to me and I started being unfair to other people. In my bitter rage I became quite cold towards others, no longer caring about their trivial problems. They complained of having a cold or a sore throat, but I didn't care. They complained of earaches or back pains, but I didn't care.

"It's not the end of the world, get over it. Do you want a real problem?" I would say to them.

I had always been sympathetic towards my friends and their problems. They used to call me on the phone for support and advice, but the calls soon whittled away. Life had no sympathy towards me and my growing problems so I had no sympathy towards others. I knew I was wrong to feel that way, but I didn't care any more. My disabilities had changed my personality. I was the last person my friends should come and moan about life to. I had too many problems of my own and was struggling to fight them. Depression was just one step away and I refused to take that step, even if it meant that I would lose friends. My emotions were hidden inside and I didn't show them to others any more. I walked around and got on with life as though I had no problems yet inside I was ready to explode. Crying was a thing of the past. Nobody could see that I was crying every day on the inside; I always put on a brave face to others. I was sad that life had handed me such a raw deal and the pressures to learn how to deal with my problems were too much. If I had given in to my emotions, I would have become depressed like a great deal of people. My friends thought that I was strong and I didn't want to let them down so I pretended to be able to cope. Maybe I should thank God for my Martial Arts because that was what helped me to deal with most problems, the only thing was that I had to deal with my disabilities on my own and my Martial Arts couldn't alter that. Sometimes the thoughts were so powerful I would feel like I was losing my mind. It could start with something simple like not being able to see a friend in a nightclub when he was standing right next to me.

"He looks like he's wearing a mask from this angle. His face is so dark, no features at all to identify him. If he were to walk off and come back without saying anything, I wouldn't know that he was the same person. His outline is so faint that it merges with the background. Why do I have to see people like this?"

"Because someone thought that it would be funny giving you crap eyes."

"But why do they have to be so bad? I can't see my friend standing right in front of me and I can't keep blaming the light."

"That's right, it's not just the light, it's your eyes."

"I can move so that the angle at which I'm looking at him changes and the light will reflect off his face."

"What's the point? What are you going to do if someone else turns up? Are you going to keep moving around like a yo-yo? And what about your hearing? People have to be on your correct side – just accept it – you're a misfit."

"This is so uncomfortable."

"Why not stay at home? You'll have fewer problems if you don't go out."

"Yes, that's what I'll do, stay at home. I wouldn't have half these thoughts and problems if I never came out."

"Yes, stay at home and become a recluse, nobody would miss you because you moan at everyone."

"No, I can't give up. Why do I have to suffer so much? My vision is so blurred and I'm also deaf in one ear, how much more am I supposed to take before I have a nervous breakdown?"

"Nobody cares so do what you like and don't worry about their feelings."

"No, I wouldn't like it if someone treated me like that, I do have feelings and emotions, I'm just confused."

"You're not confused, you're weak. Don't get all emotional on me, you're more likely to break down and become depressed and you don't want that do you? Do you want to stay in bed and moan about literally everything or become an alcoholic? And only talk about poor you, Mr Selfish? No you don't."

"No I don't!"

"Then be mean and nasty and you will cope. Don't worry about not being able to see your friend. They don't know that you can't really see them and don't be telling them and getting yourself all emotional again. Treat it like it's a game. It's your secret – you're the only one who knows that you can't see them, and keep agreeing with them because you can't hear them either."

"I can't hear or see, this is ridiculous. I feel useless. Where do I look anyway? I can't see their eyes."

"Keep looking away as if you're looking at someone passing and you should be able to see them a little clearer. If you see their eyes, remember where they are on the mask, or where they are in relation to the background, then look back towards them as if you can see them, but remember, it's your secret that you can see better from the side."

"Why do I have to do this? I feel pathetic."

The bitter thoughts continued until I spoke to my friend, but every time I listened to him talk the arguments continued in my head. It was getting out of control. It had escalated from a few times a day to every few minutes. If I wasn't busy doing something interesting then my mind would return to my disabilities.

This constant battling in my head wasn't the only problem that I had. My finances were suffering and I was getting into debt. Although looking for another job would help me with some of my debts, it also created another problem in my head. My Martial Arts was a hobby and I got more fun out of it than money. It gave me great pleasure seeing students progress from being timid and shy to being strong and confident. My day job as a Computer Technician had never paid well, but I was scared to take the risk of changing jobs because at least it was secure.

During my six-week holiday I registered at a few agencies for a part-time job. I wanted to continue to work with computers since I was already very familiar with them. I was truthful with the agencies and disclosed that I was partially sighted. I was subjected to many negative comments and attitudes, which eventually added to my hatred of the world for giving me bad eyesight. They would ask me several questions and I would answer well. As time went on they became quite relaxed with me and showed a good attitude towards finding me a job. As soon as I mentioned that I was registered partially sighted, the questions were all diverted to that. They didn't feel that they could help much and said that it might be difficult finding a job. I tried to explain that I was already in a position working with computers but it never helped. I could tell that they were disappointed. One of them even gave me a test on the computer and I found it easy with my specialised knowledge, but when I asked for help to read the questions on the small screen, they were reluctant. They said that the test wasn't available in any other format.

Another agency asked me to fill in a questionnaire, but it wasn't available in large print and they said that they would get back to me but they never did. It was obvious from the problems I was experiencing that they were not sure how to deal with someone with severe sight loss. Their system was only set up for people with normal vision. I was also told that jobs in warehouses were too dangerous.

The impossibility of the situation incensed my mind.

"I give up! It's disability discrimination."

"Why bother fighting against them? There are too many of them. You can't win."

"They were interested in me until I mentioned that I was partially sighted, and then suddenly they thought that it might cause one or two problems and employers might not be willing to adapt their workplace."

"Wait for another agency to call back."

"They won't call back. I even needed help filling in the forms and I couldn't see where to sign. The test on the computer screen was easy, I know about computers, but I couldn't finish the test because I couldn't read it properly. It's all my eyes' fault. I hate them. See, I *am* useless."

"You can't do it, so give up."

"I can't give up, I need the money."

"Those jobs are not for people with poor vision. How would you read the labels on items in a warehouse? And computer screens are too small."

"I have to find a way, but I'm not having much success with computer jobs because the screen and keyboard are too hard to read. Maybe I should give up looking for alternative employment."

"They've made you emotional again, come on, snap out of it or you'll end up depressed. Forget those people who turned you down, they mean nothing to you. Find a job without disclosing your sight problem."

"That's dangerous."

"Who cares, you need the money."

"Why can't I see? Why is this happening to me?"

"You're strong, come on, you can beat them."

The voices in my head continued until I decided on a plan.

Rather than give up and suffer more debt, I registered with some more agencies but this time I failed to disclose my disability, or should I say, disabilities. It was the wrong thing to do, but I was desperate for money. It worked and within a few days I was accepted as a warehouse assistant in a can factory. The warehouse was noisy with machines running continuously. My hearing loss prevented me from hearing people when they spoke to me, but I pretended that I just had a slight problem hearing. Someone then took me through the warehouse and showed me the different machinery. On a few occasions there were low pipes where we had to duck down to get past them. I watched the man's actions carefully and when he ducked, I followed. I walked behind him most of the time so that I was safer and I pretended that I was really interested in some of the machines, but I was actually struggling to see where to go and every so often I stopped to work out a route and memorised it. I was walking around almost blind and nobody knew.

When I was left to work on my own I looked around and checked everything out – low pipes, bins, toilets, canteen and where to sit. Half the time I guessed what to do. When I worked with others, I pretended that I didn't understand certain things so that they would show me more closely but really I couldn't see where to put things. Interesting but mixed thoughts went through my mind.

"What am I doing here? I can't even see what I'm doing."

"Nobody else knows that so stop complaining. It's paying the bills isn't it?"

"Yes, but… there's got to be another way. This is dangerous. I keep thinking that I'm going to fall downstairs or hit my head on a pipe."

"Keep holding onto the rails and walk slower. You're fooling everyone."

"I'm fooling myself. I'm struggling with door handles, I can't see them and don't know how to open some of the doors."

"Watch other people and you'll see how they open the doors. You have to keep pretending that you can see, you need the money."

"Look at everyone walking around so confidently. I'm jealous. I wish I could see like them, even for a day. I wish that I could walk around without having to worry or guess what things are. I wonder what this place really looks like. I'm useless not being able to see where to go and what to do. How am I supposed to work well seeing like this?"

"Don't start, don't get emotionally distraught, try not to think about it. Get on with your job and keep hiding and fighting your emotions."

Working in such a hazardous environment was an experience that I will never forget. It helped for a while and paid off most of my debts until I returned to my normal job. My income was still too low and I slowly got into more debt. I contemplated working in the warehouse during the evenings but decided that it would be too many hours. My hunt began for another way of bringing more money into my household.

CHAPTER 17
THROUGH MY EYES

An appointment had been organised for me to learn how to read Braille. At the allotted time, a young lady arrived at my home. She sat down and introduced herself. She amazed me just like Rita had, because she was full of life and energy but was registered blind. It encouraged me to know that there were people suffering more than I was who appeared positive and happy. It didn't matter how much I was suffering inside, I knew that I would feel much worse if I was registered blind.

"Tell me about some of the problems you experience," she said.

"I love reading for pleasure and I also need to read things at work. I need to be able to read computer instruction manuals, but I can't any more. My eyes are not just bad they're getting worse. It's like one minute I can read, then the next I can't. I'm trying my best to readjust my life to cope with the limitations of my vision, but then after a few months my eyesight deteriorates further and I have to readjust again. Most books are written in small text. Sometimes I can read them if I take my glasses off and hold the book very close to my face, but I would never do that in front of other people because it's embarrassing and must look so silly. The words in books almost appear to have a life of their own. They disappear, reappear or jump around the pages. It's very confusing and I have to read very slowly. Most words are too small to read and the ones that I do manage to read have parts missing."

"What do you mean?"

"My eyes have blind spots that are growing and slowly taking over my vision. Depending on the size of the text, parts are missing so if I was reading the word 'something', I might only see 's t ing' and then have to look several times, moving my eyes around until I slowly made up the word. It's very difficult and frustrating and extremely embarrassing when I'm attempting to read in front of others. I sound like I can't read, but I can and it makes me feel really upset."

"What about larger words. What do they look like to you?"

"If it's larger then less appears to be missing, but most large words have a part of the corner missing as though someone has bitten a chunk out of it. An 'S' may look like a backward 'C' or an 'O' can look like a 'U'; the letter 'P' can look like an 'F'; the letter 'E' can look like 'F'; 'L' can look like 'I' and the letter 'm' can look like the letter 'n'. It's very confusing and I'm sick and tired of having to guess."

I began to get a little upset as I continued. Talking about my problems for a brief moment is fine but when I go into detail it focuses too much attention on them all and I find that I can't stay detached.

"I would love to be able to read again. I wish I had read more when I was younger but like most people I took my eyes for granted. It never occurred to me that I would be struggling so much with my eyesight so early on in my life."

"What age did you start having trouble seeing?"

"It was when I was twenty-one."

"So how *do* you read?"

"When I look at a page in a book I can see where my blind spots affect the writing. Sometimes parts of a word are missing or sometimes whole words are invisible if they're quite small. It's as though someone has painted white lines all over the page and I have to work out what words and letters are missing. Most of the time, several different words could fit into the same space so it depresses and frustrates me. Pages sometimes look worse when I close one of my eyes. Each of my eyes has blind spots in different places and has a different contrast. My left eye is more visually impaired but it sees things brighter than my right eye. When I switch from left to right, it's like someone is turning down the contrast of light and then turning it back up again as I switch back to my other eye. It's very scary to experience and very depressing to think about."

"Are you suffering from depression?"

"No. I'm fine."

"You sound a little depressed to me."

"I'm fine."

"Have you got tunnel vision?"

"A little, parts of my vision are very dark but I can still see plenty of light."

"If you're that interested in reading I'd say that you would benefit from learning Braille. Would you like to learn Braille? Lots of books are available in Braille and you could start reading again."

"That would be great. I'd really appreciate it if you could teach me so that I can read books again. I'm really jealous of other people when I hear them read and wish that I could do it again too. I can't believe that some people with clear eyesight choose not to read. Don't they realise how lucky they are to have that privilege?"

"Have you tried reading with a bright light?"

"Yes; it helps but after a short while the light hurts my eyes and I have to stop and sometimes close my eyes to rest them. When I *am* able to read, it's so slow and I feel hopeless so I stop and now I hardly read at all. I've tried a few times to read to my child who is four years old but it's so difficult. I get upset not being able to read to her. She's already a very good reader, very advanced for her age and can read for herself. I hate not being able to read. Most of the time there are shadows all over the pages and that prevents me from reading as well. Sometimes I get so emotional thinking about it, I'm constantly asking myself why it's happening to me. Most of the time without the aid of a bright light, seeing to read is like reading in the dark. There are no words to be seen and the pages look blank, yet other people can take the book off me and read it easily. It's like there are shadows everywhere. Someone has to read my letters and I hate that too. It's like I have no privacy any more. It makes me feel so incapable and useless."

Then she asked me more about my eyesight and the problems it causes me at work. I explained it to her just like I had explained it to other people. Although I felt a little more relaxed talking to her, I still got upset having to repeat the same explanations.

"Can you read magazines or newspapers?"

"The pictures are interesting but I'm unable to see the writing. Sometimes I can read the titles when they're written very large or I'm in a brightly lit room. But the pictures aren't clear although I can sometimes work out what's there. A few years ago I could read newspapers but now they're a thing of the past. If nobody else wants to read them then I throw them out. They're no use to me with my poor eyesight."

"What's your writing like?"

"I hardly write at all these days. My writing is getting very messy and once I've written something, I struggle to see where I've written or what I've put. It's annoying when I write a cheque. I can't see the line or what I'm writing so most of the time I just guess where to write. The word 'Pay' is a small grey blur that I can't read, but because I know it's there from experience, I can work out where most of the other words go. Another blurred spot that I sometimes see is the pound sign on the right. Then I use a finger on my left hand to guide me where to write and I sign just below my finger. I'm surprised banks still accept my messy cheques."

"It sounds like you're experiencing a lot of problems."

"Most of what I do throughout a day causes me problems. When I'm attempting to write a cheque I have to keep blinking hard to clear away the floaters that I see regularly. They're getting quite big and move around when I move my eyes. They look like tiny dark grey clouds in my eyes. They can also confuse me when I walk and I'll stop suddenly because I think I'm going to walk into something. Then when I blink it sometimes moves. I'm having lots of trouble working out what *is* there and what isn't. It's like seeing ghosts. My vision is very foggy too and that doesn't help. I'm also in a lot of pain from the pressure of my eyes. I suffer from glaucoma and that causes me severe pain in my eyes especially my right one, but that's actually my better eye. I'm always getting headaches but I don't know whether it's from the glaucoma or from thinking too much about what I can see. I'm not one to complain anyway; the pain I suffer is nothing compared to not being able to see at all."

Then the lady took a book out of her bag and passed it over to me. It was a book written in Braille.

"There's nothing in this book, where's all the writing?" I asked jokingly.

"It's Braille; can you see any of it?"

"No; it's all the same colour as the pages. I thought that it would be colour coded."

"What's the point of colour if you can't see?"

"Good point!"

"Can you feel the different textures?"

I ran my fingers over some of the pages and found it difficult to feel the difference.

"Sorry, but it feels almost smooth like there's nothing there."

She asked me to hand the book back and then passed me another one.

"This book is to practise Braille. Are you ready?"

"I was born ready," I chuckled.

"Can you feel the big bump with any of your fingers?"

It took a while but eventually I was able to feel something.

"How many dots are there?" she asked.

"I'm not sure; it's hard to tell; I would guess that there's just one."

"Well done."

"I can read Braille!" I bellowed.

"That's just one. How many can you feel on the next one?"

Moving my index finger carefully and softly, I felt around for a while. It was difficult and although I could feel something, I couldn't feel the separations so I guessed.

"There are two this time."

"No; try again and take your time."

"Are there three?"

"Yes, that's right."

"Sorry, but I just guessed that," I admitted.

"Don't guess; feel; try the next one."

It was so difficult. I tried for ages but couldn't feel anything significant.

"I'm really struggling; I think you must need really sensitive fingers to read Braille."

"You do; I'd have thought that you would have sensitive fingers from working with computers."

"Sorry, but didn't I tell you about my Martial Arts?"

I explained that I did lots of press-ups and broke bricks and boards with my hands. She was disappointed and held my hands.

"Your hands don't feel too hard so we'll try one more lesson next week and I'll leave you with some Braille to practise on."

"That's fine, thanks."

"Don't worry; you'll get used to it."

We arranged a time for the following week and then she left.

During the week I practised long and hard at identifying the dots in the Braille book. The week went quickly and before I knew it she was sitting in my home waiting to hear how I was getting on.

"Have you been practising?" she asked.

"Yes, a lot, I really did try. It would have been great to be able to read Braille so that I can finally read some books that I've been missing out on."

"What are you trying to say?"

"My fingers are too rough and not as sensitive as I thought. It would be asking too much for me to give up my Martial Arts to be able to read Braille. It's too hard and I don't think that I'm able to read it."

"Let's try anyway."

She had endless patience and helped me as much as she could, but it was no use. My fingers had lost their sensitivity.

"I'm sorry but you really are having a great deal of trouble. It's up to you; I'll come back again if you like."

"No; it's a waste of time. It would only make me feel like more of a failure if I persisted and was still unable to identify the dots."

"Don't worry; only about 10% of blind people are able to read Braille."

I'll never know if she was telling the truth or just trying to make me feel better, which was probably for the best. My dream of reading a book was left as a dream and I had to learn to accept the fact that reading a book was a thing of the past. Unhappy with the result, the voices in my head started again.

"I guess I'll never be able to read. I'm trying so hard to beat this but every time I try harder something else goes wrong. I really wanted to read."

"You're useless. You can't read books *or* Braille. You hardly ever write anything in your own handwriting and you're even struggling to sign your name."

"I'm hopeless. Trying to cope with my deteriorating eyesight is draining me."

My faith in life had gone. Some nights I would go to bed thinking that it would be the last time I would see anything because in the morning I would wake up blind. It scared me so much sometimes I would have serious trouble getting to sleep. Although I would be happy to see the morning sun, it would still be the start of another stressful day in my head. From the moment I woke and walked into the bathroom the voices in my head would start.

"Where am I?"

"Your sight is so bad you can't even see your reflection in the mirror to comb your hair or shave."

"I won't look in the mirror then so I won't get upset. Where's the toothpaste gone again? I can't see to put the toothpaste on my toothbrush."

"You have to brush your teeth somehow. You have to get on with your life and accept that you will encounter problems."

Throughout the day my problems and thoughts would escalate out of control. Then I would go to bed worried and scared once more about waking up blind the next day. I needed help but I didn't want to trust any more people with my private life. I wanted my independence back and would try anything to keep hold of it. There was one last hope for me. In a few weeks someone was coming to see if there was any equipment that could help me at work.

This time two people turned up to see me at work. We had arranged for them to come at a time when my room was empty for a while. They hadn't brought anything with them, but they had plenty of questions. So I was forced yet again to go through some of the same mind draining explanations that centred on my disability. I hated talking about my problems, it really depressed me, but the people were there to help me so I learned to cope.

"What can you see on that computer screen?" they asked.

"I know that there is writing but I can't read it. If you were to print it out onto a piece of paper then I wouldn't know that it was writing, because that's how blurred it looks to me. I only know that it *is* writing because that's a word processing program."

"What do you see from where you're sitting, describe it."

"It looks like lots of blurred black lines with white streaks through them."

"What are the white streaks?"

"There are lots of sections of my eyes that I can't see with. They're called blind spots. There are several white streaks on the screen that I can see. Sometimes when I blink hard it helps but really it's just my eyes focussing slightly to the left or right. Everything I see has a hint of grey to it like I'm constantly looking at things through thick fog. The mist makes everything I see appear slightly grey and it's harder to see things now than when there wasn't any mist."

"Can you see the word 'File' in the top left hand corner of your computer screen?"

"No; I can't see File, Edit or View."

"How can you read the screen then?"

"I get really close to it and can guess the rest from memory and experience with computer packages."

"What about if the words were bigger; could you read them then?"

"Yes; it wouldn't be clear but it would be a great help. It would still have white lines through it, but with bigger words the lines from my blind spots take up less space. Everything would still look grey and misty."

"What size do you think you need to be able to read it proficiently?"

"Most people can read size 6 point; I need size 24 point to be able to see to read."

"That's very large don't you think?"

"It needs to be larger as my eyesight deteriorates."

"Are you colour-blind?"

"No, but unless there is a bright light I struggle with most colours. My worst colour is yellow. I could swear yellow is white because that's how I see it. In normal household light red, blue and green look like green. In sunlight I can see the colour red but I still struggle with blue and green. It makes me feel very uncomfortable when a student needs help with a colourful drawing that all appears as one colour to me. It's my job to help them and sometimes I just can't."

"How do you see to type?"

"With great difficulty! The letters on a keyboard are about size 16 point and I need 24 point. To overcome this problem I've learnt where all the keys are and I tilt my head forwards so that it's really close to the keyboard. It helps but then it gives me backache from constantly bending forwards."

"Hmm… that's very bad posture."

"I have to do it or I can't see the letters on the keyboard."

"How can you see to connect cables into the computers?"

"I don't see much. I connect them from memory and experience. Most of the computers are the same so I took a close look at mine and remembered where everything goes."

"Are there any different computers around the school?"

"Yes and I admit that I struggle with them. Most of the time it's trial and error. Sometimes I end up bending the little pins in the ends of the cables. There's a computer in a dark area that I need to use quite often and I really struggle with that one because the lighting in the room isn't very good."

"How are you with getting around?"

"Things are too blurred when they're more than about two metres away. It's difficult but I manage by walking slowly and carefully. Lots of people say hello to me but most of the time I can't see who they are. I usually wait until I recognise their voices."

"What about stairs?"

"It's more difficult to go down them than up. On the way down it looks like all the steps merge and are on one level. I can see myself falling one day, but I've got to get around."

"You don't have to take so many risks. You've got a white cane haven't you?"

"Yes, but I hate using it. It makes me feel so weak and frail and vulnerable. There are plenty of people who are considerate towards people with white canes but there are also a few too many ignorant ones. I could see myself hitting someone with it out of anger so I refrain from using it so I don't take my frustrations out on other people. I just get angry at myself."

"It's not your fault, stop blaming yourself."

They were very considerate people and I found them very helpful and understanding.

"We think that you're in need of some specialist equipment."

"So can you help me?"

"We think so. Do you have to read books too? I've noticed that you have a lot of computer manuals around."

"Yes; trying to read the books – it's just like trying to read the computer screen. They appear to have white streaks all over the words. When the words are small the white streaks can cover the entire word. When the words are larger the white streaks only cover a letter or part of a letter. It all depends on the size of the text that I'm trying to read."

"We have some equipment in the car that I'd like to show you."

"Would you like some help bringing it in?"

"No thanks, we're used to it. You can make some space on this table here though."

They went to their car and brought in lots of electrical equipment. Then they set it all up as I sat and watched. I noticed how easy they made it look, the way they would look at something and then connect it in its correct place. I could tell that they were using their eyes a great deal and I almost became jealous. Once the equipment was ready they switched everything on and began explaining what they had brought.

"Look at that keyboard. It's exactly the same as yours but it has very large letters on the keys. Can you see the letters now?"

"Yes I can see. Wow! This is amazing."

The keyboard had a dark background instead of the standard grey and the letters were white, which made them stand out and much easier for me to see.

"Try using it. Does it help?"

"Yes, it really does make a big difference."

"There may be days that are slightly darker than others so beside your computer is a bright light – try it."

I switched on the light and everything stood out more clearly.

"I can't believe this! It's brilliant! Thank you very much." For the first time in a long while joy surged through me.

"That's not all, there's more. Are you ready?"

"Yes," I said in anticipation.

"Look at your computer screen. Now type something small so that you struggle to see it."

I wrote a few sentences in a word processing program then waited.

"Is that hard to read?"

"It's *very* hard to read."

"OK, now press the control key and the plus key."

When I pressed the keys I nearly fell off my seat with amazement. My whole screen had magically enlarged. The words were bigger and the mouse pointer was bigger too.

"This is amazing!"

"Press the same keys a few times and then press the control and minus key, that will make everything on your computer screen smaller again."

Every time I pressed the keys everything on my screen grew. It went to a ridiculous size where I could only see a few letters on the screen at a time. As I moved my mouse pointer over to the word 'File' at the top left hand corner of my screen, it took up my entire screen. The magnifying package could grow to any size and then shrink back down when I pressed the control and minus keys. As I typed I could see that everything was clear and it followed everywhere I typed. Every time I moved the mouse the screen magnified where the cursor hovered and it also magnified where I typed. It was an ingeniously useful package. I felt comfortable on the magnifying level four times my usual screen size.

They then asked me to look at another monitor, which had a much bigger screen than usual.

"Do you think that this will help too?"

"A larger computer screen, yes please! That's a *great* help!"

"And here's a small torch for when you're in those hard to reach places."

The amount of equipment they had overwhelmed me. I was ecstatic. My boss had come into the room and was listening and watching intently. She was interested in purchasing some of the equipment for me. I was very grateful because I knew that not many bosses would have been so keen to buy equipment to assist a disabled person. They went on to show me a voice recognition program but it didn't work very well on our computer network. They then installed a new mouse program that changed the colour of the mouse so that I could see it more easily.

The final piece of equipment was by far the best.

"This is a CCTV, have you seen one before?"

"Yes, it's a camera for seeing people in shops and around town centres."

"This isn't the same. This is a special magnifier that enlarges the words in a book to almost any size."

"Book Reader... I can read books with it?" I asked excitedly.

"Yes; would you like to try it?"

"Of course I would!"

"Get one of the computer manuals that you struggle to read and put it under the bright light."

It was one of the most exciting things that I had seen in a very long time. There was a tray under the computer screen on which to place books. Then a bright light and a magnifying glass shone the book onto the computer screen. It had some buttons on the front of the CCTV to adjust the size of the writing similar to the magnifying package on my computer. At long last, after many failed attempts and only after sheer determination, I was now able to read books. I just couldn't hold back my excitement.

"I can't believe this! I've waited so long to be able to read a book, thank you very much."

After they left I read my computer manuals using my CCTV. My reading was slow because all the words had to be very big for me to be able to see them, but I was reading! It took much longer than normal to read books, but… I was reading. It hurt my eyes after a while because the light was so bright, but… I was finally reading books. My life had taken an unexpected turn and I was beginning to enjoy it. I started bringing in books from home and my book from my college course to read. My list was endless and I started reading everything.

Then I brought in a letter or two from home and I suddenly realised that I was able to regain some of the independence that had been taken away from me years ago. I no longer had to ask other people to read my private letters. It made me feel worthy again. I no longer felt so useless and hopeless and trapped. I could do things for myself again. The CCTV helped me read again and I was immeasurably grateful.

CHAPTER 18
CREATING A HABIT

A phone call from my brother was about to change my life forever. It was January 1994, the beginning of a new year and I was looking for a new direction in life. He called me on the telephone and said that he had a great business idea that would help me become self-employed. Since I was looking for other ways to generate more income, I was very interested in what he had to say. He turned up with a business associate called Larry. My brother sat with me as Larry proceeded to show me a business plan.

After he had finished I was very interested but like most people, I was sceptical.

"It looks great, but then why isn't everyone doing it? And where have I been? I've never heard of Network Marketing but I *am* familiar with franchising. That's how most businesses are built. Even my Martial Arts work is like a franchise."

Although Larry told me not to ask my friends for their opinion unless I knew that they were positive thinking friends, I didn't listen and asked several of them anyway.

"My brother has shown me an amazing concept called Network Marketing. It's a way of owning your own business and you can apparently make a lot of money part-time. Have you heard about it?"

I was about to find out that I had asked the wrong people so would only get wrong answers.

"Yes we've heard of it. A friend's cousin tried it for a while and said that it never worked for them. They said that you don't get anything out of being self-employed."

"Yes, but have *you* tried it?"

"No, but I know that it's no good and doesn't work and is a waste of time."

"What do you have to do then?" I asked.

"Don't know."

"Have you ever seen the concept?"

"No; nobody has approached us."

"So how do you know so much about nothing?"

It was too late, I had asked them and now they had put doubts into my mind. It took me a day or two to realise that just because their friend's cousin hadn't succeeded in owning their own business, it didn't mean that I couldn't. I discussed my options in my mind.

"I don't know now, they've put me off a bit and I was really excited before. I thought that it was the answer to my prayers. It was a way of generating enough money so that I wouldn't have to worry about my finances if I was no longer able to work because of my sight."

"What are you listening to them for? None of them are successful. How do you know that they were telling the truth about their cousin and even if they were, so what? Businesses close down all the time but it doesn't stop other ambitious people from trying. Go for it."

"The only way of knowing if something will work for me is to try it. I can't win the lottery unless I play it so why not try this."

I had nothing to lose by trying so I contacted my brother and agreed to give it a try. I was now a young entrepreneur and owned my own business.

Although I was eager to start, I didn't actually know what to do yet but I was excited! Larry came to see me and explained the Network Marketing concept and it sounded great. He then asked me why I was interested in starting my own business and I told him what most people would say.

"For the money!"

He then asked me to go into more detail about my goals and he even called them dreams.

"My goal is to pay off my debts."

"Most people want to pay off their debts but you don't see them working hard enough to achieve it," Larry said.

"What do you mean?" I asked.

"You have to make your goals so important to you that you will be willing to work hard enough to achieve them. Try not to wish like other people or you may as well play the lottery like them."

"I do play the lottery!" I said jokingly.

We laughed and then took it seriously again.

"I want to pay off my debts and be in a position of not having to worry about money when I'm no longer able to work because of my failing eyesight," I said.

"That's it! Make your goals bigger than your fears and you will succeed. Make your goals important to you."

"Thank you, I will. I'm scared of going blind and not being able to work any more. This looks like the only opportunity for me to be in a position of not having to worry about whether I can work."

It made me even more excited to hear some positive thinking coming from someone else.

"I would like enough income so that I can go on a proper holiday every year."

"Where would you go? What would you do?" Larry asked.

"I've always wanted to go to Spain and listen to the Spanish people talk. I love the accent and would love to go to their country."

"Anything else?"

"I'd love to be in a position to move house. Nothing too big, just a house in a better area."

After twenty minutes or so of dream building a weird sensation came over me.

"I've just realised that I haven't thought much about my eyesight all the time that we were talking!"

It was like a cure and a way of getting rid of the arguing voices in my head. When I thought about what I wanted in the future and built on my goals, I didn't hear the voices in my mind fighting about my deteriorating eyesight, so I kept doing it.

Whenever I had a few minutes to spare during the day, I would dream build. When I felt my mind drifting to think about my failing eyesight I fought it off by dream building. I would imagine being in a new house, with my child and enjoying life. I imagined having enough money in the bank so that I didn't have to work. The worry about struggling at work had gone and I felt free. It was a beautiful feeling that was very satisfying. For the first time in my life I felt free from worry, and free from my arguing thoughts.

Larry brought me a book on positive thinking to read.

"Why do I need to read this?"

"You'll learn how to be more positive and assertive and it will motivate you to be more productive. It will help you have a better outlook on life."

"I need that at the moment. I've been quite negative towards life lately because of not being able to see well. I think of my poor eyesight all the time and I get very emotional and then I hate life. Sometimes I think that my life is so dull and everything is going wrong for me."

"Well things are going to change for the better. Instead of filling your head full of negative things that will hold you back from finding solutions to your problems, I want you to fill your head with positive things. Keep thinking of why you now own your own business then the how will come."

"Who! How! What?"

"If your dreams are big enough, the facts don't matter and you will find a way to achieve them, so if you know why you want something, you will find a way how to get it. Try to control what you think of and don't be scared to take risks to get what you want. Fear is false. It's false evidence appearing to be real, but it's not real so it's time to take control of your life and stop waiting for things to happen… make them happen."

He amazed me with his positive outlook to life. Most people I spoke to actually have a very negative outlook. I was jealous and wanted some more of what he had.

"What book have you got there for me?"

- *The Magic of Thinking Big*

"This was the first book that I read and it opened my eyes. It tells you how some people succeed where others fail. It talks about what successful people think about and it gives you the excuses of other people for failing."

"I'll read it then. This book might tell me why so many businesses fail."

My new CCTV for reading books came in very handy – when I had spare time at work I would use it to read the book. Eventually I finished reading it and my eyes were opened once more to the world. It was very interesting and I even read it again. I especially liked Chapter Two, 'Excuse-itis' – it listed lots of excuses that people use and it made me smile when I saw a few excuses that even I had used. The book helped me to know what successful people think about and gave *me* a lot to think about. Larry came to see me several times and mostly wanted to talk to me about my goals. I enjoyed the attention and felt very relaxed around him. After a while I was really going into some serious details about my goals and I was hardly thinking of my poor eyesight and the problems it was causing me. It was my new therapy and it was working. I was happier with life and that's all that mattered to me.

The book that I read was full of positive information that also helped and I was hungry for more. Larry brought round some more books:

- How to Win Friends and Influence People
- Personality Plus
- Men are from Mars, Women are from Venus

It felt great to be able to read again and I read them all. My mind was full of positive thoughts and I had a new outlook on life. Although I would occasionally think of my problems I would mostly have a positive way of dealing with them. The books helped me to deal with the possibility of going blind and I appreciated that.

Larry came around even more and helped me to build my new business and I was very grateful. I found it very difficult to write and read from charts but Larry was there to help me. Then came the negative side and a few challenges that I had to get over. I told a few friends about my new business venture and they laughed at me and told me that I wouldn't be able to achieve anything. These comments came from some of my closest friends and it really upset me; that was until I spoke to Larry.

"My friends said that I won't achieve my goals and I feel a little sad. I thought that they would be happy that I'm trying something new and feeling more positive about things - they know that I was going through a lot with my eyes."

"You're allowed to feel sad, but tell me, did all your friends say that you would be able to teach Martial Arts even though you're partially sighted?"

"Now that I think about it; no! Many of them thought that I wouldn't be able to open my own class and I did. Then they thought that I wouldn't be able to teach because of my deteriorating eyesight and I can, so they said I wouldn't be teaching for long."

"And how long have you been teaching?"

"Seven years."

"So were your friends right or were you?"

"My friends were wrong; very wrong and I won't be giving up teaching either."

"So are they right about owning your own business?"

"No; I'm right again and I won't be giving up. My friends should be happy that I'm doing something positive with my life. They should want me to succeed and should be encouraging me rather than discouraging me. They should be motivating me and should be offering to assist me if they can. It seems like they want me to get ahead but not ahead of them, that's selfish. They shouldn't want me to fail. I wouldn't want them to fail in anything. I'm an encourager and they should be encouraging me too."

Without even realising it, the positive information that Larry and the books had given me had made me a stronger person. Strong enough not to be influenced by negative people. I quickly realised that I had some goals in life and some of my friends were not prepared to help me achieve them and that it was up to me to be persistent and consistent. Without realising, Larry had helped me build up my goals so that they were bigger than my fears. I had some goals and I was determined to achieve them. Without realising it, my personality was being reshaped again but in a good and positive way this time.

My next challenge was my brother. The books that I had read called problems 'challenges' and taught me techniques to overcome them. This was to be a challenge to remember, a challenge to see how serious I was about wanting my goals. My brother came to see me and was quite upset.

"I'm not making enough money and I want to close down my business," he said.

"I don't understand; why?"

"It's just not working quickly enough so I'm closing it down."

"What has happened to that positive thinking person? The person who wants to achieve so much, the ambitious self-motivated person? What about me? You got me started, you encouraged me and now you want me to give it all up after only six months?"

"Yes. I'm sorry but it's not working for me and I don't think that it will work for you."

"What about your goals in life?" I asked.

"I'm not worried about them any more."

It was a difficult moment in my life where I had to make an important decision. He was my older brother who knew more about life than I did and I respected him very much. I thought about how he got me started, what he told me and I thought about my own goals.

"So you lied then? When you came to me you told me that you wanted to achieve things and now you're telling me that they're no longer important to you just because you're not making enough money quickly enough. What happened to your patience? This is not a get-rich-quick business. Most businesses don't start making money for years. During the first few years you have to invest in your business and after a few years the profit will come."

"Are you going to close yours too? It hasn't helped you yet."

"Are you going to help me achieve my goals?"

"No; I don't know how any more."

"You told me that Network Marketing was the best business to be in, the only business in which other people help you build it up. I don't even know Larry, yet he has been helping me build my business consistently. Why?"

"Because he'll make money if he helps you make money."

"I'm sorry, but that sounds like a good thing to me. If he helps me make money, he makes money and if he doesn't help me I won't make money. That sounds like he will genuinely want to help me succeed and not fail. He's more helpful than my close friends. In what other line of business can you get that support? I've taught students up to the black belt level and they've left me and opened their own clubs and they no longer help me. Larry helps me and he doesn't have to and I really appreciate that."

"Well I'm closing mine down and it's up to you if you want to carry on."

"You're making a big mistake; huge! I have to carry on. It *is* working for me. It helps me deal with my eyesight problems and that's more important than anything at the moment. It's taught me how to deal with my problems positively. It's given me a new meaning in life, something else to think about and it's something positive. I hardly get any negative thoughts any more. I'm mostly dream building rather than moaning. When I looked at life I didn't like what I saw. Nothing seemed to be going well for me and I hated my life. Now I think that my life is great and my problems could be worse. How can you say that it isn't working for me? It *is* working and I'm becoming a better person and now have a brighter outlook on life."

My decision was made and after six months my brother had quit on his goals, while I was still pursuing mine. I decided to carry on building my Network Marketing business and slowly I became a more positive person.

Larry now helped me even more than ever. He took me to meet some more successful people and I met some *very* successful people. There were lots of them everywhere and they were all as positive and motivated as me. There were thousands of them and I began to think back to when I first started.

"Why did my friends try and stop me from pursuing my goals? There are many people who have succeeded so why were they trying to tell me that it doesn't work? If only my friends could come and see all these positive people! They're not moaning about life; instead they're determined to work for their goals. I like that and prefer to be around people who think the same as me."

From then I started to take it more seriously and worked hard and my business grew. More friends tried to put me off with their negative attitudes but now I knew that they had no idea of what self-employment meant and their opinions meant nothing to me. I started feeling sorry for people who moaned about their problems when all they had to do was work a bit harder to deal with them. Most problems people moaned about related to money. I now knew that successful people worked that bit harder so I followed instead of moaning. There were certain things that money couldn't cure, like some illnesses, but for most things, more money was the answer. The books taught me that there are a lot of negative people around and we just have to love them but not listen to them. I learnt that if you wanted positive information, then you have to go to a positive person. If you ask for advice from a negative person, you'll get a negative answer. I learnt that if you wanted information on how to become successful, then you have to ask a successful person. I've now got a positive outlook on life and here are some of the things that I think about regularly.

How to create a habit

- Good things come to those who wait, but they come faster to those who work for them.
- Think positive not negative.
- Everyone has problems.
- Have goals and dreams to work towards.
- Don't let anyone tell you that you cannot make it.
- Think of happy thoughts.
- Some will, some won't.
- Be a great listener.
- Everyone has choices.
- Never give up on your goals.
- Leaders lead.
- When you're feeling down, go up.

My thoughts and actions

Good things come to those who wait, but they come faster to those who work for them.

This is something that I think about regularly. It helps me to achieve more out of life. Although I play the Lottery like most people, I'm also working hard towards achieving the things that I desire. Most people play the Lottery but also say that they have no goals. What's the point of playing the Lottery if they are content with what they have? We tend to say that people who have achieved more are lucky. The people who achieve things without working for them *are* lucky, but the ones who worked hard for what they have are not lucky, they deserve it. Stop wishing and moaning and work for what you want. Write it down, organise yourself and find out what you need to do to get rid of your debts or whatever else you're concerned about.

Think positive not negative.

I always think that there are two ways to look at the same thing, positively and negatively. You can be upset with what you have yet other people will wonder what you're complaining about. Maybe you were in trouble and are complaining that God hasn't helped you yet other people will see that you are past that problem and should be looking forward to dealing with other problems. You might be negative and feel that things are not going well for you yet other people will wonder why you're moaning about something so trivial. Being negative makes you think negative. It's time to see the positive side of life like I do.

Everyone has problems.

We have a nasty habit of thinking that we're the only person who has any problems and that our problems are the worst. You do have problems but... so does everyone else. I try to accept that I will have problems and will experience more but will try my hardest to deal with them. We are all allowed bad days, maybe even parts of our lives when we experience depression but we need to work hard at getting on with our lives. Everyone does have problems. I try and say that other people are worse off than me – that helps me deal with my problems.

Have goals and dreams to work towards.

If you're happy with what you have then there's no need to dream of having more. My mind drifts and I think of my problems and what I need to be happier so I give myself goals to keep my mind busy. I hardly ever get bored because I'm always working towards something. I've thought of many goals and why I need them, now my mind works hard to find ways to achieve them.

Don't let anyone tell you that you cannot make it.

Don't let people put you off trying to achieve your goals. If you're finding it difficult achieving them, find another way, but don't let people put you off. Most successful people will tell you that on the way to success they had many people telling them that they couldn't do it. Don't listen to negative people or you will get a negative response. If you listen to a positive person who doesn't think that you can do something, they always give you good advice on another way of trying but they never tell you to give up. During my Martial Arts teaching, I have encouraged students to believe that they can achieve things. If a student is shy I take special care to encourage them to perform better. I'll tell them that they are doing well and are powerful, even when they're not doing that well. With this positive attitude I've watched students' personalities change as I encourage them to be more confident. Students try harder when I tell them that they're doing well, so I keep telling students that they're good. I see the changes almost straight away. They can be struggling, and then I tell them that they're doing well and then you see them trying even harder. It's like magic and it's wonderful to see the benefits of my positive attitude.

Think of happy thoughts.

Most of us have bad thoughts that slowly take over our mind if we let them. I force myself to have happy thoughts and they drown out the bad ones. I think of happy memories: of me, my child, my parents and sometimes my friends. I tell myself jokes or think of funny experiences. We all have them but most of us have forgotten how important they are to us. I force myself to think of what I want to think about and not leave my mind to drift at will. Like most people, I still get sad thoughts, but then I will quickly think of something happy. It's a habit that can help you in most situations. I often think of my happy thoughts to make me smile, such as when my child, Michaela, slid downstairs after doing a pooh and it ended up on every step! But it makes me laugh when I think about it even though it wasn't nice to clean up. When fighting in a training session, I kicked the wrong person but luckily didn't hurt them, the memory of that makes me smile too. Being able to see my child's school photos and pictures that she has drawn and to know how well she's doing in school also makes me smile. Talking to someone and then realising that it's the wrong person and I actually don't know them is sometimes funny. Maybe I'm easily pleased but it helps me deal with my problems.

Thinking of words, sentences or phrases that people have used brings back happy memories. People's names or certain musical tracks bring happy thoughts into my mind. Sometimes I repeat the same things in my head over and over again just to help drown out a thought that I would rather not think about. So next time you see me smile it might not be about you but about a happy thought. Sometimes

I think of confidence tricks to make me more confident and assertive. I teach people to pretend to be more confident than they really are and eventually they won't be pretending and it works. I try to control what I think about, why don't you try it?

Some will, some won't.

Not everyone will be interested in what you're doing. I've realised this and applied it to my teachings. Not everyone is interested in Martial Arts even though I think that they should participate at some stage of their lives for the self-defence and confidence aspects. When students enrol, I already assume that several of them might quit and not many of them will achieve the black belt level. Having this attitude helps me deal with people when they want to quit.

Be a great listener.

Sometimes I find myself listening to people more than I really want to. Although I have many things to say I will force myself to listen. This helps me to be a better friend towards others. We have two ears and one mouth so we should listen twice as much as we talk! It's fine to have a moan about life sometimes but try not to moan all the time, that way people won't mind listening to you.

Everyone has choices.

Some of us make the wrong choices, too many times, and then wonder why things are not going well. Some problems are out of your hands and you can't stop them because you have no control over them. I have great sympathy for people who experience these kinds of problems. There are a few people who want sympathy while they're making silly mistakes in life. We need to think a little longer before we act on our thoughts. Maybe we won't make so many mistakes in the future. I make mistakes too, everyone does, but I try not to make many and I don't moan much.

Never give up on your goals.

There will come a time in your life when you will want to quit what you're doing. It's fine to quit on things that are not important or are causing you health problems, but don't quit on things that you really want, like your goals in life. That is a major difference between success and failure. Sometimes you quit just before it was going to start working for you. There are patches where businesses don't profit as well as other times. Find out when they are and draw up a business plan. Don't keep quitting on things that are important to you. This is why I'm successful after seven years of teaching Martial Arts. I've had periods where I was losing money but I was consistent and persistent and I had a lot of patience. I've thought about quitting Martial Arts many times but I'm determined and I find other ways of motivating myself. Find other ways to achieve your goals but don't give up on them.

Leaders lead.

Be prepared to do things that your friends won't do, to have what they can't have. When I see an idea that I'm interested in, I take some risks and try it. I don't wait for my friends to try things first. This was my attitude when I first started teaching Martial Arts. It was scary and I was very nervous but I still took the risk of opening a club. The first class that I opened was in a time slot that had been used by a fellow instructor. His class wasn't going well and he wanted to close it down. I didn't take on any of his students when I re-opened and now I've been successfully teaching in that same time slot for seven years. He quit too early and shouldn't have given up!

When you're feeling down, go up.

We all have bad days; times when you struggle to even get out of bed. It's at times like this when you should turn to more positive people to motivate you. You may prefer to stay away from everyone especially more positive people because they'll make you feel more useless, but it's those same people who you need to help you. We live in a very negative and stressful world and I feel that it's important to stay positive despite the pressure to accept failure. Put your trust in other people to help you. When you're feeling low, it's just a taster of how it feels to be disabled and to have your independence taken away from you, but you expect disabled people to ask for help, so why shouldn't you when you're down? I respect psychologists. I couldn't sit there and listen to negative people all day without going mad myself! They do a good job trying to motive other people, maybe it's time we learnt how to motive ourselves. Find something that works, find something that makes you smile and feel happy and something to make you want to live again and think about it often so that it's in your mind all the time.

These are the things that I think of regularly and they help to keep a smile on my face. I now use these principals in all parts of my life.

Now that I was feeling more positive and motivated, I used the information that I had learnt from the books to encourage me to open two more Martial Arts classes. It influenced me to create new goals and I found myself pursuing my 4th Dan black belt to become a Master in the Martial Arts of Taekwondo. It opened my eyes to realise that most people are deceiving themselves. They say that they have no goals or ambition yet they gamble in the National Lottery every week, hoping to win. What would they do with the money if they have no goals? If more people were honest with themselves then there would be many more successful people but most people are afraid of failure. Many people have made a big mistake not pursuing their goals. I'm now more understanding and sympathetic towards people but I also feel sad for the ones who are negative. When I'm feeling down I go up. That means when I feel sad I will ask for advice from a more positive person and not another person who is also feeling sad.

My friends started to confide in me again. If they were having a bad day they always knew that I would try and make them feel better using my positive attitude towards life. The only confusing thing was that a few of my friends actually told me that I was lucky to be so positive and it was because I didn't have any problems! Just because I walked around with a smile on my face and never moaned about life didn't mean that I hadn't got problems. Deep down on the inside I was still suffering from my deteriorating eyesight. I still thought that I might go blind one day and it still scared me very much, I simply chose not to dwell on it or moan about it any more and to try and get on with my life.

People were still asking me how I could teach with such poor eyesight and I would answer them with a positive answer. When people told me about their troubles I would be a good listener. There were many times when I wanted to speak but I would mostly listen to their problems then offer them positive advice. I walked around with a smile on my face and if you asked how I was I rarely said fine like most people do. I used expressions like; I feel great; I feel wonderful thanks. When I answered the phone I tried to have an encouraging voice and I've been complemented for my cheerful manner. My new way of life was a habit that was now natural for me, yet I started out pretending. They were traits that I had taught my students, to pretend to be confident so that you don't get bullied and then eventually they became confident. Maybe it was all textbook, maybe I was false and full of pretence, but it worked for me and eventually it became me. Although I was going through many changes in my life, mostly trying to cope with the stress my deteriorating eyesight was causing, I would always try to have a smile on my face. We don't know what other people are going through when we walk past them. Just because they're smiling doesn't mean that they have no problems, it could mean that they're learning to deal with them. Next time you moan to a happy person, remember, they might have cancer but haven't told you! Sometimes I could feel people's problems. When I walked past an elderly person who seemed to be struggling to walk and yet they said good morning to me so cheerfully, I knew that they were in pain but chose to hide it. Fill your mind with happier thoughts, that's what I do, and that's why I appear to be happier.

That year ended very happily with the birth of my second daughter. She was born on the 9th November 1994. Her name is Jasmine and just like Michaela, she too keeps me happy.

CHAPTER 19
THIS IS MY STORY, THIS IS MY SONG

Every Christmas since my father had passed away my mother always said that it would be her last. All my family got together at my mother's house to celebrate Christmas. We started early with a big fried breakfast of eggs, sausages, bacon, baked beans and toast. We used special Jamaican bread called 'hardough bread' for our toast, which is much thicker and softer than normal sliced bread. Then we helped ourselves to Jamaican 'bun', which is a very tasty cross between bread and cake. It's brown with currents and generally served with cheese, jam or just with butter.

Then my older sisters prepared the dinner. My mother used to do it, but by that time she was too ill and frail to do much. We always had a choice of three meats; it would sometimes change from year to year but we still ended up with three, generally chicken, pork and beef. Sometimes we would replace one of the meats with spicy mutton or curried chicken. We ate the dinner and looked after our mother, and then we worried what the New Year would bring.

My mother was very ill and had been that way for years. She still hadn't got over the sudden death of her husband and said that she should have died first. It was always difficult trying to convince her that she was wrong and had many more years to live.

This Christmas proved to be different. She had caught the flu and was struggling to be rid of it. We were all very worried but somehow she made it to the New Year. Her breathing got worse and she complained that her chest was hurting a lot so we admitted her into hospital. It wasn't a nice way to start the New Year but she had lasted through Christmas even though she was already suffering badly. The doctors did many tests and put her on a machine that assisted her breathing. We visited her regularly and were very worried. More thoughts rushed through my mind.

"Is this it? She isn't looking well at all."

"She's strong, she'll make it."

"I'm not so sure this time. I'm scared and not ready to lose her. Please help her God."

"She's struggling so much to breathe. Can't the doctors do something about that?"

I would sit and talk to her and she would struggle but manage to talk back, but deep down I was really concerned.

After a week she was came home. It was more her decision than the doctors'.

"Why didn't you stay in hospital until you fully recovered?" I asked.

"I don't want to die in hospital; I want to die here at home with my family," she replied.

"Don't be silly, you're strong and you're not ready to go yet."

"That was my last Christmas, I can feel it. God is ready for me."

"You're always saying that. Don't you realise that you say that every year?"

"Yes, but I feel it this time. I'm not getting better and I'm really struggling to breathe. My time is up."

"No! God isn't ready for you yet. Stop talking like that, you're making everyone nervous."

"I should have gone before your father."

"But you're too strong. You have a few years left."

I hated hearing her talk like that, it made me very nervous. She was so relaxed and serious when she said it as if she wasn't afraid of dying. Although her breathing became more difficult and louder she continued to make us all laugh with her humour. She loved to watch television and her favourite show was Colombo. She called Colombo 'dirty raincoat' because his coat always looked dirty. She also loved her grandchildren and wanted to see them all the time because she thought that she wouldn't be around to see them for much longer.

Within another two weeks she was rushed back into hospital suffering from severe breathing problems. I visited her every day but I felt very uncomfortable being in the hospital. It was only a few years since my father had passed away in the same hospital and I was still suffering from vivid memories. As I watched my mother struggling to breathe I became tearful. The noise of the machine breathing for her was too loud and disturbing. Her chest would rise and fall vigorously as the machine pumped air into her lungs. After a week or so she was unable to talk and I would visit her and talk to myself hoping that she could hear. It became too much for me and I would go for walks to the hospital canteen to get away without actually leaving her.

She was in the hospital for weeks and the doctor told us that it would be very unlikely that she would get much better. They told us that her major internal organs were failing one by one and if she ever came out of hospital she would always need assistance with breathing. Things were not looking good for my mother and my emotions became overpowering.

"She can't talk and it looks like she isn't even breathing for herself. She's going to die. I don't believe it; I'm going to lose my mother too. No, I won't accept it. She *will* pull through; she has to. She's strong; no, it's not her time. Please God, not yet, don't take her yet, I'd miss her too much."

Being so upset made me struggle to work by day and teach by night. My boss was very understanding when I told her that it was unlikely that my mother would survive and gave me time off so that I could be with her more often. Larry agreed to take over my Network Marketing business and I asked a fellow instructor to teach my Martial Arts classes. The rest of my family were also suffering from emotional torture. My sister Carline had come from London to be with our mother every day. The only person who wasn't with us was my sister Jennifer. She was on holiday and refused to believe that mother would die. Each night I would go to bed wondering if I would get a phone call during the night to say that she had finally passed away. It was a very intense time of my life where my nerves were tested to the full. My other sister, Angela, was great. She was nervous and slightly depressed, but was still there with our mother to the end. She would stay at the hospital and sleep on a chair overnight just to be near her, she never left her side and never showed how much she was hurting, but I knew. Only a year ago she had decided to stay in Rugby and nurse our sick mother. During that time her boyfriend had mysteriously died and she was heartbroken. Also her eyesight had deteriorated quickly and was now as bad as mine. She was suffering inside and covered it up by looking after our mother. I felt that if mother died, she would probably feel the most hurt; she had given up her social life to nurse her and wasn't ready to lose her too.

After a week my mother seemed to make a miraculous recovery. She was able to talk but still wasn't well enough to leave the hospital. We were weary but a little happier to be able to speak to her. She talked about organising her funeral and sorting out our family matters. We thought that she would slowly get better but she was still sure that God was ready for her, even to her final hours she was still very religious. After a day or two of seeing her grandchildren and other family members she slowly slipped back into a deep sleep and the machine would once again pump hard to assist her breathing. The doctors told us that her condition wasn't going to change so we had a few family meetings. We discussed whether to admit her into a care home if she was released from hospital or whether to have her back home with the machines to help her breathe so that we could care for her. Looking after her at home night and day would be a demanding and tiring job and we couldn't reach a decision. Most of us were working and it would have caused major problems to care for her so much and work at the same time. We also didn't want to leave it all up to Angela who had already given up most of her life to care for our mother and was suffering more and more from her deteriorating eyesight. The discussions went on for a few days and many of us became very emotional.

Then late in the evening on February 19th 1995 I received that awful phone call that I had been hoping to avoid. My mother had passed away quietly while holding Angela's hand in hospital. It shattered my heart and I broke down in tears.

Although I had been expecting it to happen, it hurt just as much as when I lost my father suddenly. One long, slow and emotionally draining death, and one sudden. Now with only a few years separating them, I had lost both my parents.

The next few months were difficult for us all. I kept myself busy so as not to centre on the depressing part of my life but it kept coming back.

"I've lost my mother and father? What am I going to do? How will I ever learn to cope without them both?"

"You have to cope. Keep yourself busy and you will think of them less."

"I'm upset. I've got to think about my loss."

"Yes, you can think about it, but you have to be strong. Tell yourself that it happens to everyone eventually and try not to get too upset."

"It's sad, I miss them both so much."

"Think of the happy memories."

It was the only way I learnt to cope. Every time a sad memory came into my head like the sound of my mother struggling to breathe in hospital or the sound I heard upstairs in my father's house just before we found him, I would fight in my mind to think of something positive. There was a complex web of thoughts in my mind and I had to learn to control them or I would be lost to the ever-growing depression that was taking over so many people. It was so hard to fight the sad thoughts and I could feel my mind drifting backwards and forwards from sadness to happiness. All it took was to see a television show that my mother had liked or hear a song that they used to sing in church and the memories would come flooding back. There were plenty of good memories that kept me going and slowly I learnt to control some of my thoughts.

My sister Carline from London began to suffer from depression and really struggled to come to terms with the loss. My mother had been the only one holding our big family together. There were too many of us and there was generally an argument somewhere, but when my mother was alive she always found a solution. Now that she was gone our family slowly drifted apart. My sister Jennifer, who was on holiday at the time of our mother's death, was also suffering from depression; she hadn't been there when her mother died and it was haunting her. I watched everyone as they struggled to get over the loss and I didn't like what I saw. I was still only one step away from giving in to depression and I fought off the multitude of thoughts.

"You don't want to suffer like them do you?"

"No way! The depression has changed them and they're mostly sad and always complaining about life. I don't want to be like that. I'm already on the verge of depression as a result of my deteriorating eyesight, so I have to keep fighting."

"Look at them blaming themselves for the loss, blaming themselves for not doing more for their mother while she was alive, you did what you could."

"I think I did. I was always there for her. I'd visit her regularly and bring my children to see her. If we argued I would swallow my pride and make it up to her. When I thought that she was wrong about something, I would respect her enough not to argue even though I thought that I was right. But I still miss her."

"Just you remember that you were there for your mother and your father to the end."

"Yes I was and I can't believe how well Angela did. She's suffering so much with her eyesight yet she tries to do everything. Life isn't fair. There are three of us now with eye problems and I've lost both my parents. I can't take any more challenges, there are too many."

"You can do it; you have to learn to cope with all the stresses of life."

"There are too many. It's too hard."

"Think positive, come on, you can do it. Think of something happy, a good memory."

Sometimes it would be so hard not to think about them even though the thoughts upset me. I felt a little sad for the others who had not been there for our parents as much as they could have been. It's so easy to wrap yourself up with work and with your own life and children that you accidentally neglect your parents. I knew that they were getting old and would not be here forever so I worked extra hard to please them and see them as often as I could. Sometimes I got tired of taking my mother places or tired of checking up on my father, but I knew that it was my job as a good son to be with them and look after them to the end. I've watched so many other people have trivial arguments with their parents and not see them for months, but I couldn't live with myself if they died during an argument and I hadn't seen them for a long time. They could pass away before you have time to say sorry. It's amazing how much you miss someone when they've gone, yet when they're here we take them for granted and sometimes can't be bothered to see them. Since I lost both my parents I've always told my friends to see their parents more regularly because they might regret it if they suddenly passed away. Most arguments mean nothing to me when they involve parents. We always think that our arguments have good ground and we're justified to take a stand, but other people don't see that and that's why I always tell my friends to forgive their parents and go to see them regularly. Part of my life is empty without my parents and I really do miss them. I would probably be suffering from depression now if I hadn't been talking to either of my parents before they died. It's hard enough putting up with the thoughts of their deaths; if I thought that I could have done more, I would be constantly thinking of that too and that would be too much for me to handle.

Although I still have some vivid thoughts of their deaths, I mostly have happy memories. My mother liked to tell jokes and ghost stories a lot. She was very superstitious and had many stories from when she lived in Jamaica and she always used to tell us about her dreams and what they all meant. She told my sister that she was pregnant with Dyonn before my sister even knew because she had dreamt it. I don't know if she guessed or really had some sort of gift; I guess I'll never know now. She did get many things right throughout her life. Whenever I watch a ghostly program, I think of her. When I hear hymns, I think of her. When people talk about the Bible, I think of my father. I had my own way of dealing with their deaths and it helped me cope. Sometimes I would leave the room if I saw a television programme where someone had collapsed on the floor and needed hospital treatment. I would do the same whenever I saw a programme where someone was struggling to breathe using the same kind of machine that my mother had used.

It comforted me that I had done all I could for my mother before she passed away. You should have seen how happy and excited she was to see and touch a snake. She had many stories about them but had never actually touched one until I took her to a reptile exhibition. She was ecstatic. I remember the first time I took her to the cinema. Sometimes she would cook coconut drops – everyone liked them, everyone apart from me! They were too sweet. She loved to wear hats to go to church; both my parents were very religious and while they were in good health, they attended church regularly. I feel that it was my religion that taught me good morals and I've never been against any church. I had a slight lapse of faith and avoided church while I tried to learn to cope with my own problem of going blind.

My father was a funny man too. He never felt the cold and his house would sometimes be freezing. He also liked to exercise, although not as vigorously as me! He would stand on the spot and pretend to lift up weights, but I don't think that he ever entered a gym in his life. Another great memory of my father is when we were sick. It didn't matter what was wrong with us, whether we had a tummy ache or whether we had the flu, he always said that a drink of Guinness would cure us. Sometimes he would mix Guinness with some thick milk to make punch. It tasted lovely but I don't think that it ever cured me!

He worked at Ford Motors for most of his life. He also worked at Thomas Hunter and the Railway Station for a while. We had a big family and my father used to buy things by the dozen so that we wouldn't run out. He used to buy trays of eggs and ten or more tins of baked beans at a time. (Now that I think about it, so do I!) He always wore a suit as if he was going to church and would explain everything by referring to his Bible. My parents were so religious that I'm almost embarrassed to admit that none of us have followed in their footsteps. We've been caught up in the fast moving world and are struggling to keep up and not leaving any time to go and thank God that we are still alive.

Dealing with the loss of my mother brought on some very confusing thoughts.

"Why is this happening to me? I'm so sad about my mother and I don't know what to do. She took ages to die and after so long I don't know if I have the energy to do anything. First my father and now my mother have left me and now I feel so alone. They were the only ones holding our family together. We're surely going to drift apart."

"You have to be strong. It's fine to be sad."

"But it hurts so much. Part of my life is empty without them. I have nobody to guide me any more."

"You're more positive now, you have your books to help you cope; you can do it, just be patient."

"It's so hard and I feel so weak. I even struggled to bury her. It was so hard not being able to see where to shovel the dirt."

"You did it though. Don't worry about your eyesight. The loss of your mother is more important."

It was a tradition to bury our dead ourselves – most Jamaicans did so. It saved the funeral companies lots of work. We would sing church songs, and the family would fill in the hole where the coffin was placed. It took ages and sometimes we had to do it in the rain but we would sing, song after song until all the dirt was back where it belonged. Then we put flowers on top. I've kept the spade that I used to bury my mother. Both my parents had extra deep graves so that one of us could be buried on top. I've always said that I would like to be buried with my dad. I was called 'Daddy's son' and that made me feel so special.

Another Jamaican tradition was to have nine nights of mourning. It was called 'Nine Night' and people would come and pay their respects. Throughout the nine days and nights we had to provide food and drink for our guests, traditionally Jamaican curried goat and spicy chicken, rice and peas. It's a long time and obviously sad, but there were happy moments too when our friends recounted their happy memories. It's intended to give us more happy memories to help us deal with the loss. We know that everyone will die one day and there is no way out so we all have to learn to accept the inevitable.

CHAPTER 20
YOU ARE BLESSED

Despite the recent traumas in my life, over the next few months I coped. Although the loss of my parents was still quite fresh in my mind, I kept myself busy and tried not to dwell on the pain. It was as though someone was testing me, seeing how many challenges it would take to push me over the edge. The memories of my parents were still in my mind, but I was able to remain a positive person and seemed to get on with life.

There were other things on my mind now. It was only a few months after the death of my mother and it was time for my next eye appointment. It was at the new Eye Hospital and was very difficult to find but as usual I took a friend along to help me. We drove to Birmingham this time instead of travelling by train. We arrived and I registered with reception. All I had to do now was wait.

It took ages before I was called for my first test and in that time I began to get nervous. The conflicting arguments started in my mind.

"This appointment better go well."

"How can it? You do realise that you're coming to help the doctors find a cure in the future but there's nothing that they can do for you."

"Maybe they've had a break through in technology. Or maybe my eyesight has stabilised."

"Be realistic. You know that your eyesight has become progressively worse, you just don't know by how much."

"Everything will be fine."

"There's nothing you can do to help, your eyesight is out of your control so whatever happens… happens, just accept it."

"I don't want it to get any worse, it's too hard for me to get around as it is. Everything I do is becoming more difficult. It's not fair, I want it all to stop now."

I followed the doctor into the room and took a seat.

"That board looks slightly further away than the other one," I thought to myself. "Either that or the letters are smaller because everything looks slightly more difficult to read."

The doctor told me to cover my left eye and to start reading from the board.

"This is a joke!" I thought. "The letters look more blurred than ever, maybe my glasses are dirty or maybe my eyes are cloudier today."

After cleaning my glasses and blinking quite vigorously to clear my vision, I proceeded to read from the board.

"The first letter is... A."

"Yes; go on."

"Are you sure that the board isn't too far away?"

"No, it's not, why?"

"Well... that's all I can read. I can only see the first letter, all the rest look too blurred and distorted to identify."

"Are you sure? Can't you see any of the next line?"

I took a good, long, hard look.

"No; that's it. That's all I can read."

"Can you try and guess any of the letters on the next line?"

"They all look too distorted, I'm sorry but I can't."

My heart began to beat faster as I became more nervous. After a few seconds of entering the room I was already aware of the rate of deterioration in my right eye and I felt extremely uncomfortable.

"Would you like to try again using these dark glasses with pinholes?"

They passed me a pair of dark glasses similar to those I had used when I was learning to walk with a white cane. They had small holes in the lenses to help me focus on specific objects. It gave a tunnel vision effect so everything else was blacked out apart from the letter I was trying to read.

"No; they don't help, I can't read any more with these. It's actually worse because everything appears even more distorted."

At that moment many thoughts raced through my mind.

"What! I don't believe it. That's all I can read? That's just the first letter, the big one on its own; surely I should be able to read more than that. My eyesight hasn't become that bad has it? No! This is my good eye and it can't have deteriorated that much. It's as bad as my left one."

"If your right eye is that bad, maybe your left is worse too."

"No way; I don't want to think about it. There is no way my left eye is worse. It was bad enough. No... no... this isn't happening."

"Pull yourself together. It won't be that bad, stop worrying so much. Wait until you know how bad it is."

"My right eye is so distorted; I can't believe it has deteriorated so much. If my left eye is worse, I don't think that I can cope with knowing. I knew that I shouldn't have come. There's nothing that they can do to help me anyway. I'm just a guinea pig, someone to do their tests on. Don't they realise how much this is breaking my heart to be told that I can hardly see?"

"Try to relax."

"Can you swap and cover up your other eye please?" the doctor asked, breaking into my thoughts.

The moment had come to see or rather to find out if my left eye had deteriorated much. It was a very intense moment and I hesitated before covering up my right eye.

"Here goes," I thought hysterically.

"It's... it's..."

I blinked vigorously and tried to focus more clearly. Then I opened my eye wide and tried again.

"It's... too blurred. I can't read anything, not even the top line; the big letter on its own. Everything is out of focus; everything looks too blurred."

"Are you sure that you can't read anything?" the doctor asked.

I tried once more but was disappointed again. I felt a tear building up in my eye.

"No; nothing. I can't read anything; I can't believe it."

My heart sank and I became overwhelmed by emotions.

"My left eye can't see anything, I feel so hopeless. I can't see or read anything, what's happened to me? I must be able to read something, one letter, just one, please."

"You can't see out of your left eye. Your left eye is very bad. Nothing is clear, nothing! What a great life you've got ahead of you. Nothing is going to be easy to do now."

"I hate my eyes, they're so useless. They can't even see enough to read anything. I hate them, I hate them and I hate my life."

"Can you see any clearer with the dark glasses on?" the doctor asked.

Nothing seemed clearer with them on. Everywhere was too dark and too distorted.

"No; it doesn't help. I can't see enough to focus on anything."

"Can you see me waving my hand?"

He began to wave his hand near my face to see if my eye had any response to movement.

"Yes, but it's not clear."

"Try this. I'm going to hold a card up and I want to know if you can read anything on it."

He held up a card and slowly walked forwards towards me until I was able to read it.

"Yes, I can read it but it still isn't clear. It's the letter 'C' isn't it?"

"Yes; that's correct. Thank you. Please follow me out to the waiting room."

After I found my seat my mind drifted.

"What has happened to my eyes? Why is this happening to me? Why do they have to be so blurred and so useless?"

"Your eyes are getting worse and there's nothing you can do about it."

"Why does this have to happen to me? I don't want to lose my sight. I don't want to go blind."

It was an upsetting moment and I became uncomfortable and agitated.

The next test was my field test where I had to look into a satellite dish and signal whenever I could see a small light that was moved around slowly. I put my chin on the rest and looked into the centre of the satellite dish. While keeping my eyes in the same position I had to press a beeper every time I saw the light. It was something that I was used to doing now but it was an uncomfortable test. Over the years I'd noticed that the light had become harder to see and reappeared less frequently. This test made it obvious that my eyesight had deteriorated further. I could almost feel the blind spots taking over my field of vision. It was clear to me that they were a lot worse and I almost became hysterical. After the doctor confirmed that the blind spots were increasing, the conflicting thoughts in my mind started once more.

"Why are there more blind spots? Why do my eyes have to get worse? Why can't they stay the same now, I've had enough challenges in my life. I don't know if I can cope if I go blind. No, it can't happen to me. I can't take any more stress."

"There are many parts of your eyes that you can't see with now. The blind spots are growing and it's only a matter of time before you go blind."

"No! I'm not going blind, I won't accept it. It's too much to cope with. This isn't happening to me. Why does my eyesight have to be so cloudy, why… why?"

I was sent back to the waiting room to await my next test. While sitting there I was almost in tears as my emotions got the better of me. I was ready to explode and I wanted to scream 'WHY ME!' but somehow I contained myself.

The next test was to check the pressure in my eyes and also to look at the back of my eyes with an ophthalmoscope for any obvious signs of deterioration. They checked the pressure first and then put some eye drops in to dilate my eyes to get a clearer look. Then I was sent to wait while the drops took effect. The world slowly became more distorted as pictures and people became harder to recognise.

"Here we go again. I'm finding it difficult to see anyway and yet here I am watching even more objects in my world disappear. I hate this feeling. Nothing is recognisable. It's making me feel so scared. I'm worried about what it's going to be like if I go blind. It will be too much to cope with, I give up; life stinks."

"Think of something happy or positive."

"What's the point? Things are getting worse and I've run out of strength. You win. I give up. I haven't got the strength to fight any more."

Some tears appeared and began to run down my face. It was too much for me to comprehend and I sat there weeping.

My eyesight became so distorted that I had to be assisted back into the room, a nurse linked my arm and slowly guided me in and helped me to my seat. It made me feel so frail and useless. The doctor gave me a tissue to wipe away my tears and then proceeded to finish the test.

"There's a lot of scarring on the discs in your eyes," he said.

"I know; the doctor at the other Eye Hospital said that too."

"Do you experience problems with objects disappearing?"

"All the time; I can't see coins unless they're in my hand. If I drop money it disappears even though it could be right by my foot. Sometimes I get embarrassed having to ask someone else to find money that I've accidentally dropped in a shop. Also parts of people's faces are disappearing. Unless I'm standing right next to someone, they look like they have parts of their body missing. People look like ghosts and it's pretty scary to see."

"Do you have tunnel vision?"

"No; I don't think so. I see things fine if they're close to me and I see lots of light."

"What about at night?"

"I experience many problems at night-time. I've got night blindness."

"Yes; I know. Do you use eye drops?"

"Yes."

"There's quite a lot of pressure in your eyes. Do you do anything strenuous?"

"I used to lift heavy weights but I've stopped now. The last doctor told me that it was dangerous to put additional strain on my eyes."

"Do you experience any other problems?"

"Like what?"

"Is your vision cloudy?"

"Yes… why?"

"You have a small cataract in your eye which would give you cloudy vision. Your eyes are very dry and that would cause it too. I'll prescribe you some tear drops to moisten your eyes."

"Cataract? How did I get that? My eyes are bad enough, I don't need that too."

"It's only small, you should be fine."

"Why don't you operate on my eyes to get rid of the cloudy vision? It causes me so much distress; it would help me a great deal if you could at least give me clearer vision. It's horrible; it's like looking at everything through thick fog and the fog is getting denser.

Sometimes I wash my eyes several times hoping to clear the fog, even just a little bit. It's so uncomfortable."

"I'm sorry, but there's no way that we can touch your eyes. They're too delicate and we don't know enough about your eye disorder."

"I don't care any more. I want to see clearer. I've had enough of having bad eyesight so if you can get rid of the cloudy vision that would help a great deal."

"Use the tear drops and see if they make a difference."

I became very distressed. One by one more things were going wrong with my eyes and there was nothing that I could do about it. There was too much wrong with them now. It wasn't just one thing, there were several and I became emotional.

"I can't believe this. What's happening to my eyes? Why do they have to be so poor? It's too much to comprehend. It seems like everything is going wrong in my life."

When I entered another room for more tests there was only a doctor present. I was told that there were no more vigorous tests for me. The doctor was a specialist who had taken over from the professor. She introduced herself and then began reading my notes.

"Can I have a look at the back of your eyes?"

"Yes."

As she approached me a thought came into my mind.

"Why is everyone so fascinated with my eyes? It's like they've never seen my disorder before."

She then had a look at the back of my eyes with her ophthalmoscope.

"There's got to be something seriously wrong," I thought to myself. "This disorder is no longer new so they should know enough about it by now."

Then another thought came to me.

"Unless *my* disorder is new. They said that my sister shouldn't have had any problems, yet she seems to be losing her eyesight too."

Although I was feeling very emotional, I was also feeling confused.

"If my sister has RP and she shouldn't, then maybe we haven't got the strain of RP that they thought we had. Maybe they don't know what's wrong with our eyes. Maybe that's why they're so fascinated by what it looks like. I could be right because they're not sure why I'm also deaf. Well… I guess if they don't know what's wrong then I should be grateful that they're all so interested in finding out more."

She finished looking at my eyes and then asked me a few questions.

"Can you see my finger?"

She held up her hand and was waving some of her fingers to check if I could see them.

"I know that you're holding up your arm but I can't see your hand or any fingers. Your arm looks too blurred and you're too far away from me to see your hand."

She came closer until I was able to see.

"Can you see now?"

"Yes I can see your hand but not clearly."

"Keep your eyes focussed on my finger and follow wherever I move it."

When she moved her finger I stayed in the same position. Then I noticed that her arm had moved so that meant her finger must be somewhere else so I looked around until I focussed on it once more but every time she moved her finger I could feel a delay before I was able to see it again.

"Where does her finger keep disappearing to?" I thought. "It's hard to see. I'll watch to see when she moves her arm and then I will look around until I can focus on her hand."

"Your hand keeps disappearing," I said. "I can see your arm even though it appears distorted and when I look to where your hand should be it's vanished. It's taking me a while before I focus on it but then when you move it, your hand disappears again. It's too difficult. I don't know where to look."

She then sat back down to ask a few more questions.

"Yes, there's a long delay before you focus on things," she said.

"That's because I was struggling to see your hand, so I was watching the movements of your arm as it's much bigger and easier to see, even though it also appears blurred to me."

"Your eyesight is very poor."

"I know; that's why I'm here. Have you discovered a cure yet?"

"We will soon."

"Not for me though. I won't be cured. By the time you discover a cure, I'll be too old to care or already be dead. I'm more worried about our next generation just in case any of them get it."

"Are you working?"

"I'm a Computer Technician working with lots of small computer screens that cause me a great deal of distress."

"Have you any specialist equipment to help you manage?"

"Yes; I have a keyboard with large letters; a large monitor; magnification programs and a CCTV to help me read. It's a great help to me but it doesn't help when I have to help someone else on their computer. We have over fifty computers at my workplace and I wouldn't expect my boss to adapt all the computers to cater for my needs."

"Do you go out at night?"

"Sometimes but I struggle more at night to see. People have to be right next to me for me to be able to identify them and that still depends on the amount of light. Most of the time I guess, or recognise them from their voices. It's very frustrating but that's the only way that I see people. Sometimes I force myself to go out even though I know that it's going to make me feel very uncomfortable."

"You've lost a great deal of vision and your eyes are showing lots of signs of tunnel vision."

"How much vision have I lost?"

"I would say... 95%."

"Pardon? Sorry, but how could I have such little vision and still be getting around so well?"

"I'm afraid that we're going to have to register you as blind."

For a minute I was lost for words as I tried to take in what she had just said.

"Your eyes have deteriorated considerably since your last appointment."

"Blind? But I can see."

"You can only see things that are very close to you. Many blind people can see a little. You don't have to be totally blind to be registered as blind."

"I don't want to be blind."

"Walk with me."

She walked off around the room and I followed. Then she went out of the door, along a corridor and back into the room and all the time she was watching my actions closely. It wasn't clear to me where she was going and I couldn't see if there were any obstacles in my way so I followed behind her carefully, rather than walking with her. We then returned to our seats.

"You see, you followed me, you didn't walk with me. You looked very unsure of your surroundings because it was all new to you. The way you walked like you were thinking so hard about each step, told me that you couldn't see."

"My sight isn't clear enough for me to walk beside people so I tend to follow then. I've done this for a long time and that's why people think that I can see more than I really can but I never dreamt that I've been walking around practically blind."

"You have and you're doing well but you need more help and I think that it's about time that you used a white stick. If you like I won't register you as blind if it upsets you, but you are and you can receive more help that you need."

I was in shock and hesitated before answering.

"Blind!" I thought to myself. "Oh my God, I'm blind! What am I going to do? I wasn't supposed to be blind, not yet. How will I ever cope? It's too much for me to handle. I can't be blind. I don't want to be blind. My whole life has just ended. I hated the feeling of imagining how it would be if I became blind and all this time I was already... blind. No, this is a dream – a nightmare. This isn't happening to me. No, I refuse to accept it."

My body was numb as I sat there wondering what to do and what to say.

"Shall I sign the form to say that I'm registered blind? How will I tell everyone? This is going to be so humiliating. I'll lose students at my Martial Arts club; nobody will want to train under a blind instructor. They'll say that I can't see if they're doing something right or wrong. I don't know what to do."

"Sign the form and accept help. You've done well to get this far on your own, now it's time to ask for help and to trust other people."

"Maybe I'll sign, but I'm not telling everyone, I can't, I can't take it, no, it's too embarrassing."

It took me a few moments while I contemplated what to do in my mind, but finally I made a decision.

"Yes, I'll sign the form to say that I'm now classed as blind," I answered, feeling defeated.

She approached me and showed me the form to sign.

"Where should I sign?" I asked.

"Here; where my finger is."

She even moved my hand to the right position so that my pen was near her finger.

"She's right; I can't see," I thought as I struggled to sign. "I'm fooling myself. How long haven't I been able to see? How long have I been blind without knowing? How embarrassing, having to be helped to sign my own name. I'm completely useless and I didn't realise. It's finally happened, I'm blind."

My appointment was finally over and the specialist led me out to my friend who guided me out. The hospital was new to me and I wasn't sure how to get out. I felt disorientated and very confused. We had to stop whenever I thought that I was going to bump into a wall or collide with someone. We also had to stop when I wasn't sure whether there were steps. I was feeling very uncomfortable and fragile. I was no longer sure about anything and didn't feel confident in my steps. As soon as we got outside I was met by the blinding light from the sun. I wasn't thinking straight so I'd forgotten that everywhere seemed brighter when I had the eye drops in. It was bright in a bad way because it irritated my eyes so much that I could hardly keep them open due to the pain. Then I remembered that I'd brought along some sunglasses for this very reason, so I placed them on my face and got into the car.

We set out on our way back to Rugby. Still feeling useless, I sat in almost silence all the way back home. It became too much for me to hold back my emotions and the tears began to fall from my eyes. My mind became cloudy with thoughts.

"Why is this happening to me? Why do I have to be blind? Why?"

More tears dropped from my eyes.

"Why do I have to suffer so much? I don't want to be blind. How does my brother cope so well? I don't think that I can. I hate my eyes; I wish that I could see. Now I'm going to have to tell all my friends that I'm no longer partially sighted, I'm blind! How embarrassing. I hate the world and I hate my crap life."

I was so upset that the tears continued to fall for most of the journey back to Rugby.

After explaining to my friend that I was now registered blind I returned to suffer in silence.

"That felt awful telling my friend and now I'm going to have to tell everyone else. How embarrassing. I can't do it, I really can't. And how am I going to tell my students? I can't handle it; it's too much to cope with. They won't want to train with me. They might think that I can't see to teach. If I lose my students it will be all my fault for going blind. No, I might as well quit Martial Arts now. My whole life is a mess – it's over. Everything that I've worked so hard for, I'm now going to have to give it all up."

"You can't give up yet, there must be a way."

"Does this mean that I'm going to have to use my white cane more?"

The thought of me walking around using my white cane scared me.

"I can't do it, I can't… I can't."

The confusion in my mind grew.

"My world is fading away and there's nothing I can do about it. I've suffered too many challenges and I give up. I don't care about anyone or anything any more. I hate my eyes and I hate my life."

"You can't give up."

"I'm not fighting any more. I've changed my life so much to prevent this from happening but I've still become blind."

"Try to relax and control yourself."

"I'm not in control of this, there's nothing I can do but wait and take whatever life wants to throw at me. My life has ended. I'm a misfit. I can't see or hear properly. Why is this happening to me? I've got an eye disorder that has no cure, but I've also got glaucoma and a cataract, and cloudy vision and my eyes hurt from the pressure. This is too much, it's a joke; someone's having a laugh at my expense."

We arrived back at my house and I was still feeling very sad so I lay on the settee and closed my eyes. Although there were still plenty of things rushing around my mind, I seemed to think slightly less with my eyes closed.

"I'm so pathetic and I feel useless. My friend had to guide me out of the car, into the house and tell me where my own settee was, I'm hopeless."

"You can't do much so you may as well just lie here until the eye drops wear off."

"I'm no use to anyone blind. What am I going to do?"

"You're going to have to learn to cope."

"I can't; I can't cope any more."

"Yes you can and… you have to. You can't give up, not now, not after what you've gone through. You're strong."

"Life's too hard, I've lost the test, there were too many challenges and I lost against them. The fight is over now."

"No; don't give up, not yet."

"It hurts too much to suffer like this. I feel like I'm going to have a nervous breakdown."

"You're strong, you can beat this."

"But why did I have to go blind? Why?"

"You can still see something."

"But it's so little, so blurred and so cloudy."

"Think of something else to cheer yourself up."

As I lay there feeling sorry for myself, I couldn't help feeling emotional. The thought of going blind had scared me for years.

"I wonder how long I've been walking around technically blind?"

"Who cares? It's happened and now you have to learn to deal with it."

I lay there, with my eyes closed, hoping for a miracle.

The miracle never came and the next day I was confronted with yet more challenges. The eye drops hadn't worn off and I was unable to see so I lay around for most of the day. I didn't even have breakfast until the afternoon, knowing that I would only struggle more trying to do things while the effects of the eye drops were still present.

"I'm hopeless. I have to lie here and wait for the drops to wear off before I'm able to do anything. I'm not ready to ask for help so I'll just stay here and suffer."

"You have to ask other people for help, that's your future."

"I'm too embarrassed and I feel useless. My independence has been taken away."

"No; no; this can't be happening. I want my independence back. I don't want to be blind. I hate my eyes."

The eye drops eventually wore off later on in the day. Then I was back to my real challenge.

"How am I going to tell everyone that I'm registered blind?"

CHAPTER 21
RETURN OF THE GHOSTS

The stress of knowing that I was now registered blind almost became unbearable. A serious battle was on the way to deter me from the thoughts that could render me helpless.

"I'm blind? I can't believe it. I can't see anything clearly. There goes my life and my training. There's no way that I can go for my 4th Dan black belt now! Not now that I'm registered blind. It's all over for me. It's all downhill from now."

"You can't give everything up. You've worked too hard."

Then I became emotional.

"What's the point? Everywhere looks too blurred. I hate my eyes. I feel like an invalid."

"Why not try using your white cane? You should go out and use it how it's supposed to be used and not carry it folded up."

"No way; it's too embarrassing; I can't do it."

"You have to or else you'll become a recluse. Is that what you want?"

"No; I suppose I should give it a try."

Somehow I was able to convince myself to go out during the day using my white cane at its true length.

After stepping through my front door, I first straightened my cane. Then I looked around at my blurred world and was unhappy with what I saw. People were walking around with even more parts of their faces missing. When they were at a much greater distance away from me, they looked like their heads were missing. The ghostly figures of people were back and scarier than before. They now looked like ghosts with disfigured faces. Some of them appeared to be walking around without legs. The blind spots in my eyes were growing and my world was slowly disappearing. The confusion in my mind started again.

"People look scary. They appear to be walking around without heads and sometimes their legs disappear. How am I going to cope?"

"You can do it. Don't look at them."

"I can't help it! Maybe I should go back inside and wait for someone to help me."

"You still want your independence, don't you?"

"Yes, but at what price? People have to be close for me to see them more clearly – they look so scary. People no longer look like people. They really do look like ghosts. The parts of them that are missing change depending on the distance I am away from them. It can start off as their whole head and as they get closer only their mouth is missing. I feel so hopeless. My eyes are useless."

"Then walk on and look at people as you pass them."

"That will make it more difficult to recognise my friends from their outlines."

"You're the one who can't see, let them recognise you first."

After a few seconds I plucked up the courage and started on my journey into town.

Using the skills that Rita had taught me, I walked on cautiously. Tapping the ground gently I moved my white cane from left to right to make sure that my path was clear. The ghostly figures of people walked towards me and slowly emerged as humans with all their bodily parts back in the correct place. They sometimes moved out of my way and sometimes they walked straight towards me as though they hadn't seen me. I had to move out of the way of some children who were walking with their parents.

"They should have moved those children out of my way. I could hardly see them. Why did I have to manoeuvre? Suppose I was totally blind and was unable to see any movement, I would have walked straight into one of them. People should be more considerate. I would have felt awful if my cane had hit a child."

"Be careful and walk slowly."

After a while I came to a road that I had to cross. I stood and waited.

"This feels weird. What must the drivers be thinking? I've got my white cane now so it wouldn't look good if I took too many risks. I'm going to have to wait until I'm pretty sure that the road is clear."

A minute or so passed and I was still waiting for a clear gap in the traffic. It wouldn't have looked good if I rushed across, just missing a car, like I usually did, so I waited. Then I listened carefully with my good ear.

"Now I'm confused. I've got my white cane that says that I can't see and I'm also deaf in one ear so I can't hear clearly when it's safe to cross the road. I'll wait until the sound of the car engines are nearly silent then I'll cross. Let's hope that there isn't a new car with a quiet engine!"

It was difficult to identify all the blurred images. The air became almost silent and I couldn't see any obvious blurred images moving. The road appeared to be clear, but then I saw a bicycle pass. It appeared from nowhere. They were very hard for me to see because bikes are small compared to the larger blurred images of cars. If I were to wait until I was sure that it was clear then I would be waiting all day. I had to take a risk.

"You're still going to have to risk it. Hold your breath and cross or you'll be standing here all day."

So that's what I did to cross the road. Although it appeared to be clear, I wasn't sure and pushed my cane out in front before walking across.

It wasn't long before my confidence was tested. A ghostly figure approached me and I was unable to identify them from their outline.

"Hello," a voice said.

Their voice wasn't familiar to me so I was unsure of who they were.

"What should I say?" I thought. "They said hello as though I should know them but can't they see my white cane? Well if they can't be considerate enough to tell me their name then I'll pretend that I know who they are."

"Hello," I answered. "I haven't seen you in a while."

"I haven't seen you in a while because I *can't* see you," I thought madly. "Now talk to me until I work out who you are."

"How are you?" the voice asked.

"As you can see, I'm blind thanks," I thought, hysteria threatening to engulf me. "No, I won't say that. I don't know who you are yet."

"I'm fine thanks and getting better," I answered.

"Why, were you sick?" the voice replied.

"No; I just like to say that rather than just say 'Fine'. It makes it sound more interesting," I remarked.

"You seem very cheerful," he said.

A few names flashed through my mind as I attempted to find the identity of this person. After a few more seconds I decided who I thought he was, took a risk and began to talk about his interests. He answered and from that moment I knew who he was. We had a general chit-chat, and then I proceeded into town. A few things crossed my mind.

"Was he blind too? He didn't even mention my white cane and why I was using it. Maybe he didn't know what it was."

"Yes he did; but he didn't know what to say to you so he ignored it."

"I'm not sure how to take that."

"Who cares? You didn't even know who he was until you recognised his voice after a while. If he didn't know that you had sight problems in the past, he does now, he saw your white cane."

"Maybe it was the red stripes on it that confused him."

"Maybe he didn't know that the red stripes mean that you're also deaf but he saw your long cane. Stop making excuses."

A few minutes later I came across another road and experienced some more problems while trying to get across.

"I don't know when to cross. Some of the cars are going too fast and I would look silly walking out in front of a car. If I didn't have my cane I could pretend to be a pedestrian in a hurry and rush across. This is very uncomfortable and I feel vulnerable."

Then a car flashed its lights; I think.

"Was he flashing his lights at me?" I wondered. "What should I do? In theory I'm blind so didn't see that. He's probably waving his hand at me to cross but I can't see through car windows. I can't see anyone. He could be flashing his lights at something else. Drivers don't know what to do with a blind person crossing the road. I'm going to risk it and cross."

So I crossed in front of the car that had slowed down. Then I walked on.

I came across another road and waited until I could hear that it was clear. That too made me think.

"I didn't realise that I used my hearing so much when I cross roads. Although I've only got one good ear, I'd be lost without my hearing. If I were totally deaf too I really would stay in my house. It must be so hard for other people to come out and take more risks to do normal things."

I held my breath and walked across quite hastily.

"It really scares me when I cross a road. I'm sure I'm going to get run over one day. Maybe I should ask other people to drive me around. Suppose there was a motorbike or a cyclist? I wouldn't see them because they would look too distorted to focus on. I'm fearful crossing roads."

"You want to rely on other people? I don't think so. They all have a life and you would have to manage around their schedules. No, do it yourself. You might want to go somewhere and they won't be able to help you until it's too late."

I walked slowly on.

It was obvious to me that I was walking much slower when using my white cane. The feelings that I experienced were overpowering and made me feel much worse than usual. Without the cane I could pretend to be clumsy and get away with walking a touch faster and accidentally bumping into people. I was used to it now and was very apologetic when I did collide with someone. Now that I was using my cane, I didn't want to walk faster and accidentally bump into someone, I would feel inconsiderate. So it felt natural to walk much slower. It also helped to avoid lamp posts and other obstacles that would normally frighten me. They still appeared out of nowhere but my cane found them before I hit them and if a dark spot was just a shadow then my cane would pass through it.

As I waited patiently to cross the next road I noticed ghostly figures approaching me then standing beside me waiting to cross. Even though I had a long white cane that indicated that I was blind, I had other senses that worked well. Some people ignored my disability and crossed the road. I almost followed them but I felt that the road wasn't totally clear. They weren't being at all considerate because I could have followed them and been hit by a car. I thought that they could at least have indicated in one way or another that it was safe to cross. This also happened later on when I was waiting to cross a road with traffic lights. People seemed to be in such a hurry that they didn't give a thought to the safety of other people around. I could have thought that the lights weren't working and followed them across.

Then I came across another person who knew me. As I approached, their distorted outline became clearer, but not enough for me to know who they were before they acknowledged me.

"Hello. How are you?" they asked.

"Let me think," I pondered. "Yes! I know who that is, I recognise their voice."

"Fine thanks and getting better," I replied.

We had a small conversation and then they asked.

"What's that stick for?"

"Here we go," I thought. "Surely they know what it's for, but I have to tell them I guess. Here goes."

"I've got very bad eyesight and sometimes I need this cane," I replied.

It didn't come out. I'd tried to say that I was registered blind but it wasn't ready to reveal itself.

Now I felt nervous but I knew that I had to reveal my true identity soon. Even though it was obvious from the length of my cane that I was blind, people wanted me to admit it.

The next person I met I knew that I would have to tell them. After a brief chat without them acknowledging themselves by name, I took a deep breath and prepared myself to speak.

"What's that for?" they asked.

"I have to use this cane now," I answered.

"Why? Has your eyesight got worse?"

"Yes… I'm registered blind now."

"Blind? But you saw me and you can see me now can't you?"

"No; you spoke first and I recognised you from your voice. That's how I knew that it was you."

"What do you see?"

"You appear to be wearing a mask. Unless you turn your face into the light, your features are too hard to identify and… you look like a ghost."

A tear came to my eye. It just appeared from nowhere. I didn't realise that I would feel so sad after explaining that I'm registered blind. I suddenly felt useless speaking about how bad my eyesight had become. As I walked on, I found myself explaining the same thing to another friend. Admitting that I was registered blind was draining me of my energy. It was making me feel worse than knowing the truth and pretending to others. Explaining to other people made me realise how bad my eyesight really was.

There were several situations that I struggled to deal with. A ghostly figure stopped to have a chat to me and I was unable to identify them from their voice.

"Do you know who I am?" the voice asked.

"No, I can't see properly," I answered.

"Maybe I should leave this cane at home next time," I thought to myself. "Some of my friends are ignoring it anyway. How am I supposed to recognise someone if I clearly can't see them?"

Maybe they weren't thinking straight when they asked the question but it still made me feel as though my white cane was invisible.

Then someone else called me and I wasn't immediately sure of their voice. I looked around at the unfamiliar ghosts but neither of them revealed themselves. They could have been anyone. I watched and waited for the owner of the new voice to identify himself. Eventually a blurred image stood in front of me and began to talk as if I knew who he was. After a short moment they were gone, back into the cloudy mist of ghosts. I was still unsure who they were and yet I had my white cane in plain view.

"What's the point me using this cane that makes me feel so uncomfortable, to help other people know that I have a serious sight problem if they're just going to ignore it?" I thought in frustration.

"Most people don't know how to deal with someone who has a disability."

"It's embarrassing using this cane and it makes me feel totally useless."

"Don't use it then. You're used to the town centre and know where most of the obstacles are. Maybe just use it in unfamiliar places."

"Who were those people? Why should I have to ask for their names? It's happening too many times and it makes me feel really uncomfortable."

"Just ask a few people for their names so that you don't feel too useless."

"But when I talk to someone who's partially sighted or blind, I always tell them my name first. Why can't other people do that?"

"They're not doing it on purpose, they really don't know what to do. They need to try and see situations from different perspectives to understand how it feels. But people don't think, do they?"

Although I was a little upset with the situation, I also felt sorry for some of the people. It was obvious that they didn't know what to do or say to a blind person. Some of them had probably never come into contact with one before and it was a shock to their system. It was also partly my fault. I shouldn't be embarrassed of what I am and shouldn't get emotional having to explain my disability to others. It was all new to me too and I hoped that I would learn to deal with it but at that time I was a little angry at life.

When I got back home I became dizzy with thoughts.

"That was just awful. I felt so embarrassed using my long cane in front of my friends. Some of them asked too many questions and I found myself repeating the same disturbing facts that make me realise how bad my eyesight has become. I can't deal with it."

"Don't use your cane any more. It's making you feel worse. You feel more incapable when using it."

"But I have to use it. I have to get used to the feeling of using my cane."

"Some of those people didn't care about your cane. Some of your friends didn't even mention it so why put yourself through that pain and torture over and over again?"

"I can't keep pretending. I can't see and people need to know. Some of my friends were fine with it."

"And some of them were not. One of them even admitted waving at you from across the road. Didn't they see your cane? Haven't you already admitted that you were partially sighted to them?"

"Yes; that's true. It was like I had to repeat the same things to the same people too. Are they deaf? Aren't they listening to me? Don't they realise how much this is hurting me?"

"They don't really care. They want to talk about their problems but they don't want to listen to yours."

"Don't they realise how fortunate they are? They don't have real problems. They complain about trivial things like their hair doesn't sit right or they have a spot on their face and feel embarrassed to be out in public, or their ear feels blocked and they feel like they're going deaf or do they look fat or that girl over there has a big bum. Who cares? If they couldn't see then they would realise that most of the things that they complain about are not really that important. I can't see spots on people's faces so they always look good to me. I can't see if someone's having a bad hair day. If they couldn't see then they would realise that it's not that important. There are more important things to worry about in life."

"Some people like to moan about nothing. They don't really realise that things could be a lot worse. They could be permanently disabled, completely disfigured or even dead. They're lucky. They should be grateful that they still have the ability to do normal things and see the true beauty of the world."

"Don't they realise how difficult life is for a disabled person?"

"No; they take everything for granted, that is until they lose that ability."

It upset me to know that normal people were walking around thinking that they have a serious problem yet there are so many other people who wish that they could just walk again without the use of their wheelchair or have the ability to talk or see or hear.

"Maybe people should visit hospitals more to see real sick people, some of whom haven't left the hospital for weeks or even months because of an illness. I bet that they would like to swap their illness for an earache."

I tried to think of some happy memories; something positive that would take my mind off my problems.

Then I had a phone call. It was my friend John who phones on a regular basis to see how I am.

"How was your eye appointment?" he asked.

"Terrible. My eyesight has become worse. They've registered me as blind and I feel like someone else is in control of my life."

"Are you sure they're that bad?"

"Yes; I suppose I knew that it was coming but I can't accept that it has happened. Why me? Why did it have to happen to me? I don't want to be blind."

"You're the strongest and can cope with the most. I don't know what I would do if I lost my eyesight. I rely on it a lot. How would I be able to drive to work?"

"Exactly; it holds me back from achieving many things and I hate my eyes for that."

"I don't know how you can do it, but you can cope."

"This is too much for me to cope with. I had so many things planned to do in my life, but now that I'm registered blind, they will be impossible to achieve."

"Don't let your disability hold you back."

"How can I continue to try to achieve my 4th Dan black belt? It's too hard. It's too late. I'll never do it."

"Look how far you've got with your limited ability. Who else could have done it?"

"But there are no 4th Dan black belts who are blind. Doesn't that tell you something? It's too hard."

"Then you will be the first. Imagine that? You; the first blind Master of Taekwondo in England."

I took a few moments to imagine.

"It sounds great but it would be very difficult. I don't want to be given the belt out of sympathy and compassion, I want to work for it, but I'd be against some of the best fighters in the country, WTF Olympic fighters who could knock me out with one kick. Supposing I didn't see a kick coming because of my lack of sight?"

"I believe that you can do it. Go for it. Let your disability be your drive to prove to others that you deserve the title; Master."

I'd already given up competitive fighting because of the risks of injuries. It had been a difficult decision and here I was literally in the same position once again.

"Do I give up?" I thought to myself. "It would be a serious risk. If any of them were blindfolded I could and would kick their ass, but here I am almost deciding to do the same thing, to go in for my 4th Dan almost blindfolded. I don't know; it would be so easy to quit now while things are good. Is it really that important to me? Do I really want it?"

"Yes!"

"It's going to be difficult," I cautioned myself, "but I'll do it. Life will be hard though. I'm going to have to study hard and study people's actions and reactions when they fight."

"I'm glad you chose to carry on," John said when I told him of my decision.

"It hurts to tell other people about my disability. First I told people that I was partially sighted but now I have to tell them all that

I'm registered blind. It's too much. I hate it so much. I hate my eyes, they're holding me back."

"People will understand."

"They don't though. Some of them wave their hands in my face and ask me if I can see their hands or reckon that I saw them first. Some of them say hello to me from across the road without telling me who they are or even have a conversation with me when I've no idea who they are."

"That's very inconsiderate of them."

"Why should I have to keep asking them their names? If they feel uncomfortable telling me their names, can't they imagine how I must feel having to ask nearly everyone I talk to?"

"It is bad."

"I guess most of the time I get used to people's outlines but I sometimes get it wrong. Sometimes I think that I'm approaching someone who I know and as they get closer it turns out that it's not them. They appear so distorted to me and they have parts missing off their anatomies. They all look like ghosts when they're just a few metres away. It's so hard to describe but even harder to live with."

"It must be difficult. I think that you've put up with a lot."

"I might as well close my eyes when I talk to someone because I'm mostly using my hearing to recognise their voices. That's how it appears like I can see; I'm just not totally deaf and am quite perceptive."

"That's good."

"That's nothing. Some people don't move out of my way when I'm using my cane and I have to manoeuvre out of *their* way. It's so frustrating. It's so hard crossing roads. Did you know that nearly every time I cross a road I hold my breath and cross, thinking that I'll get hit by a car?"

"You're crazy. Why don't you ask other people for help?"

"I don't want to be a burden on anyone and sometimes people can't help me when I need them the most. When that happens I feel so useless and hopeless and wish that I could do things for myself. Then I realise even more how useless my eyesight is and it upsets me further."

"You have to ask your friends for help and support."

"I can't. I hate feeling like an invalid. I enjoy my independence and I'm finding it very difficult to adapt to rely on others. I feel less humiliated if I try and do things for myself."

"You're going to have to learn though."

"How? Why? Why is this happening to me? I can't do it. I can't ask others to put toothpaste on my toothbrush, check that I have shaved correctly, feed me because I can't see my food, read menus and letters for me, show me where the toilets are wherever I go, take me places so that I don't take risks crossing the road, cook for me, clean for me and organise my life and assist me at work! It's too much. I have no life. I'm blind and I feel useless."

"I'll help you as much as possible."

"Thanks."

"Now you need to tell your other friends."

The phone call was over but it signified the beginning of the long quest of sharing my disability with others.

CHAPTER 22
I'M NOT A ROBOT

Most of my friends were now aware that I was registered blind. It was a very uncomfortable experience having to inform twenty or thirty people about something that made me slightly depressed every time I mentioned it. Several of my students, mostly the seniors who knew me well, were also told. I chose not to tell the other students because of fear of lack of knowledge and fear of losing them. Although I had proven that a person who is registered blind can teach as well as any other Martial Arts teacher, the majority of people would find it hard to comprehend. It wasn't worth losing students by trying to prove that I could teach proficiently even though I was blind. If I came across a student with a problem that they felt would hold them back from performing well then I would tell them more about my disability to encourage them to try harder. There were several students who I encouraged.

"Can you take your glasses off when you're fighting please?" I said to one student. "You need to learn to fight without them just in case they get knocked off your face when you're in a fight."

"Oh, please can I keep them on sir?" he asked.

"Why? How bad is your eyesight?" I asked.

"It's really bad, sir."

"How far down the chart can you read when you go to the optician?"

"Without my glasses I can't read the last three lines, but with them on I only struggle with the last line."

Then I prepared myself for my response.

"Should I tell him that I'm registered blind?" I asked myself. "No, that sounds too drastic and he might quit. He knows how much difficulty he's experiencing so if I say that I'm blind he might find it too hard to imagine."

"With my glasses on, I can't read any of the chart at the opticians," I answered. "Yet you see me taking my glasses off to fight, so why don't you?"

"Yes sir."

"I know that it feels very uncomfortable for you to see without your glasses, but please try to get used to it."

The student then removed his glasses and fought. Over the next few months that student became much more confident fighting without his glasses on.

There was also another student who I helped overcome his disability. He was registered partially sighted and was on the verge of quitting for years but I kept him going by telling him that I was registered blind. I told him that if I could do it, he could too. He came to me for extra practice and I taught him how to use his other senses to compensate for his disability. He lasted about five years with me before he finally quit. He was just one belt away from his black belt and it was a sad thing to see, giving up at the last hurdle.

I used to see him around after he had left and we remained friends. When we met it was always quite an interesting experience because we were both guessing whether it was the other person.

One day, as I walked towards his blurred ghostly outline, I noticed that he appeared to be observing my actions. I slowed down as he approached and a few names went through my mind.

"That looks like James or Simon," I thought. "I'm not sure so I'll walk a little closer to see a bit clearer."

When the figure was only about two metres away, I decided that it was Simon.

"I'm sure it's Simon," I thought. "I'll smile like I know it's him and see if he answers."

"Hello," the blurred figure said.

"Yes, it sounds like Simon too so it must be him; I think!"

"Hello Simon, I haven't seen you in a while," I responded.

"In fact, I hardly see you at all," I thought to myself jokingly.

"I wasn't sure that it was you," Simon said.

"I guessed it was you from your voice," I replied.

That was how we usually saw each other on the street.

It was now 1996 and there was only a year left before I was going to take my 4th Dan and I found myself practising long and hard. I'm not sure how it happened but the more I practised the more energy I appeared to have. Sometimes I would go to the gym for a light session with my friend John who would help change the weights for me. At night-time I still wasn't tired so I would look for other things to do and would sometimes still be up at 2 am, pottering around my house, tidying up here and there and generally making myself useful while I still had the energy. I started to notice that I was losing weight easily but I put it down to the excessive training. My Wing-Chun instructor had moved away from Rugby and his school had closed down. With the extra time on my hands I began to train under a Taekwondo instructor who I had trained with years ago.

One day my sister from London, Carline, came to visit us in Rugby and saw how active I was. She complained that I had too much energy for someone who was doing so much during a typical day. She was a trained nurse and had only recently changed her job but she still had her skills of observation.

"Come here to me," she said.

"Why; what have I done now?" I asked.

"Nothing; I'm just curious. I want to have a look at your eyes."

"What for? I know that I can't see."

"No; I think that there's something else wrong, I sense it."

"More wrong? I think that I've had enough problems with my eyes to keep me going for years thanks."

"Let me look at your eyes," she insisted.

So I went closer and she made her diagnosis.

"Your eyes are bulging out. I've got a feeling that you've got a thyroid problem," she concluded.

"A what?" I asked, feeling worried.

"That could explain why you appear to have loads of energy. You're too active, something's definitely wrong," she answered.

"No; it's the pressure of my eyes from the glaucoma. My eyes are always in terrible pain from it, I've got eye drops to relieve some of the pressure."

"It could be but what about your weight loss? You look like you've lost a lot of weight lately."

"I've lost over 7kg, but that's because I train so hard."

"Why not make an appointment to see your doctor? Let him have a look at you."

I agreed and was referred to the Rugby St Cross Hospital to see a specialist called Doctor O'Hare.

While I was waiting to be seen a few things came into my mind.

"Well, I hope that my sister is wrong about me having a thyroid problem."

"You *are* quite active lately."

"It's because I'm training so hard, it gives me more energy during the day."

"Haven't you noticed that you're finding it hard to sleep too?"

"I've had enough problems, I don't want any more. My eyes *are* quite large; they do appear to be popping out of my head. Maybe I have got a thyroid problem. I do lose weight a bit too easily these days."

"Don't you think being blind is enough to cope with?"

"It's more than enough. I have to hide my emotions from other people or I'll lose it and become depressed."

"Think of something happy and stop concentrating on your problems."

I found another happy memory to keep my mind busy until I saw the specialist.

The doctor called me into his room and began his tests. He read through the results of a recent blood test and also the results of my blood pressure and took my body weight. Then he had a look at my bulging eyes. He also felt around my neck for my glands and asked me to swallow. Then he asked me to hold out my hands. They were trembling slightly, I could feel them shaking but I thought that was because I was nervous. Then the questions started.

"Have you got an eye disorder?"

"Yes; I have RP and glaucoma and a small cataract."

"RP? That's fascinating. Can I take a look into your eyes?"

"Help yourself; everyone else does."

He looked at the back of my eyes with his ophthalmoscope and said, "Wow; it's incredible. It would be better if your eyes were dilated but they're very interesting."

"I've had more than my fair share of eye drops to dilate my eyes thanks."

He proceeded to ask about my eye condition before turning back to my immediate problem.

"You have hyperactive thyroids," he announced.

"How come?" I asked.

"There are many ways that they can flair up. Your heart is working too hard like you're constantly exercising and we need to slow it down before you have a heart attack. I'm going to prescribe you with two different tablets that will help to control them."

"Will I have to use them for the rest of my life?"

"Maybe."

At that moment I felt like I had gone into shock.

"More problems?" I thought to myself. "I'm now in danger of having a heart attack? I can't believe this is happening to me. I'm so lucky that Carline is a nurse and spotted it or I would still be racing around until all sorts of hours in the morning. Then I might have had a heart attack. I really am a misfit; my body is falling apart. I won't be donating any of my organs now, it wouldn't help anyone."

Doctor O'Hare told me that I would have to have regular appointments every four months to check that the amount of tablets were sufficient to slow me down and stabilise my thyroid.

When I got home I became confused.

"Why me? Why is all this happening to me? I'm registered blind, isn't that enough?"

"Oh no! You have to have more problems to cope with until you go mad."

"I've adjusted my whole life around my eyesight and now I have to readjust my life around my thyroid problem?"

"Those tablets are going to take away all your energy and slow you down."

"How am I going to train hard for my 4th Dan black belt now? I don't want to have a heart attack."

"Think of happy thoughts. Don't get too emotional."

I became emotional, sad but angry at the same time. I knew that I had to conquer my emotions for fear of giving in to depression. It was a fight that I had to continue but the way things were going it would only be a matter of time before I exploded. I had plenty of emotions but hid them well. People still saw me with a smile on my face but underneath I was hurting and beginning to boil. When friends asked me for my opinion on things I would answer with an almost cold expression.

"Have you heard that your mate is in hospital with liver failure?" a friend asked me.

"He shouldn't drink so much alcohol," I replied without concern.

"That's not very nice."

"I don't know him well anyway, it's not my problem."

"Yes, but you could be a bit more sympathetic."

"I am sympathetic to people who have problems through no fault of their own, but he drinks a lot, he brought it on himself and now has to suffer the consequences."

"That's cruel. He could die."

"We all have to die sometime."

"Don't you care? Have you no compassion? Haven't you got any feelings?"

"Yes I do have feelings, but I didn't tell him to drink so much so what can I do?"

"You're really cold. You're like a robot with no emotions."

It was too difficult for me to explain to my friend what I've been through and what goes on in my head. I did have feelings, of course I did, but I knew that I had to learn how to control them or I would fall apart. Rather than trying to explain my actions and making myself feel upset from reliving the truth of how bad my eyesight was, I chose to ignore them and leave them to their own conclusions. Talking about what I see would lead me to become too emotional and that would be too much stress for me to cope with. I didn't want to be reminded of how poor my eyesight was so I became silent and hardly had an opinion about other people. On the outside I appeared cold, but on the inside I was beginning to boil and was an emotional wreck.

Over the next few months I felt myself slowing down. The tablets for my hyperactive thyroids sometimes made me fall asleep in the early evening. They were only short naps, but sleep it was. For a few years I was an insomniac and never realised it. There were so many different sports that I took part in and I thought that they were the reason why I had so much energy. It seemed that I'd had hyperactive thyroids for years and I'd never known. If it weren't for my sister warning me I would probably have had a heart attack eventually. That scared me and added to my chain of thoughts. Then I had my second shock that year that deterred me from thinking about my thyroid problem.

My sister Angela, who had devoted her life to looking after our mother and us, came back with some crippling news. She had also been registered blind by the Birmingham Eye Hospital and was very upset and was finding the news hard to deal with. It was a shock to us all.

"I can't believe this," I thought. "Three of us, all registered blind, that's ridiculous. Three of us in the same family! That's a lot to deal with. Why is this happening to us? Maybe we *are* cursed."

"No; you don't really believe that, do you?"

"Then why is it happening to us? The doctors still aren't sure which strain of RP we have, they said that my sister should have been a carrier and only the male line could develop it, but now she's blind too."

"She said the doctors told her that we all have a 50% chance of getting it. That's one in two of us so who else has it?"

Then a weird sensation came over me.

"If my sister can get it then… maybe my two children can. They're both girls and should not be able to develop RP but now I don't trust the doctors. They don't know enough and don't know who else could also have it. No… that's too much to think about, please no; not my children."

"Think of something else, quickly or your emotions will get the better of you. Think of something quickly before you break down and cry."

Angela became emotionally distraught and was soon housebound. When she was young she had been very outgoing, now she is a depressed recluse who hardly leaves her house and most of the time she doesn't want to see anyone.

"I have to be strong," I thought to myself. "I don't want to become depressed and be housebound like my sister. I need to fight this, whatever it is that's eating away at us. I can't give up."

Secretly the knowledge of having three blind members of our family began to eat away at the rest of my brothers and sisters who thought that they were fortunate to have avoided the curse. They started to talk about it more and when I heard them, I realised that it wasn't just the three blind members who were suffering, we all were. They found it hard to accept and they also thought that it was possible for their children to develop RP, but they were still too scared to be tested.

A few months later I decided to get away from the stress and take my children away on holiday. It wasn't much of a holiday though because it ended in disaster.

We went to Butlins, a holiday park where there are lots of activities aimed at families. It was in this country so we didn't have to travel too far. We went by train for the first part of the journey and then a short bus drive. I had taken my cane with me but refused to use it opened out (silly me!). Sometimes I carried it half open and sometimes I never carried it at all. I was back to my guessing game where I would act clumsy and guess whether there were obstacles or not.

I went swimming and everything was fine. We also took along my nephew Dyonn and he wanted to stay in the swimming pool a little longer, so I said that I would make my own way back to my room (big mistake!). On the way out, I didn't realise that I used a different door from the one we had gone in to the swimming area by. I had a rough map in my head of the route to take and where the obstacles were on the way. As I walked out of the door to proceed on my way, I tripped down some steps and fell to the floor. There were about five steps and I had literally missed them all out and tried to walk as though the ground was flat. My left ankle gave way as I stepped with my left foot. There were several people around and I heard a few laughs so I quickly picked myself up and tried to walk away as fast as possible. I had lost the feeling in my left ankle and every time I tried to take a step, I almost fell over once more. I was badly hurt but didn't want to show it in front of anyone so I stood still for a few seconds while I concentrated.

"There is no pain," I thought to myself. "You can do it. Walk away like you didn't hurt yourself."

After a few seconds I limped away hastily.

The pain was almost unbearable but I had to walk on and pretend that I was clumsy but feeling fine after my fall. When I got around a corner, away from the original crowd of people who had seen me fall, I stopped to compose myself. My left ankle was swelling up and I could feel it throbbing. After a short while I took some more steps closer to my room and then stopped again from the excruciating pain.

After another short while I walked on again until I finally made it back.

I lay on my bed in pain for hours thinking of what to do.

"You're crazy. Go to see the first aid person."

"No; I'm too embarrassed to say what happened and to say that I'm actually registered blind and should have used my cane."

"You're in a lot of pain; you have to go."

Eventually I persuaded myself to go and they said that I hadn't broken my ankle but it was badly sprained. They strapped it up with a bandage and said that I would have to rest it for a few weeks.

When I hopped back, I lay down and wondered what to do.

"I can't rest my ankle, I'm on holiday. I have to do things and go places and somehow enjoy myself."

"You've messed up your holiday now."

"I'm still going to enjoy it. I'm going out tonight and I'll just have to put up with the pain."

"Next time slow down. If you were more careful you would be fine now."

"How did I confuse the way I entered the swimming pool to the door I used to exit?"

"There are no roads and the surroundings all look the same. It was an easy mistake. Be more careful next time."

"What about when I get back to Rugby? How will I get around?"

"You can't see and you'll be walking or should I say hopping with your white cane. You're going to look like a mess."

"How humiliating. How will I be able to teach Martial Arts?"

"By hopping and guessing. You have to teach but you won't be able to kick with that ankle."

"This isn't happening to me. I came on holiday to get away from the mental torture of my family problems and now I've created another one."

"It's the risk you take from not using your cane. Your cane would have found the steps so it's your own fault."

"I know but I can't do it. I want to be normal. I don't want to have to use a cane for the rest of my life."

That night I ignored the pain and went out. Although I should have rested my ankle I hopped along to a show bar where children were allowed. This time I used my white cane and it was out at its correct length and not folded up in my hand. I was even more wary of steps now and I didn't want a repeat of the same thing. There were plenty of people already there waiting for the show to start.

"It's a bit dark in here," I said, feeling worried.

It was too dark for me to see any empty seats so I had to follow Dyonn as he guided me to one.

"How did you know where to sit?" I asked.

"Although it's a bit dark, I could still see where there were some empty seats," Dyonn answered.

We sat down and then Dyonn went to get us some drinks.

After a while the show started. The performers were dancing and singing and entertaining us. We were quite close but I could hardly see. They looked like ghosts with masks on their faces and clothes that blended in with each other so that I was unable to identify them. Dyonn kept referring to their facial expressions and commented a few times on their clothing.

"I can't see anything," I thought to myself.

Their faces looked blank. There were no eyes, noses or mouths to be seen yet Dyonn could see them all clearly. As I looked at the performers I felt a little emotional. I wanted to be able to see them too, but I couldn't.

"It's not fair, I want to see what they're doing too," I thought sadly.

"Don't get emotional, look at something else and listen to them sing or you'll feel sorry for yourself," I warned myself.

All night I kept looking in different directions every time I felt myself getting emotional from not being able to see. It worked and I managed to enjoy myself.

The next day we went out for lunch. I must admit that for the rest of the holiday I used my white cane! I was in unfamiliar territory so I didn't know where all the obstacles were. Dyonn guided me to a seat and then someone came over and handed us some menus.

"We only need one menu. I can't see to read," I advised.

A simple statement like that made me feel as though I was a failure. Then I quickly thought of something cheerful to take my mind off my problems.

After a while our food arrived and I had to be told where everything was on my plate. The lighting wasn't brilliant so everything appeared to be one pile of blurred mess. Sometimes when I looked at the food my mind would begin to wander again but then I quickly thought of something positive. I was determined to enjoy my food despite not being able to see it.

Later on that day we went to the cinema. On the way in the hall was very dark so I followed Dyonn hesitantly. He showed me to a seat and we prepared to watch the film. The screen was big and we were sitting pretty close to it but as the film got underway, it became apparent that I couldn't see what was going on. Occasionally I saw people's faces but it was like they had bigger masks on. Most things blended in and my frustration grew.

"Look how big that screen is and you still can't see it," I thought to myself.

"I really am blind. I'm a waste of space."

"You couldn't even read any of the writing and now you can't see what's going on. You may as well sit here and just listen."

I sat there for an hour and a half, listening to what was going on and trying to picture the action in my head.

"That was a good film wasn't it?" Dyonn asked, beaming widely as we emerged from the cinema.

"Well; it sounded good," I answered creatively.

A few days later I tried to play football with Dyonn. I'd never been very good at football and hadn't played for years. My nephew insisted that I try because he said that nobody knew us and I could make a fool of myself without feeling too bad.

"Like when I hurt my ankle," I thought with mirth.

It had been years since I'd played because of my lack of sight. Footballs appear to be almost magical in my eyes. They could disappear and reappear depending on the state of my blind spots.

We played for a while and I admit that I was terrible. I would sometimes kick the ball, then start running after it (or hopping) then suddenly it would disappear and I didn't know where to look. Dyonn would then run in another direction and I soon realised that the ball was somewhere else completely. Most of the time I couldn't see it and my nephew thought that I was quite amusing.

Then he put me in goal and hit the ball towards me to try and score. When the ball was low I could time it quite well and saved a few goals. He was amazed that although I could hardly see the ball, I appeared to be stopping him from scoring. He tried different ways of getting the ball past me. Then Dyonn found my weak spot and it came as quite a shock to me. He began kicking the football high over my head and every time he did so it disappeared.

"Where's it gone?" I wondered as my nephew laughed once more.

"Goal, goal!" he shouted.

"How did you do that?" I asked. "Do it again."

He kicked the football over my head and... once again it disappeared. I heard the ball in the goal behind me before it had reappeared in my eyes. My nephew had stumbled upon something quite amazing. I knew that I had blind spots but I hadn't realised the extent of them. He repeated it over and over and each time the football disappeared. It was like magic.

Although I tried to see the funny side like my nephew, it also created some negative thoughts.

"Literally everything above my eye level is invisible. I didn't realise my eyesight was that bad. Every time Dyonn made the football go above my eye level it disappeared. That's awful. Maybe I've got more tunnel vision than I realised."

"He took advantage of your weak spot. You're more disabled than you think."

"He's my nephew so it doesn't matter. I wonder how many of my friends know my weak spots when they see me from across the road. They know that I can't see them, so I wonder how many of them are ignoring me knowing that I won't see them?"

"Probably lots, but who cares? Do you want to feel sad? Do you want to get emotional again? It's too dangerous to get stressed. If you let your emotions get the better of you, then you'll eventually become depressed."

"Why am I going through so much? It's one problem after another."

"That's life, get on with it."

"Why did I have to go blind? What am I missing seeing out there? I want to see, I want my eyesight back, surely there must be a cure, there must be."

"There's no cure; you'll have to learn to accept it and live with it."

"It's so hard. Nearly everything I do uses my eyesight in one way or another. I hate my eyes."

"Stop thinking so negatively. Think of something positive or even a happy thought!"

"Like what? Like three of us are now blind?"

"No; something happier."

"It's so hard not to think of negative things."

"You have to think positive or you'll have a nervous breakdown due to emotional overload."

"I have to be emotional or people will think that I'm cold and that I have no feelings."

"You have plenty of feelings, but if you lose control you will become depressed."

The battle continued until I eventually found something else to take my mind off my problems.

On the way back home I used my white cane to search out those hidden steps. But when I arrived back in Rugby I reverted back to my old ways. I was familiar with Rugby and felt that I was safe without using my cane.

CHAPTER 23
CRYING FOR RECOGNITION

With only a week to go before I took my 4th Dan black belt exam, the pressure was really on. My ankle was still hurting a bit and the more I trained the more it hurt. I noticed that it hurt most when I spun around to kick with my right leg, twisting fast and hard with my left foot to execute a reverse kick with my right. This was one of my best techniques so I was unhappy having to avoid using this kick. The accuracy of my breaking had improved although this used to be one of my worst techniques due to my poor eyesight. My fighting skills were not improving due to the recent changes to the training hall. The hall had been divided into two because it was such a large area. Half had been converted into a good-sized gym that I used on a regular basis and the other half was where I taught Martial Arts. They had installed mirrors, improved the lighting and the floor and walls had been decorated with brighter colours. Although these changes were improvements, they caused me severe problems. The suits that we wore were white so with the bright blue walls and bright green floor, people were almost invisible to me. It was frustrating trying to fight someone who I could hardly see. They kept blending in with the background colours and I had to move around until I found an angle that I could see them from. After a few seconds they would move and disappear again so I would constantly have to try to keep them at the same angle as well as actually having to fight them.

Next I practised fighting against two black belts at the same time and a web of thoughts went through my mind.

"This is going to be difficult; they're so blurred and faint that they're blending in with the background."

"Keep them facing away from the mirror."

"Now there appear to be more than two of them. I'm confused with which blurred images to fight against. They all look the same, including their reflections in the mirror. There are four blurred people to fight."

"Turn them around so that their back is facing towards the wall."

"Now they've disappeared. Their white suits are blending in with the bright blue walls. Which way should I go to be able to see them clearer?"

"Get them away from the mirror so that you can't see their reflection."

"I see them now but they keep moving to an angle where I can't see them any more."

"Try to keep manoeuvring them back to the position where you *can* see them."

It helped a great deal to be able to see something when fighting against them. I didn't have much time to think of blocking or what techniques to employ, my main thoughts were to keep them in a position to be able to see who I was fighting against.

The practice for my exam was over and I was now on my way to the real thing. It took about two hours to get to the venue by car. Being scared of travelling fast, I was unable to relax or have a sleep during the journey. Although we got slightly lost on the way, we arrived before 9 am so we were still early.

When I entered the sports hall there were already about fifty black belts in their suits warming up. I stood and watched them for a moment.

"Wow!" I thought to myself. "Some of them are very impressive. I wonder which ones I'll be fighting against."

"They won't all be going for their 4th Dan black belt so stop worrying."

"I can't see them clearly, but some of them appear to be tall and very fast. If I could see them clearer I would know who to avoid."

My helper then found the changing room for me. The small label on the door was too blurred to read so I was glad that I had brought someone to help me. The examiners were aware that I was registered blind but I had kept it a secret from the other black belts just in case they tried to take advantage of the situation. After getting changed I made my own way back into the sports hall to practise.

After about half an hour of warming up, someone came into the sports hall to organise the order of examination. I was pleased to see that the majority of people were 1st Dan black belts. When they called for the people who were going for their 4th Dan, I lined up. There were only four of us so I was relieved to see that there wasn't too much competition. I watched them as they walked off because I wanted to try and observe them training but then I heard the names of the people who were going for their 5th Dan black belts. There were only two and I was very familiar with one of them. He had trained with me and gained his 1st Dan black belt from my instructor. Then I proceeded to observe the other black belts.

"They're good you know," I thought to myself. "Maybe this wasn't such a good idea coming here to compete against them. I'm going to get my ass kicked. They're all very good at kicking and if one of them catches me, I'm finished."

"Think positive!"

"I'm positive that they will knock me out if I don't see a kick because of my blurred vision."

"Be serious. If you could see clearer, you wouldn't be worried would you?"

"Nope; technically I'm as good as they are or I wouldn't be here."

"Then prove it. You can do it. This will be your greatest achievement if you pass your 4th Dan Masters degree."

After a while of practising my techniques over and over, the person who I had trained with approached me. He was assisting the examiners and wanted a quiet word with me.

"Hello," he said.

"Hello; nice to see you here. I didn't know that you were going for your 5th Dan black belt."

"Yes I am, but I have some bad news to tell you."

"What's happened?"

"The Grand Master doesn't want to accept your 1st Dan black belt certificate because your instructor isn't a valid member of the WTF Taekwondo organisation."

"Are you joking?"

"Sorry, but no."

"I've travelled over two hours to get here and now you're telling me that I can't proceed to the next level?"

"Yes, I'm afraid so."

I was very upset and began to take my anger out on him. I knew that he held a high position in the WTF and had the power to influence the Grand Master. I became suspicious that he was a little jealous that I had achieved so much.

"You are joking," I said. "Do you realise how hard it's been to get to this level with my limited eyesight?"

"I know about your poor eyesight," he stated.

"I'm registered blind and none of you could cope with the stress I've had to put up with to get this far. Well, I have a message for your Grand Master. Tell him that if he refuses my certificate because my instructor isn't valid, then he can dismiss yours and several other people's here that I also know gained their black belts from my instructor. Did you forget that my instructor used to be your instructor?"

"No."

"Then tell him I'm not going home and if he doesn't like what I've said then he can ask me himself and I'll tell him all about you. Just because you've changed associations from your original instructor doesn't mean that you're any better than him. What's happened to all that discipline and respect that you were taught? Don't ever put your instructor down, it's very disrespectful."

"I'll talk to him," he concluded.

Now I was even angrier. I needed to calm down. My blood was boiling and I wanted to hurt someone.

"If they agree to proceed with my application, I want to fight *him*," I said to myself. "I'm going to kick his ass and make him look dismal when going for his exam."

After a while he came back and told me that the Grand Master had agreed for me to proceed. Then I sat around, relaxing, conserving energy for my confrontation.

After a few hours we were finally called in. They had graded the 1st Dan and 2nd Dan students first and it seemed to take forever. I followed the other three people into the other grading hall because I knew that I wouldn't be able to see clearly enough to lead the way. It felt very uncomfortable having to pretend that I was shy but it felt better than feeling useless. We entered the grading hall and waited for our instructions.

We were first asked to perform patterns. There was only one of them that I was worried about performing. It involved moving my hands in slow motion while balancing on one foot for eight seconds.

Being deaf in one ear causes me to occasionally lose my balance on my left leg especially when I'm moving my hands. Also my dark vision made me feel disorientated. Knowing this in advance, I had practised it even more to eliminate the problem. My other problem was my left ankle that I had damaged a few months ago when I fell down some steps. The extra practice paid off and I was able to keep my balance.

Next, we had to do a series of techniques. The only problem I had this time was with the knife defence.

As I looked at one of the other competitors who I knew had a knife in his hand I thought, "Where *is* the knife? How am I going to defend myself against something that I can't see? The lights in the hall are off and the light from the sun shining through the windows is creating dark areas."

"You could ask him to turn around so that he's facing the light from the sun, then you'll see brighter images."

"No I can't do that. This could happen on the street at night. Maybe I should ask them to turn on the lights."

"No; you can cope. Assume that the knife is quite long and watch for when he moves his arm."

"I wish I could see better. This is going to be hard with what little vision I have left."

"Concentrate!"

It was difficult but I managed to avoid his arm and thus avoided the invisible knife. I then blocked his arm as though he had no knife in his hand.

The next section was the fighting. We had to fight one against one with another person who was taking their 4th Dan exam. We were told to get some body armour on so I knew that it was going to be full contact. I removed my glasses and prepared to start.

"I can't believe that I'm really going to do this," I thought. "Maybe I *should* ask the examiners to put on the lights in the hall."

"You'll manage. You have over fifteen years experience so you should be used to fighting in poorly-lit areas."

"But these fighters mean business. They're going to try and kick my head off. They don't know that I'm registered blind. Maybe I should tell them so that they take their time on me!"

"Concentrate; you can beat them. You're going to deserve your new black belt level."

"These guys fight in the Olympics. They're top fighters."

"Concentrate; you can do it."

The first fight began and many things went through my mind.

"He's good, very powerful."

"Hit him harder. It's full contact. Now move around so that he can't get you."

"I can hardly see what he's doing. He's blurred and sometimes invisible."

"You know what the blurred bits represent. Keep moving and guessing."

"He's almost invisible now."

"Move him towards the light so that you can see where to hit him."

The first fight was over and it was almost time for my second.

"He was good but I survived," I thought to myself.

"See; you're as good as them. Get ready for your next fight."

"This guy looks slimmer so he'll probably be faster."

"If he's faster then you need to hit him harder."

The fight began and just as I thought, he was much faster and more furious.

"He's trying to knock me out!" I thought to myself anxiously.

"He's not scared of you."

"He's faster on his feet than I am so I'll have to perform several techniques with a lot of power so as not to give him a chance to execute his techniques very often."

It worked and I was able to control the fight, but the extra power that I used wore me out.

During the last fight, I took my time slightly, moving around a great deal more and trying to regain my energy before hitting back a few times.

The fights were over and I was tired but then a group of people who were taking their 3rd Dan black belts came in. Two of them paired off with each of us.

"Two people?" I thought. "Two fighters, either one of whom could probably knock me out. I must be crazy coming here. This is going to be really hard, fighting against two people who I can hardly see."

"You'd better move around a lot because they're going to be out to get you."

"It wouldn't be so bad if I could grab and sweep them onto the floor but it's not allowed here. I'll have to control my techniques."

The fight started and they were straight in to get me.

"They're both fast so I'll use side kicks to keep them away from me," I thought cunningly.

"Keep moving around and concentrate. Any of their techniques could knock you out if you miss one due to your lack of sight."

The fight continued and I became much more tired.

"Come on!" I encouraged myself. "You can do it. Don't let them hit you. Keep moving around and pick them off one by one."

"I'm struggling to see them again. Their images are so dark and blurred that they keep going invisible."

"You can do it. You've got the experience to turn them towards the light."

"They're moving around too fast. They're a bit nifty on their feet."

"Don't give up. Concentrate."

The fight was over and then we had to fight against another two black belts. After we had finished we were excused to rest for a while in the sports hall.

"Where's the exit?" I wondered. "Everywhere looks too blurred and I can't see clearly enough."

"Don't be the first one to leave the room. Follow everyone else."

I followed them out into the other sports hall that we were allowed to rest or practise in. I went over my performance in my mind.

"That was hard. It was so difficult for me to see. They were so distorted or too dark to see. I could hardly see their hands and legs. I must be mad to be here."

"You did it. That's probably the hardest part out the way."

"I can't believe that I've just fought against other instructors and a few Olympic athletes."

"And you could hardly see them!"

"I should tell them at the end that I'm registered blind. I bet that would surprise a few of them."

"You've got to pass first."

"Some of their kicks were so fast that I had to use my instincts."

Then someone came and told us that our next fights would be against the two people going for their 5th Dan black belts.

"I'd better get my breath back," I thought wearily. "I'll be against my friend next and I want to fight him hard."

"Put him under a lot of pressure until he can't keep up."

"I still can't believe he didn't want me to grade."

"Concentrate and get your breath back."

After a while we were called back in.

They asked us to fight in pairs against them. They had already fought against some other black belts and were having their final fight against us.

"That's not fair," I moaned to myself. "I wanted to fight him on my own. I'm really disappointed now. He's got no chance against two of us. I'm not satisfied with this."

I was put against the other black belt going for his 5th Dan first.

"Now he's going to have another excuse. He's going to be tired from his first fight and it won't give me the same satisfaction battering him when he's already tired."

We bowed and the fight started.

There was a lot of aggression and plenty of noise while we fought.

"Wait for him to kick my partner then I'll kick him before he can put his foot down," I plotted. "He's finding it difficult to fight us both, he's almost running away. I don't blame him really; I would find it extremely difficult too."

"Conserve your energy for the next fight."

"He's moving so fast that he keeps disappearing from my view."

"Manoeuvre him to face the light."

"I'm struggling to position him because my partner's doing his own thing. I'll let him off. I won't pressure him too much."

I did just enough so that we controlled the fight and looked good for the examiners too.

Then came my final fight. The fight that I had been waiting hours for. We first bowed and at the same time a thought flashed through my mind.

"I wish I could see his face now, I hope he's worried."

In no time at all the fight was underway. He came straight in with some rough and powerful techniques. My partner hit him from the left and I hit him from the right so he began to back off.

"That stopped you didn't it?" I thought to myself nastily. "I'm as rough as you mate! You wait until I catch you with one of my side kicks. I want to knock you down."

Every few seconds he would hit us with some powerful techniques, then back off. I caught him a few times but he was yet to go down. After a while he began to tire and backed off even more.

"All I need to do now is get you in the right position to see you a little clearer so that I might see the expression on your face as you go down."

"You need to position him towards the light."

I kept trying to face him towards the light but I was struggling. My partner was fighting as hard as me and wasn't bothered about the light, he could see.

"Come on!" I thought excitedly. "I'm going to get you, just one kick will do. Now face towards the light!"

A few more kicks went in but still he hadn't gone down. Even I was getting tired now.

"I'm going to get you," I thought as I manoeuvred once more to force him towards the light.

I couldn't believe it. Time had run out and I hadn't been able to kick him to the ground. I was immensely disappointed.

"I'll let you off," I thought. "You're so lucky that I couldn't see clearly enough and had to have you in certain positions because you became almost invisible. I hate my eyes for that."

We were told to return to the sports hall to remove the body armour and prepare for our last section, which was breaking boards. Once again I waited for the other three people to lead the way and I followed. When we arrived we sat on the floor and got up in turn to have a go at breaking the boards. Everyone's kicking techniques went well, including mine. I was especially impressed with a few people who performed some remarkable breaking techniques. There were lots of jumping techniques to break two different boards before landing. I chose a flying side kick on two separate boards and only managed to break one. I watched carefully to work out what each blurred person was attempting to do. There were some double spinning techniques that I admit that I couldn't execute.

The last technique was a 2-inch hand break. This board was thick and tough and gave a few people trouble. Then it came to my turn.

"What technique shall I perform?" I thought to myself. "A few of them tried to impress the examiners a bit too hard and weren't successful at their breaking techniques. This is my last break so I want to succeed but at the same time I don't want to execute an easy technique. I think I'll try a reverse knife-hand strike."

I performed the reverse knife-hand strike by opening my hand and touching all my fingers together, tucking my thumb in front of the palm of my hand. Then I positioned the side of my index finger against the board so that the back of my thumb was also nearly touching the board. If this is executed incorrectly then it can be a very painful technique to perform. But if successful, it's pretty impressive. Not many people like it so I was the first here to try.

The board was set into position and I was ready to break.

"This is your last technique," I thought to myself. "You have to break this. If it breaks, then it won't hurt your hand but if it doesn't, it will hurt."

"Concentrate... now hit that board *hard*."

I paused for a few seconds while my hand was against the board, focussing my attention. Then I pulled my arm back to get as much momentum as possible and hit the board as though I wanted to hit the people holding it. My hand smashed through the board and nearly hit them too. The board was broken and I was impressed with my performance. Then I bowed and returned to my seat.

After everyone had finished their breaking techniques we sat for a few minutes while the examiners discussed our performance to make a decision on whether we had passed.

"I wonder if I've passed," I thought to myself. "I think I did pretty well. There were some excellent black belts but they all had sections that they struggled with."

"You performed as well as anyone else so if they fail you, then they had better fail some of the others too."

"It was so difficult to execute techniques that needed good eyesight."

"But you managed it. If you were to take away some of their sight, they couldn't have performed as well as you."

"I wonder if I've failed. I'm an outsider and have only been an instructor under them for a few years."

"If they fail you, don't worry about it, you know that you deserved to pass."

After a few more minutes one of the examiners began to read out the results in order of grade so I had to wait quite a long time before they finally reached the 4th Dan list.

"Here goes," I gasped.

"Vendon Wright… you passed; congratulations," an examiner said.

"Yes! I did it," I shouted in my head. "I'm an official Master, a Master of WTF Taekwondo. I achieved it and I could hardly even see. I'm impressed Mr Wright. I thought that I would get my ass kicked by a couple of the Olympic fighters but I survived. I'm the first blind Master in England!"

A big smile appeared on my face. I felt ecstatic. It felt great to finally achieve a goal that I thought wasn't possible due to my lack of sight.

After the whole event was over, I received a huge compliment. The Chief Examiner, a Grand Master from Korea at the 9th Dan black belt level, came straight over to me.

"Congratulations!" he said.

"Thank you sir."

"You were amazing. We couldn't tell that you're blind, the way that you performed, you looked just like the rest of the black belts."

"Thank you sir."

"I don't know how you cope, to train and teach without being able to see. I rely on my eyesight so much and you've achieved more than I could if I had limited vision."

"I love Martial Arts and what it does for everyone; that's what drives me to carry on teaching. I've wanted to quit many times but seeing what I'm doing for other people keeps me going. It makes me so happy to see a student go from being shy to being very confident. Without my students, I would have quit a long time ago."

"It was an honour meeting you."

"No sir, it was an honour meeting you."

I was completely taken aback to know that I was respected by probably the highest standard Martial Artist that I will ever meet.

"Wow!" I thought confidently. "He respected me for being able to get to this level? I can't believe that he wouldn't have carried on training if he was registered blind."

"Doesn't that tell you something?"

"Yes; I've got nothing else to prove. Taking this exam for my 4th Dan black belt was very hard with such limited vision. Now that I'm a Master of Taekwondo, there's nothing left to prove. I don't need to take any more exams."

"You can hang your belt up and be very proud of yourself."

In July 1997 I became the first official registered blind 4th Dan Black Belt Master of Taekwondo in England.

CHAPTER 24
DOWN BUT NOT OUT

After my eye appointment in 1999, it was obvious that my eyes were continuing to deteriorate. Although I expected to hear that they were worse, I was scared to find out by what degree.

My right eye, which I still referred to as my good eye, had deteriorated to the same extent as my left and I was no longer able to read anything from the eye test chart with either eye. So for the first test the doctor held a card with a very large letter printed on it and moved slowly towards me until I was able to focus on it. I already felt weak at the knees.

"When is this going to stop?" I thought to myself sadly. "How many more of these appointments with disappointing results am I able to cope with before I reach my limit and burst into tears?"

"It's always bad news. Every appointment that you attend clearly shows that your eyes are deteriorating constantly."

"Am I supposed to just watch my world disappear forever?"

"Yes; there's nothing that you can do about it. You're going to have to accept it and live with it."

"But I can't accept it. I don't want to go totally blind. Why do I have to go blind?"

"Change the subject. Think of something cheerful."

"There's nothing cheerful about going blind. I hate my eyes."

I became overwhelmed with emotions.

The next test showed a significant change in the amount of blind spots. They were growing and taking over my eyes. My body felt numb after that test but I managed to hold my emotions in check. However, after the next test where they put the eye drops in to dilate my eyes, the tears steamed down my face. I could hardly see without the eye drops, now it was like looking through binoculars that were extremely out of focus. There was nothing that I could recognise and I was sad and scared.

"I don't want to go totally blind," I thought to myself. "Everywhere looks so distorted that it's scaring me to look at things. Why can't I see something? Can't I see normally just for a day? It's too much to cope with not being able to see clearer."

After my final test the specialist told me the usual news about my eyes. Then she told me that she had received the results of some tests that I had undergone in London with another specialist. I was informed that I had Ushers Syndrome, which linked my eye and ear disorders. My confidence was shattered once more. She explained that Ushers Syndrome could cause you to go both deaf and blind. Then she told me that it originated in the Alps in France.

"How can this be?" I asked. "I'm not French, I'm of Jamaican origin."

"I don't understand it either, but that's the conclusion of your tests."

"I guess I'm French then."

"Nobody understands what we have," I thought to myself. "Maybe my mother was right and we are cursed."

I was then guided out of the Eye Hospital like an invalid. The tears were streaming down my face.

After I returned home, I couldn't help feeling sorry for myself. It felt like I was attending my eye appointments for the sole purpose of receiving bad news and to become emotionally drained. There was never any chance of going there for good news and so I felt useless and hopeless.

"What's the point of attending the appointments?" I thought to myself sadly. "I always come out feeling worse than when I went in."

"There's nobody to help you but you can help other people that may develop your eye disorder. They're learning a great deal from studying your eyes."

"But what about me? It's destroying me. It's taking all my strength to hold on and not allow my emotions to take over."

"You have to hold on. You can do it."

"I'm not sure that I can any more."

The constant memory of not being able to read any letters on the chart at the Eye Hospital weighed me down. Whenever I was unable to do something because of my lack of sight, the memories of the blurred chart would come flooding back.

Although I had specialist equipment to help me at work, my struggles continued. Part of my job was to help other people on their computers but I was unable to see clearly enough to help them efficiently. Most of the time I stood beside people picturing what was on their screens in my mind and then tried to help them from memory. It was working less and less and I was beginning to make too many mistakes. The tasks that I was struggling with began to build up and I was having difficulty coping with the stress it was causing me.

"Why couldn't I see the yellow on that student's screen? He said that it was in plain view."

"You're blind and no longer any use to people at work."

"I can do it. I'll learn to cope by adapting my teaching methods."

"Until when? Just face it; you can no longer cope. You need your eyes to work in this field and they're just not working for you."

"My boss is compassionate; they'll buy more equipment to help me."

"It's not them; it's you that's the problem. You feel useless and incapable of doing your job efficiently now."

"I'm hopeless."

I struggled but eventually found ways of coping.

A short while later my boss left and she was replaced with someone who I felt was less compassionate and understanding. Although he was told that I was registered blind, he urged me to do more difficult jobs. He asked me to read all the serial numbers of the computers myself even though I told him that I physically wouldn't be able to do it, but that I had prefects who could help me. He seemed to ignore my disability; he wanted me to do the job myself. After a short while he even took away my prefects so I had nobody to help me do the difficult jobs. There were many tasks that I was asked to perform and my job became too much again. I felt as though he was ignoring my disability and wanted me to do my job or leave. The pressure was on and a job that I had previously looked forward to doing became a nightmare – it became an extra strain on my mind and added to my problems. We argued and almost came to blows but he was my boss and had the power to influence other managers. After a while I felt as though I had to drag myself into work every day – I no longer looked forward to going there.

Around this time my sisters added to my emotional strain. Angela found a lump and was worried so she asked my other sister Carline to accompany her to the hospital for tests. Angela was fortunate and the lump turned out to be benign. While in the hospital, Carline decided that she might as well undergo tests too. She was less fortunate and was diagnosed with cancer. When she told us we were devastated. We couldn't believe that Angela was fine but Carline had cancer. It added to my growing depression and I was slowly becoming superstitious. For years my mother had said that someone back in Jamaica must have cursed us, but I never believed her. With the growing problems my family were experiencing, I was beginning to change my opinion.

Not being able to perform my job efficiently and the growing problems my family were experiencing finally became too much for me. My negative thoughts overpowered me and I had to make an appointment with my doctor. After I explained my feelings he decided to sign me off work with depression. He hoped that the break from my stress of not being able to cope with my job would relax me enough to put me in a more positive frame of mind.

A week soon became a month and I had not returned to work. I was still showing no signs of improvement and sank further into depression.

"I'm hopeless," I thought to myself pathetically. "I can't see clearly enough to do my job."

"Well you tried. There's only a certain amount of pressure anyone can take before they crack. You've reached your limit."

"And I used to think that I was so strong."

"Not any more."

There were no words of encouragement in my mind and I sank deeper and deeper.

"Why can't I see clearer?" I thought sadly. "I want to see more. Everywhere is so blurred and I hate it. I hate my eyes. Why are they so useless? It's so hard to keep concentrating so much to be able to see. My eyes hurt from the pressure and everywhere appears so cloudy; this is pathetic. How is someone supposed to remain happy seeing what I see through my eyes? I give up; I can't cope any more. What's the point with struggling to work with my crap eyesight? My boss doesn't seem to care that I can't see. He seems to be purposely giving me tasks to do that he knows I can't perform – he's trying to get rid of me. I feel useless and it's all because of my eyesight. I give up trying. I'm going to stay home and suffer by myself."

It got to the point where I was hardly able to leave my house. I had to get one of my assistant black belts to teach my Martial Arts classes and I could no longer be bothered to train at the gym. I was a nervous wreck.

My doctor noticed the change in my personality and referred me to a psychiatric therapist. Sometimes I would attend my appointments and not smile or take off my hat, or even unzip my coat. I no longer cared about anything or anyone. I was clinically depressed. The one thing that I'd been trying so hard to avoid for so many years had finally won. Sometimes I would sit in almost silence and other times I would say a few words but my therapist slowly got me to open up and admit what was wrong.

"How are you today?" my therapist asked.

"Fine."

"Do you work?"

"Yes."

"What do you do?"

"I'm a Computer Technician."

"Do you enjoy your job?"

"I used to but I don't care about it any more."

"Why?"

"Because I can't see enough to do it properly any more."

"Does your boss know about your eyes?"

"Yes, but he doesn't seem to care. I feel as though he's putting too much pressure on me to perform tasks that he knows I'm unable to do. I don't think he likes me or blind people. I think he's trying to get rid of me – force me to resign."

"Is your eyesight that bad?"

"Yes; I'm registered blind and I hate my eyes. I can't see to do anything."

My therapist was very smart and at first she didn't refer to my eyesight much. She would ask a few more questions each month until she found things that I enjoyed talking about – something to relight the positive fire that had accidentally been extinguished.

"Have you any children?" she asked.

"Two."

"Boys or girls?"

"Two girls."

"How do you cope with two girls? With all those hormones running around your house, I bet you feel terrified! You're very brave being the only male!"

"Yes; they are scary. They get the better of me and I feel like I'm never right. They get in silly moods and are so difficult to work out."

"But I bet that you love them."

"Yes; even though they can be a handful, I enjoy having them around."

As time went on, I became more relaxed about sharing my thoughts and problems with her. Several months had gone by and I was still not well enough to return to work.

"I bet your children keep you busy?" she asked.

"They're quite a handful. My eldest demands a lot of attention but my youngest finds her own ways to entertain herself."

"Have you got any hobbies?"

"I used to do Martial Arts."

"Which one? How long did you do it for?"

"Taekwondo and for about eighteen years."

"I'm impressed! That's a very long time."

"I taught it too."

"You must be very good."

"Not as good as I'd like to be."

"Why not?"

"Because my eyesight is so poor that I struggle with everything."

I felt more emotional thinking of my sight loss but she still slowly squeezed it out of me.

"What level are you?"

"I'm a 4th Dan Master."

"Why stop now? You've already achieved a level most normal sighted people would struggle to gain. Do you enjoy it?"

"Yes; I used to love it but I haven't got the strength to teach it any more."

"Why not go and watch once a week. You don't need to teach, just be there where you used to feel comfortable. If you don't feel up to it that's fine but there's no harm watching."

"I might try it one day."

After a while I began to watch my assistants teaching but still didn't feel comfortable. She was yet to find out how to cure me.

"How do you feel about work?"

"Whenever I think about how hopeless I am at work I feel more stressed."

"What is it about work that you don't like?"

"It reminds me too much of how useless my eyes are. Nearly every moment that I'm at work I think about a task that I can no longer do because of my eyes. It's so hard. I don't want to be blind. I'm struggling so much at work. I feel that I'm not getting enough support from my boss and he's making me feel more of a failure. I'm under so much pressure that I can't take it any more."

"What about having someone guide you and assist you with your job?"

"I can't do that, I've tried to imagine it but I can't bring myself to accept help. I want to be independent and not look like an invalid and I don't think that my boss would help anyway."

My therapist tried several different ways to help me out of my depression. When she realised that she had exhausted all her outlets to help me back to work she decided to ask me a few crucial questions.

"How would you feel returning to your job part-time?" she asked.

"That would make me feel even more like a failure. Every time I imagine myself there, in certain situations, and not being able to see clearly enough, it makes me feel like disappearing under a rock, never to be seen again. I can't do it; I can't face my job any more."

"Deep down in your heart, what are you feeling?"

"I would feel better if I never had the stress of my job to think about. The constant reminder that I'm a failure is haunting me. I'm not sure if I can ever face going back. Every time I looked at someone there, I would be thinking that they're wondering why I even come into work if I'm no longer capable of doing anything. They all know that I'm hopeless. They probably talk about my poor performance in the staff room. I can't face them any more."

"Go home and think about it and next time we meet you can decide what choices you have."

At my next monthly appointment, now over six months after my therapy started, I finally gave my decision about my job.

"So, how are you?" she asked.

"Fine," I replied.

"Have you trained yet?"

"I've watched a few Martial Arts classes but I haven't returned to the gym."

"Why not try the gym once and see how you feel?"

"I don't feel like doing anything. Sometimes I don't even feel like getting out of bed. I used to be such a morning person but now I can't be bothered. I don't like seeing things or looking at people any more. I prefer to close my eyes so that I don't see all the distorted images. It upsets me when I realise how bad my eyesight really is and I hate talking about it, that's when I feel worst. I wish I could see. I wish that I could see what everyone else sees."

She then started on my vision and slowly opened my eyes as I started to dream build again.

"Wouldn't it be great if they found a cure?"

"Oh yeah; I would be so happy."

"What would you do?"

"I would admire flowers, birds and trees. Study the details of things. Maybe become a photographer and admire the details of photographs. It would be great to see what my children really look like. I'd give up my job and become a taxi driver. It would be so great being able to drive."

"Do you like travelling?"

"I'd love to be able to travel, even travel alone but it's too difficult when you can't see. I would need a guide and that would remind me of my disability."

"Where would you go if you could see better?"

"I'd love to visit my friend Jean-Seb in France or my family in Jamaica. I'd also like to go to Spain."

"Have you ever been on an aeroplane?"

"No; it makes me nervous not being able to see where I'm going – and all those steps, and I'm scared of travelling fast."

"What else would make you feel happier?"

"I no longer like where I'm living and would love to move house."

She knew that I was feeling much more relaxed so she finally asked about my stressful job. It was obvious that it was the main cause of my depression and it was time to decide whether to give it up so that my health could improve.

"What about work? Have you made any decisions?"

"I would feel less useless if I didn't have to go there day after day struggling to see. The constant reminders of how incapable I am are draining me. Maybe I would be better off not working there any more. Maybe I would feel better in myself not having the pressure to perform in front of so many people."

I resigned from work and returned for my next appointment with my counsellor.

"How do you feel today?" she asked.

"Fine."

"Do you feel any better now that you've resigned from your job?"

"Yes; I feel as though a weight has been lifted off my shoulders."

"Are you up to talking more about your eyes? If you feel uncomfortable we can stop at any time and resume next time."

"I'll try. At least I don't have to worry all day about not being able to work up to standard because of my deteriorating eyesight."

"How are your children?"

"They're fine. They keep me going because they're very funny."

"What funny things have they done?"

"I could write a book on the excuses my eldest daughter Michaela uses for not going to bed. She comes back downstairs after being sent to bed and says that her nose isn't working. A few minutes later she comes back down again and says; 'Night night, love you, see you in the morning. Night night, love you.' Then she comes back down for a drink, then to bring the cup back down, then to ask for a tissue, then she thinks that her nose is bleeding, and then she wants the nail clippers to cut her fingernails. She uses so many excuses that she makes me laugh."

"What about your younger child?"

"She makes me laugh too. Jasmine played a game called 'I spy with my little eye' and we had to guess what she was thinking of that was in our living room. She said that it began with 'H' and we went through everything in the room but couldn't guess it. When we gave in and asked her to tell us, she pointed to the rug on the floor and said 'Hug!' – she thought that a rug was really called a hug!"

"Well it's nice to see you smile. You need to think of things to cheer you up. Have you been out with your friends lately?"

"I can't be bothered to go out any more. It's too hard getting around when everything is so cloudy and distorted."

"Have you tried going back to the gym?"

"No; I don't feel like I've got the energy to go."

"Maybe you'll feel like you have more energy after you go. Why not try it?"

"OK, I'll try."

After a week or so I forced myself to go to the gym. I wasn't in the mood for training and didn't want to do anything but I was willing to listen to the positive advice I was given. Once I got started it became easier. First I tried one exercise machine, then thought that I may as well try another and soon I felt energy returning to my body. Before I knew it I had been at the gym for more than an hour and was enjoying myself again. Some positive thoughts returned to my mind.

"That felt great. I didn't even want to come to the gym but once I got here and did something, I didn't want to stop. I'd forgotten how great this feeling is."

At my next counselling session I was much more cheerful and almost back to my old self.

"Good morning," I said.

"Well, you look a bit more cheerful today. What have you done to make yourself smile?" she asked.

"I forced myself to go to the gym and I felt much better. I really didn't want to go but because you advised me to try it, I did and it worked."

"I'm glad. Now don't overdo it, but keep going. Maybe just once a week for a while until you feel like going more often."

"Thanks for the advice."

"How are things at home?"

"Terrible. I'm becoming obsessed with everything."

"Like what?"

"Like making sure that the kitchen worktops are always clear – making sure that things are straight and hygienically clean. I'm always wiping my shoes on every mat I come across, including when I'm walking in and out of shops, to make sure that they're clean and haven't got dog muck on them. I even wipe my feet before entering the shopping centre. Sometimes I smell dog muck all the time in the air but part of me knows that it's just in my mind. I'm becoming too obsessed and I don't know why."

"What else are you doing that you feel is obsessive?"

"Washing my hands. Nearly every time I touch something I wash my hands. I can't help it. I now sit down to have a wee on the toilet because I'm worried that I will wee on the floor if I stand up."

"Why do you think that you're doing this?"

"I don't know."

"Why do you wash your hands?"

"To clean them."

"Then why do you think that they've become dirty again?"

I paused and thought.

"Because they might still have germs on and I can't see clearly enough to be sure so I wash my hands again," I answered.

"Why do you like your kitchen surfaces clean and clear from clutter?"

"Because you shouldn't leave a mess in the kitchen."

"But the mess does no real harm does it?"

"Yes! I might knock something over and I don't want to break anything because it will make me feel useless not being able to see it."

Although it should have been obvious to me, I didn't realise that I had become obsessed with everything due to my failing eyesight. I was trying to organise things so that I wouldn't accidentally knock them over. Because I couldn't see marks and stains from all sorts of things, I would wash my hands repeatedly to make sure that they were clean. This also applied to wiping my feet obsessively. It was almost impossible for me to see whether I had trodden in something nasty so I wiped my feet over and over again to make sure. As my therapist went on she helped me find reasons for more of my obsessions.

"Your deteriorating eyesight is the main cause of your Obsessive-Compulsive Disorder and you need to learn to deal with it," she said.

"I can't stop; I'm obsessed and out of control."

"Accept that your eyes are the main cause and if they were better then you wouldn't have to worry as much about trivial things."

"So I need to learn to control my OCD?"

"Yes."

As time went on I slowly began to get back on my feet. Going to the gym once a week became twice a week and then before I knew it I was training regularly again. The more I trained the more my energy levels went up. I was now back at the gym several times a week and back to teaching Martial Arts.

At my next counselling session I was very relaxed when talking about my problems.

"How are things going?" my therapist asked.

"Much better. I'm training regularly and feel quite positive again."

"What are you going to do during the daytime?"

"I think I'll return to college and study. I like teaching so maybe I'll study to become a Computer Teacher or a Fitness Instructor."

"It's nice to hear you talking positively again."

"The less I do the more I think of my lack of eyesight and the problems it causes me. I feel much better keeping myself busy. When I get negative thoughts I try to think of something to cheer myself up again."

"That's great. How are your eyes?"

"Terrible, but that's life! I'm getting used to accepting my poor sight but what I struggle with is telling people that I'm registered blind. I hate using that phrase and it makes me feel emotional and incompetent so I avoid using it."

"You're going to have to learn to accept that too."

"I know, but it's so hard. I use all my energy telling some of my friends that I'm registered blind but then some of them forget or ask too many questions and it make me feel emotional so I avoid it by just saying that I have poor eyesight. I can cope with that but I can't cope with using the word 'blind'. I guess I'm in denial but I want to avoid being depressed again so I think that I'll avoid using that word whenever I can."

"Why not carry your cane?"

"I do sometimes but it makes me feel so vulnerable. I know I need to use it more often and I know that I need to tell people that I'm blind but they should also learn to be more considerate to disabled people. I was talking to a friend the other day and she asked me if I knew who she was. She hadn't told me her name so I assumed that it was someone who didn't know about my eyesight. After I told her that I had very poor vision and couldn't see, she replied that she already knew. Now why didn't she just tell me her name in the first place instead of highlighting my disability?"

"Some people don't think before they speak – they don't mean to be rude."

"Well it hurt me and I felt uncomfortable having to explain my visual impairment again. That's why I don't like to tell people that I'm blind because some of them forget after a few weeks or months and I don't see why I should suffer the humiliation of explaining it again. Other than that, I'm fine!"

"Don't feel pressured to have to tell everyone. It's up to you. If you want, tell people that you would rather not talk about it."

"I really don't like talking about it because I feel uncomfortable showing my emotions in front of people. Most of the time I can think of cheerful memories that drown out my negative thoughts but when people ask me to talk about what I see or tell me how much more they can see, I feel useless and struggle to contain my emotions."

Then came the news that I'd been waiting for.

"It sounds like you have a firm grip on life again," she said.

"Yes; there will be times when I'll be down but I'll bounce back. I keep telling myself that there are people out there worse off than me. That makes me feel more fortunate again."

"I can say that you're no longer depressed."

"Thanks!" I said ecstatically.

"If you ever feel that you're getting down again, please don't leave it too late to make another appointment. Don't wait until you're too low because that's when you won't want to listen to other people's advice that will help you."

"Thank you for helping me get back on my feet to face the challenges of life."

I left my therapist and returned home. For several months I had suffered from clinical depression but now, I was back!

CHAPTER 25
CHARLIE'S ANGELS

In 2000, I managed to move house and now live at 93 Grosvenor Road in Rugby. It's a three-bedroom house with two reception rooms downstairs. One is the living room and the second I use as a computer room. At the back of the house there was a small kitchen with two more small rooms behind it. The house was in need of serious work. We knocked down the walls behind the kitchen to make one big kitchen, then we had the house rewired and a new central heating system put in. It took a little time but it looks great now.

Feeling more cheerful I went and enrolled on a college course. I decided to train to become a Computer Help Desk Specialist and learn all I could about the different software packages. I was told to enter the course on the higher level because of my previous skills. The teacher said that I would first be taught a few things that I already knew and used to teach when I was working fulltime, but would soon progress to the stages where the course could help me. Although it felt difficult I informed them of my disability. After specifying what equipment I would need to attend the course, I returned home and looked forward to studying again.

On my first day I entered the classroom and was shown to a computer. When I sat in front of it I noticed that there wasn't a keyboard with large letters on like I had requested prior to enrolling on the course. After a few discussions, I was sent home for two weeks while I waited for the college to organise their equipment. I wasn't too worried about missing out on two weeks since I already knew the things that they would be covering during those weeks, but when I returned to the course, it took half the lesson for them to find the keyboard. Then came my next problem. I had a keyboard that had large letters and a lamp to make everywhere brighter, but they hadn't installed a magnification program to make the letters on the screen bigger as I'd requested prior to the course! I felt awful and humiliated. There was a class full of people watching me struggle like an invalid, yet with the correct equipment, I was worthy of teaching the course. I felt like a special needs person who was not being assisted. The lack of equipment made me miss out on assignments. It took another few weeks for them to organise the equipment and I had to stay at home during this time… again! I still wasn't too bothered because it gave me a chance to practise on my computer at home, which had large labels on the keyboard and magnification software.

After a month or so, I returned to the computer course and was relieved to see some of the equipment that I needed. The teacher was now starting to teach work from a textbook and the writing was too small for me to read. They offered to enlarge the manual while we waited for the arrival of a CCTV magnification book reader, but the text was not bold enough for me to read. I returned home (again!) for another month, waiting in anticipation. Frustration began to set in.

"How have other visually impaired people managed to study at the college?" I asked myself. "It's taking weeks for them to purchase equipment that should have already been available. I'm capable of studying this course without any problems if they had the equipment that I need. I'm beginning to lose interest in it now because it's causing so much trouble and it's humiliating."

When I returned to college and saw all the equipment that I needed, I soon got on with my work. I resolved to try my best to catch up on the work that I'd missed, but then the teacher came to see me.

"I'm afraid that you're too far behind and you won't be able to catch up on the missed assignments. You'll have to enrol on this course next year."

"Next year?" I answered furiously. "I am not going to wait another year to do this course. It's not my fault that the college didn't have the equipment to aid visually impaired people with their education."

"It wouldn't be fair on the other students because you would need my assistance to help you catch up."

"I don't need your help. I'm very familiar with most of the packages and can work on my own. I'm here for an up-to-date qualification."

"I've been told that you have to enrol next year."

This was exceedingly unfair and I felt very angry.

"I'm not waiting another year because of your incompetence. Why don't I just sit the exam? I used to teach ICT and need the certificate to prove it."

"Sorry, I can't allow you to sit the exam without taking the course."

The teacher wouldn't change his mind and I had to return home. Many thoughts came to my mind that day.

"Why me? Why do I have to be blind? Why do I have to have a disability that hinders everything I try to do?"

"You could have *taught* that course and now you feel like you were pushed to the bottom of the class."

"It was so humiliating to be treated like that. Now I feel hopeless again. Having poor eyesight makes me feel so useless and no good for anything. At this rate, I'll never get another job."

"You'll find a way."

"I should complain about how I was treated. Visually impaired people won't be encouraged to attend college if they haven't got the right equipment to help them."

"What's the point of complaining? Forget them and get on with your life."

"It made me feel as though I know nothing about computers yet I've been working in that field for ten years. How do other blind people cope?"

"You'll always run into obstacles. Be prepared next time."

"There won't be a next time. I don't want to return to college knowing that they think so little about the visually impaired."

It was a difficult moment in my life that drew me close to depression once again. I had to fight off the negative thoughts. Although I managed to avoid becoming depressed I still lost interest in a lot of things and needed more motivation.

Then came my guardian angel. My friend Charlie came to save me from sinking too low. He called around to see if he could persuade me to go out.

"I hear you're feeling a little down at the moment?" he said.

"Yep. I can't go to college because of my failing eyesight. I feel so hopeless."

I became emotional but there were no tears. Anger was mixed in with my feelings of dissatisfaction.

"Let's go out for a beer," Charlie suggested.

"I can't be bothered. I'm not up to socialising yet."

"Why not?"

"Everything looks too dark and depressing. It's so difficult to recognise my friends with my blurred vision."

"I'll help you and tell you who they are."

"Maybe another day."

"Come on; let's go out, I want to party and cheer you up."

"I don't feel like partying."

After a while Charlie realised that he needed to try a different approach.

"I know what will excite you and bring a smile back to your face," Charlie said enticingly.

"What?" I asked curiously.

"I know what you need. I'm sure that it'll bring a smile back to your face."

"Tell me then!" I pleaded.

"I'm going to take you to a pole dancing club. I guarantee that you will smile."

"I'm not going to a pole dancing club! Anyway, I won't be able to see much."

"I've been told that they come so close to you that they almost touch you! I bet you will be able to see something and anyway, we'll be having fun. Come on, let's go."

I took a few moments to think about it.

"It might not be bright enough so I probably won't be able to see anything."

"Let's just give it a try and if you can't see then we'll leave early and return home. Come on, let's do it! Come on, it's different from clubbing in a nightclub and maybe that's what you need to cheer yourself up."

"Oh, all right then," I answered, my curiosity getting the better of me.

We prepared ourselves, I combed my short hair and off we went.

We arrived at about 10 pm. The club was called 'Legs 11'. I'd never been to a club like that before and wasn't sure what to expect. As we walked through the entrance we were met with a dazzling display. Gorgeous women of all nationalities were walking around looking beautiful. Charlie struggled to compose himself but I was yet to see anyone in great detail and find out what all the excitement was about.

There were about twenty beautiful women dressed in glamorous outfits similar to what women would wear in some nightclubs but maybe slightly sexier. Some of them had trousers with slits all the way up their legs and others had sexy short skirts on. That's what Charlie told me but I couldn't quite see clearly enough… yet! There were about thirty men sitting around drinking and I bet smiling too! As I looked around I wasn't sure whether I would stay because the lighting was similar to a nightclub and that meant there were dark areas. The women were too far away from me so they still had ghostly appearances. Then out of nowhere a glamorous lady came up to me.

"Hi there; would you like a dance?" she asked sensually.

She was standing so close to me that I could see her. Obviously not in as much detail as my fortunate friend Charlie, but clear enough! She brought a smile to my face.

"I've only just got here. Come back in a few minutes after I've got myself a drink," I answered shyly.

After agreeing, the young lady walked elegantly away.

"What do you think so far then?" asked Charlie.

"Well; I wasn't expecting them to be so brave and approach us first. She was beautiful and very pleasant."

"Will you have a dance from her?"

"I don't know; I'm shy so she'll have to ask me again. Why don't you go first?" I suggested.

"I'll have a dance later," Charlie answered.

She was in my mind as we waited to get served at the bar. She was dressed in a gorgeous little black dress and knee length boots. Her hair was long, dark and wavy. From what I saw, she was a very pretty lady. We took our drinks with us as we went to find somewhere to sit and chat.

We picked an area that was quite bright and under a spot light.

"There's someone pole dancing over there," Charlie said with a cunning smile.

"Where?" I asked curiously.

"In the distance, to your left."

Unfortunately she wasn't very clear to me. I was only able to see a ghostly figure dancing around the pole. It was brightly lit but too far away from me to see clearly.

"I bet you can see her in detail can't you?" I asked.

"Yes; would you like me to describe what she's doing?"

"Yes please!" I thought to myself. "He might make me feel too jealous so I'd better say no."

"No thanks," I answered. "I'll use my imagin-ation!"

After a while Charlie squeezed my arm.

"What's wrong?" I asked.

"That woman's coming back over," he said excitedly.

"Really?" I replied nervously.

"Yes; she's approaching from your left."

"What shall I do?"

"Ask her for a dance!"

I took a quick sip of my drink. It was a soft drink and nothing that would get me drunk.

"No, I can't! I'm a chicken!" I whispered.

"Too late, here she is," said Charlie.

As I looked I saw this ghostly figure coming closer and her outline soon became much clearer. Closer she came until she was standing right in front of me. Her details soon became more apparent.

"Wow; she's beautiful," I thought to myself. "She's… stunning."

"Hello again," she said.

"Hello," I replied nervously.

"So are you ready for your dance yet?"

I paused before replying.

"Err, not quite yet."

"OK, no problem."

She then sat down on the other side of me to where my friend Charlie was sitting. I grew even more nervous. I didn't know what to expect and would have preferred it if Charlie had a dance first. We had chosen a good place to sit and the light in that area was reflecting off her face.

"So what's your name?" she asked.

A cunning thought came into my mind.

"I don't want to use my real name. It's too unusual and I don't want anyone to remember it."

"My name is… Eddie," I replied craftily.

"Hi Eddie, I'm Rachel."

"I bet she's using a false name too," I thought to myself.
"You've never been here before have you?" Rachel asked.
"No; this is my first time."
"I can tell because you're very tense. Try to relax. Where're you from?"
"Maybe I shouldn't tell her where I'm from either," I thought.
"Coventry," I replied.
"What do you do for a living?"
"I'm a Computer Technician."

Before long, we were sitting having a general conversation but I was still nervous because I wanted her to dance for me but I didn't really know what to expect.

"She's stunning and has a great personality," I kept thinking to myself.

Charlie kept nudging me to urge me to ask her for a dance but I didn't know how to ask.

"Are you ready now?" Rachel asked.
"Yes," I replied joyfully.
"Come with me over there."

She got to her feet, held my hand and led me to a room at the side of the dance floor. There were several bouncers waiting outside the room. We went in and I saw several seats, most of which had men already sitting on them. The men were laughing and enjoying themselves because they had a dancer performing for them already.

"Where would you like to sit?" Rachel asked.

I looked around for the brightest area.

"Over there," I replied.

She walked me to a chair and I sat down.

The chair was leather and very comfortable. As I sat there I could still see some of the other men with their dancers.

"Amazing!" I thought to myself. "Those men are so lucky. Those women are beautiful too and very sexy dancers."

"Put your hands to your side and no touching! Now open your legs," Rachel commanded provocatively.

I sat in silence, nervous but curious. She spoke to me for a short moment and said that she was waiting for the beginning of the next song and then she would start dancing. I sat in anticipation. Then before I knew it, the next record had started and she was now standing right in front of me.

"Here goes," I thought to myself.

She stood there dancing similar to but more sexy than women dance in nightclubs.

"Wow! My own private dancer," I thought happily.

Then out of the corner of my eye I thought I saw another dancer take her top off and I turned my head to look.

"Maybe I should be over there," I wondered to myself.

Rachel saw me looking at someone else and grabbed my chin and faced me towards her again.

"Keep your eyes on me!"

She continued dancing and after a short while she sat on me and then lay in my arms.

"I'm in love!" I thought to myself.

Then she got up and bent down so that her bum was facing me. She lifted up part of her dress to reveal her bum.

"Now I really do wish that I could see more clearly."

She then slapped her bum with one of her hands and I struggled to refrain from bursting out with laughter and excitement. At that moment I was extremely happy and had the biggest smile on my face.

Then she stood back up and lifted one of her legs up into the splits and placed her foot on my chair at the side of my head. I wanted her to stay like that forever, but then she brought her foot back to the floor and carried on dancing. She moved her face close to mine. Her lips were nearly touching my lips. Then she moved her head around so that her hair went into my face.

"This is exciting!" I thought to myself as she began to strip but then the record ended! She got dressed again. I was still sitting there, frozen, with a permanent smile on my face.

"Did you enjoy that?" she asked.

"Oh yes; you're the best," I answered.

"Thank you."

"When I came here I was slightly depressed but now... I'm gratified. You've made my day and cheered me up. This is a very happy moment in my life that I will never forget. Thank you."

She held my hand and took me back to Charlie. After I told him how much fun it was, he went off with a few private dancers himself.

Then at midnight all the dancers disappeared and emerged ten minutes later in different sexy outfits. There was a cowgirl with a hat on, an angel, a policewoman, a nurse and even a French maid. They were gorgeous and I couldn't resist asking the French maid for a dance, as that was my favourite fantasy and that night, I was fulfilled. To my surprise, Rachel came back over to me later and we sat talking for ages. I was very flattered. She cheered me up and I felt comfortable sitting with her. That night I didn't felt useless or hopeless at all – I felt excited!

After that night, as time went on, I would sometimes think of how happy I felt at the lap dance club. It always brought a smile to my face and was a special thought that always cheered me up when I felt a little down. My friend Charlie calls me sometimes and if he thinks that I'm in need of cheering up, he finds something to say that will make me laugh. Sometimes it would be as simple as saying that we should go and play Bingo because my lucky number is eleven. It helped me to overcome some more difficult times in my life and I will always remember the warm feeling that it gave me.

Feeling more outgoing, I decided to respond to a request to have my Martial Arts club travel to Germany for a friendly competition. Rugby twins with a town called Ruesselsheim in Germany and we agreed to represent the Martial Arts in the sports twinning. Previously I had travelled there by boat but this time my students wanted to go by aeroplane. I had to overcome my fear of flying to be able to go. I'd never been on an aeroplane before – I'd always been afraid of the speed.

"I can't do this," I thought to myself. "I'm afraid that it will go too fast and crash."

"Flying is safe. You can do it."

"Why can't we travel by boat?"

"Your students want to fly and you can't let them down."

Finally I agreed to travel by aeroplane and I booked our tickets.

All was arranged and we set off. There were twelve of us and we travelled in three cars to London. Then we left our cars in a short stay car park where they could remain for the four days that we would be away. As soon as we arrived the questions started. I had only told certain people about the extent of my disability so there were a few students who didn't know. As I stepped out of the car into unknown territory, I opened my cane to its full length.

"What's that for?" a student asked.

"I've got very poor eyesight and I need to use this sometimes."

"How bad are your eyes?"

"Here we go with the questions," I thought to myself. "I hate all these questions. They make me feel so incapable."

"I'm partially sighted," I replied.

"How can you see to teach us?"

"That's it," I thought, "I've had enough questions now."

"I'm used to it and I know all the moves off by heart," I replied calmly, managing to retain my composure.

"What are the red stripes for?"

"I'm deaf in one ear."

"Now I feel embarrassed to have had to admit that as well," I thought in disappointment.

We made our way to the shuttle bus where we lined up to get on. Although I had my cane, people were still pushing in front of me to get on the bus. They even pushed in front of children.

"Many people don't even have the manners to let children and disabled people on first," I thought. "They're so ignorant and inconsiderate. It's like my cane is invisible."

I had to stand on the bus all the way to the airport. One of my students who was already aware of my disability helped me manoeuvre around objects and guided me up and down steps.

"This is a little embarrassing," I thought, "I'm the Instructor yet I'm the one being guided like an invalid."

We booked in and went to wait in the bar area.

I had a beer, or two, and chatted with a few students. By now most of them had separated and gone to look in the various shops. We spoke about my fears of flying and they tried their best to assure me that I would be fine. We weren't quite sure how it happened but after a while we heard our names being called on the loud speaker. The voice said that it was the last call for our flight. We must have been sitting drinking beer for longer than we thought, we'd checked in but not gone through to the secure area where they scan for weapons.

We jumped up and rushed towards the gate. It was a long distance away and it took us several minutes to get there. I was being dragged at the same time as being told to watch my step. If I'd been able to see, we could have run much faster so I was slowing us down. Now we began to panic. When we got to the gate we spoke to a security officer and he told us that we were too late to board our flight so my students casually blamed it on me. They told the security officer that I had got lost and they were looking for me. They rambled on with their story and I stood there innocently. The security guard radioed in to the captain and relayed our story. Somehow we were able to make them feel compassionate towards me and they let us in. My students guided me at the steps and we entered the aeroplane. As we walked down the aisle to find a seat, everyone on the plane began to clap and cheered us as we made our way to our seats. It was a very embarrassing moment!

As I got strapped in, the excitement of rushing to catch our flight wore off and I remembered that I was afraid of flying. Gradually I began to get nervous again. Just then, a young lady airhostess came to my rescue. She was stunning (even though I shouldn't have been looking).

"Would you like any assistance when we arrive at Frankfurt-Hahn?" she asked.

"My students can help me," I thought to myself, "but I'd prefer you to!"

"Yes please," I answered hastily.

The engines started up and the aeroplane began to move as it taxied into position at the start of the runway. After a while it began to speed up.

"Hold on tight," the student sitting next to me advised.

"Why?"

"It's going to accelerate at great speed in a moment."

I closed my eyes and prayed. The engine noise increased to a roar as the plane began to accelerate and my head was thrown back with the force. It felt like a rocket. My heart was pumping hard and I was very scared. Then it lifted off the ground and I became frantic. After a moment or two we levelled out, the engine noise subsided a bit and all was calm.

"That wasn't so bad was it?" the student asked.

"I didn't think that we'd make it. It felt like we weren't going fast enough to take off. It was exciting but scary all at the same time."

After two hours we prepared for landing. This felt worse than the take off. The aeroplane was shaking violently and I was praying again. The plane leaned from left to right as it prepared to land. It seemed to take forever to touch the ground and I wasn't sure how much more excitement I could take. I wanted my feet back on solid ground and to get out of there. Then things felt even worse. The aeroplane touched down and now the runway felt too rough and we shook even more. I thought that it would never stop, but just as I began to feel hysterical, everywhere went calm again and we travelled slowly towards the terminal. Landing was one of the scariest experiences I'd ever had. I felt like we would run out of space to be able to slow down.

Then that gorgeous young lady came back and I glowed with happiness. She asked me to remain in my seat until everyone had left. As the last few people were disappearing out of the plane, she linked my arm as though we were married and walked me to the exit. I was ecstatic. It was too hard to hold back a big smile on my face but my moment of pleasure was cut short. At the top of the plane's steps a man was waiting to take over from the airhostess and help me into the terminal. I was so disappointed but it had been fun while it lasted. He took me to a buggy and drove me into the baggage claim area. As we passed some of my students, I heard them laughing. They found it funny that I'd got a male assistant instead of a female one. He found my bag for me and helped me carry it until my students stopped laughing and took over. I was very impressed with the service at Frankfurt-Hahn Airport.

Then we caught a bus to another airport called Frankfurt Flughafen.

This is classed as one of the busiest airports in the world. We then went looking for our German friends and found a group of them waiting for us. There was Angela, Thorsten and their instructor, Markus. The instructor is married to Kerstin who is also an instructor. We were given a warm welcome. Meeting and organising the twinning with Markus felt special. Both Markus and I had been students when we'd met ten years ago and now here we were as the instructors of the twinning between Rugby and Ruesselsheim, Germany. Markus showed great consideration towards me and helped assist me around

Germany. I didn't like being blind but I was very grateful for the kind support I had. I had the privilege of staying at Markus and Kerstin's home.

The demonstration and competition was held at the Walter-Koebel-Halle. I taught part of their Taekwondo class and was then asked to perform a demonstration, following which my students participated in a friendly competition. Although I felt a little uncomfortable not being able to see clearly, I still managed to enjoy myself by thinking of cheerful thoughts and appreciating the wonderful hospitality. Afterwards we went to a restaurant and Markus told me when to step up and down steps and also helped me with my food. Later we went to a nightclub and my students guided me around obstacles and down steps. They even showed me where the toilets were!

We were also shown around Ruesselsheim and Mainz and were taken to the famous rivers Main and Rhine. I used my white cane to get around safely and my students helped to guide me. Everything around me appeared to blend in so much that I struggled to identify objects.

"I didn't realise how many objects I recognise from memory," I thought to myself. "In Rugby, I walk around quite confidently. I seem to know where lamp posts and boulders are. Here in Germany, I'm not used to the place so I can't even judge where the pavement starts. I don't seem to see the lamp posts and I have to walk very carefully."

Even goods and ornaments in the shops lost their shape and appeared to be more blurred than usual. It was because I knew where certain items were in the shops back in Rugby. Times like this made me realise that I appeared to see things when really I didn't – I would just be remembering where most things were in the shops. That's why I'm lost when a shop decides to move their products around.

On the last day we all had dinner together. There were loads of us because all our hosts were present too and we met up with the people from the other sports who had travelled to Germany for the twinning. I was unable to identify any food so my students got my food and drinks. I really appreciated all their help even though I felt like a burden.

"This is so humiliating," I thought to myself. "A Martial Artist yet I have to be assisted to the toilet; people put food on my plate and have to tell me what it is. I appreciate the help but I still feel useless."

So many people had helped me during our stay that I felt quite sad to have to leave Ruesselsheim.

Our friends from Ruesselsheim had also organised a barbecue for us at one of their homes. They gave us too much to drink and we got a little drunk! The party went on through the night and we didn't bother to sleep, as our flight was very early in the morning. They drove us to Frankfurt Flughafen Airport where we had to wait for a bus to take us to the next airport over an hour away. Frankfurt Flughafen is huge and we were drunk. It was dark and there were a lot of buses passing through the huge bus lane so I asked some of my students to look out for the right bus. They kept looking and then playing around, as you do when you're drunk! Some of them were racing up the escalators the wrong way and one of them lay on the floor and allowed someone else to drag them by their feet around the airport. They had fun but at a cost!

They still hadn't seen any sign of our bus and it was now an hour late. I went with a student into the airport to complain because we didn't want to miss our flight at the other airport but they assured us that the bus had turned up on time and had now left. So I asked them to show us where the bus had stopped and it wasn't near where my students had been looking out. We had missed our bus link to the next airport. We asked the officials how much it would be to catch a flight from Frankfurt Flughafen but they insisted that they would have to charge us the full price. We began to panic. (We sobered up pretty quickly!) Someone suggested calling our German friends. It was almost 6 am and I felt cruel but we didn't want to miss our flight back to England so I asked them nicely if they could do anything. They were very helpful and a few cars came to pick us up even though they had to go to work in a few hours. They drove us to the next airport, an hour's journey away. We rushed through the main doors to check in but were told that we had just missed the last call for our flight and it was preparing to depart. I tried everything but they couldn't stop the aeroplane and offered us another flight, which was departing a few hours later instead. We would have to pay forty pounds each, but this was a greatly reduced price and our only option, so we took it. But my ordeal wasn't quite over yet!

As we waited I heard my name called over the load speaker system, asking me to see the airport security. Someone guided me to where I had to go and we found two airport security guards waiting to take me away. They took me into a room where they searched my bag and found the weapons that I used for my demonstration and were clearly not happy with the discovery. I kept explaining that I had been invited to Germany to perform a demonstration for Ruesselsheim but they wouldn't accept it. They told me that it was illegal to have any weapons without permission. They were ready to take me away so I emptied my bag and showed them my black belt with my name on, my Martial Arts suit and my licence. After about half an hour they agreed to let me go but wanted to confiscate my weapons. Although I was grateful for escaping being locked up, I was furious about the possibility of losing my weapons, so I took a gamble and continued to argue, refusing to leave without them. Remaining calm and reasonable, I politely begged them and I could feel that they were hesitating. Fortunately one of my students had a German newspaper clipping that featured our demonstration. I was allowed to call my student in and he produced the newspaper. They took a good long look and then agreed to let me have them back but warned me never to bring them into the airport again.

As we embarked on the journey back to England, I felt a little fearful again. As the aeroplane lifted off, my praying began and I closed my eyes tightly until I felt the plane level out. I felt fine for the flight itself and was quite relaxed for the two-hour journey. During the flight I thought about the twinning and how the demonstration had gone. I thought that we were slightly ignorant towards our German friends because hardly any of us could speak German, yet they were very proficient at speaking English. During my stay I had learnt some important German phrases, like: hello; what is your name; my name is; please can I have some food and where is the toilet! I had also promised to learn German when I returned to Rugby.

The scariest part of flying was still the landing. During the flight I had become very relaxed and had almost forgotten about the landing but as soon as the plane touched down, I was shocked and grabbed the hand of the student sitting next to me. I was very scared and thought that we were going to crash, but we came safely to a stop and our journey was over.

Flying to Germany had been the first time that I had ever been in an aeroplane. At long last I had overcome my fear of flying. Although I was still not comfortable flying, I was prepared to travel by aeroplane again some other time!

CHAPTER 26
THE FADING SUN

My next holiday was to Paris in France. I'd dreamed of going for a few years since a close friend of mine had moved back to France, but every time I thought of travelling my fear of flying would return. In the end I had to find another way to get there.

My French friend, Jean-Seb, had stayed in England for a few years and I'd missed him since he'd returned home. He's also a black belt in Taekwondo and we trained together during the years when he was in this country. He was a great help to me and understood the limitations imposed on me by my disability. When we went out clubbing he helped to guide me around. He helped me play pool and sometimes helped to position my cue to get the right angle on the white ball. Sometimes we had fun as he first watched me line up to hit what I thought was the white ball, then he'd quickly inform me that I was about to hit the wrong colour. Somehow I managed to beat him on a few occasions. I've also beaten a few of my other friends too – they're amazed that I can play. It takes a lot of concentration and I also need to be playing the brighter colour. If the colours are red and yellow, I always try to play yellow even if I'm told that a red ball is near a pocket. I struggle so much to see the red that it's sometimes a waste of time me playing if I have to play that colour. The yellow balls look white but at least I can see them. Jean-Seb realised this and when we played he also tried to play yellow, which didn't exactly make it fair but we sure had a lot of fun playing.

My goal was to visit Jean-Seb in France, but I wasn't ready to travel by aeroplane again so I decided to travel using the Eurostar. My friend John had agreed to travel with me but it took me a while before finally deciding to go. The Eurostar train travels through the tunnel below the sea which links England and France. I was afraid of flying and now I was terrified of drowning. It's a strange feeling to travel below so much water knowing that if anything went wrong then I would surely drown. I knew that my days of travelling were limited and that one day my world would be too dark to feel comfortable travelling anywhere. My days were already darkening due to my failing eyesight so I had to force myself to enjoy life as much as possible while I was still able to have fun. The dream of travelling to France was also bigger than my fear of drowning so I eventually went.

After booking our tickets at the local train station, I asked the man to put everything in one envelope so that I wouldn't lose anything. Still trying to hold onto my independence, I checked the tickets myself when I returned home. Then Jean-Seb sent me some tickets for the Metro tube station in France and I put them with my other tickets but then he sent me some more up-to-date ones and I became confused. So I swapped them over and left them on my computer. The train tickets and the Metro tube tickets looked similar to me but instead of asking for assistance, I thought that I could distinguish between the tickets myself. (But I was grossly wrong!)

On our train journey from Rugby to London, we were beginning to relax when a ticket collector came round. Confidently I passed him our tickets and resumed my relaxed position.

"Tickets please," he asked.

"Here are our tickets. They're all in that envelope," I said.

He rummaged through the different tickets and seemed confused.

"Sorry, but there are no train tickets here," he said.

"Everything is in there," I replied. "That's how I was given the tickets. I asked them to put everything in one envelope so that it would be easy for me to find because I'm registered blind."

I showed him my white cane that was still opened at only half the size but at least I had managed to persuade myself to bring it along.

"I'm sorry, but I still can't find any train tickets so you'll have to pay again."

Everyone around us was looking now and I felt a little embarrassed. I was no longer relaxed, maybe slightly worried. My friend John took the envelope and checked. Fortunately our Eurostar tickets were in there with a receipt showing that we had paid for both train tickets and Eurostar tickets at the same time. John told me this and I passed them over to the ticket officer.

"You see. I paid for our train tickets and Eurostar tickets and these are all the tickets that I was given so if there's any mistake, then it's down to the Rugby Train Station," I said becoming annoyed.

"I can see that you've paid for the train tickets but because they're not here, you will have to pay again."

I became frustrated.

"I'm not paying again! When I get to London I'll be making a complaint. I asked them to put everything in one envelope because I was afraid that I wouldn't be able to see the difference between the tickets, and I trusted that they did as I asked. This is disgraceful. You can see that I've paid for our tickets but they didn't put them in the envelope. I'm disgusted and will be taking it up with a higher authority when we arrive in London."

My friend John kept quiet and left me to fight for our rights. Eventually the ticket officer agreed to let us off.

"I'll let you off but you will have to inform the Customer Service Centre at London of the mistake because you have no train tickets for your return journey."

We sat in silence for a while before John decided to ask me if it was possible that either of my children had tampered with the envelope at any time.

"I'm sure they didn't touch it," I replied. "It was in the exact position that I had left it, on my computer."

Then suddenly a vivid thought flashed through my mind.

"You swapped over the Metro tube tickets. Maybe you left your train tickets instead of the old tube tickets."

"Check to see if our new tube tickets are in the envelope," I said.

John rummaged through the contents of the envelope and then looked at me with a confused expression.

"Only the old tube tickets are in here," he replied.

"Only the old ones? Where are our new tube tickets that Jean-Seb sent…?"

I hesitated as another shivering thought flashed through my mind.

"Instead of leaving the old tube tickets, I left the new ones and they were with the train tickets so I must have left them on the computer too!"

I whispered my thought into John's ear so that nobody else could hear. Then without hesitation, John began to laugh and I nervously joined in.

"You left the wrong tickets didn't you?" John asked.

"Sorry, but yes, it appears that I must have. What are we going to do?"

"Well, I'm not paying again," said John.

"We'll have to tell the Customer Service Centre that I made a mistake and left the wrong tickets."

"They won't care. They'll say that we have to pay again," John concluded.

"Whoops!"

"And you blamed Rugby Train Station for your mistake! You are terrible."

We laughed quietly all the way to London.

The train arrived in London and we hesitantly made our way to the Customer Service Centre.

"Have you thought of what you're going to say to them?" John asked.

"I'm going to have to go on with our story or they'll no doubt charge us again," I replied.

We entered the Customer Service Centre and I approached the help desk.

"Can I help you?" a man asked.

"Here we go," I thought to myself feeling slightly worried now whether I'd be able to brazen this out.

"Here is an envelope with all the information that the Rugby Train Station put in when I purchased my Eurostar tickets to France," I moaned. "The ticket officer on the train said that the train tickets are missing but there's a receipt in there that shows I paid for both train tickets and Eurostar tickets together. I'm registered blind and told them that I was unable to see the tickets so kindly asked them to put everything in one envelope. The tickets are here for the Eurostar but not for our train journey and I'm exceedingly disappointed in the service and the mistake that has obviously been made."

"I'm very sorry sir, I'll ring Rugby Train Station to check," he replied.

I stood there and began to worry because I knew that the tickets were sitting on top of my computer at home and I had forgotten them but I was determined to bluff my way to France.

After a while the man at the information desk returned and agreed to issue new train tickets. I felt ecstatic. After thanking them for their kind help, we swiftly left and hastily disappeared out of sight.

"I can't believe it!" I laughed. "We got away without having to pay again."

"I can't believe how you were able to keep a straight face through that ordeal," John said.

"I know! But I didn't want to pay again even though it was my mistake!"

"You were so good that I was beginning to believe your story too," John laughed.

Feeling very pleased with ourselves we made our way onto the Eurostar. It still cheers me up every time I think back to what happened that day!

Our train started on its adventure to France, but as the Eurostar entered the Channel Tunnel I became restless. Thoughts rushed through my mind and I became paranoid that something would go wrong. As I was thinking of different disasters and ways that the water could get into the train, we emerged out of the other end of the Tunnel. It was a quick journey under the sea, maybe only twenty minutes or so, and thankfully not long enough for me to build up complex thoughts that could lead to paranoia. The longest part of the journey was on land, but now that I had braved the Tunnel, I was prepared to do it again.

Jean-Seb was waiting for us as we walked from the Eurostar. It wasn't easy to miss him, as he's very tall – six foot six inches. As we walked out into a new country Jean-Seb started helping me straight away.

"There's a step coming up," he advised.

"Thanks," I replied.

"Step down... now."

"Thanks again!"

Jean-Seb looked after us very well and was excellent at guiding me around.

He showed us all the beautiful sights of Paris during the day and the night. We went up the impressive Eiffel Tower; visited the Louvre, the most famous museum in the world, which houses the Mona Lisa; saw the Arc de Triomphe, built to commemorate one of Napoleon's victories and looked around Notre Dame Cathedral, made famous by the author Victor Hugo who wrote 'The Hunchback of Notre Dame' and 'The Sacre Couer'.

Whenever we ate Jean-Seb relayed what was on my plate. Most of the time, I drank beer because when I had water, my glass seemed to become invisible before my eyes. I even trained with some top Taekwondo students and was treated as their special guest.

When I returned to England I felt more positive again. I had gone away on a proper holiday abroad and even there I hadn't been able to resist doing a bit of training. The holiday to France made me feel like I had achieved another goal. However, there was something in the back of my mind that had been there for a while and kept eating away at me – I wanted to return to college to enrol on another course but I was afraid of encountering any more disappointments. Although I wanted to stay in the computer field, I was afraid of equipment not measuring up to aid my disability so I decided that it would be best to stay away from computers! The only other thing that I was good at was teaching so I looked up a few courses and eventually decided on a Sports Science course that would help me become a Personal Fitness Instructor.

I had a difficult time persuading myself to actually enrol.

"What if they haven't got the special equipment that I need?" I thought to myself. "It was so humiliating to be treated unfairly in front of other students on that computer course. Do I really want to go through that trouble again?"

"You won't need much equipment this time. You should only need a book reader."

"I don't think that I can manage the pressure with my disability."

"You can. You're supposed to be the strong one. Do it to show other people that those with low vision are capable of many things."

"How am I going to be able to give people personal fitness training anyway? This is going to be a waste of time and effort."

"You're practically doing it already. Swallow your pride and give it a go."

At the meeting to enrol, I was asked if I had any disabilities or special needs. I felt embarrassed having to explain my problems but I knew that I had to do it for my own good. Then I felt even more embarrassed having to be shown where to sign. I had to put my pen where their finger was and then hope that I was signing in a straight line. Then I had to show my card to prove that I'm registered blind. It felt like a very degrading moment.

"That made me feel very uncomfortable," I admitted to myself. "They had to point and leave their finger on the form so that I could sign it, then I had to produce my registration card. I'm not sure that I'm going to be able to cope."

"You have to do it. Try not to think of the way it makes you feel. Think of a happy memory."

On my first day, I walked into the classroom and there were already a few people sitting down.

"Where do I sit?" I thought. "I can't see clearly enough to see whether people are sitting in all the seats."

"Walk slowly forwards until you see an empty seat."

"Supposing there aren't any? I'll feel so embarrassed having to walk back and then around to the other side of the classroom."

"Trust yourself, just walk."

So I walked forwards carefully until I thought that I saw an empty seat. I put out my arm and grabbed the back of the chair with my hand. I applied a little pressure to move the chair slightly knowing that if someone were sitting in it then the chair wouldn't move. The chair moved easily so I manoeuvred myself to sit on it.

I sat and listened to some of the other students' conversations. Most of their voices indicated to me that they were much younger than me. Then I looked around to draw a picture in my mind of what I thought they all looked like. A few of them spoke to me and noticed my folded up cane.

"What's that for?" they asked.

"I hate having to explain about my disability," I thought to myself.

"I've got poor eyesight and I use it to get around," I answered.

"No; you were supposed to say that you're blind," I thought, disappointed with my lack of courage.

"You don't look blind," someone said.

"What are blind people supposed to look like?" I thought.

"Can you see me?" someone else asked.

"Please; no more questions," I thought.

"Yes I can see you, but not very clearly," I answered, remaining calm.

"Can you see my face?"

"No; you look like a ghost to me," I thought.

"Yes I can see your face, but it's very blurred and distorted," I answered.

The teacher entered the room and the class began.

He asked us to write down what he was saying so I got out my big bold black pen and began writing in my notebook.

"How embarrassing," I thought. "Look how big and bold I have to write. I bet everyone can read it from where they're sitting. Even the teacher must be able to read it from where he's standing. My writing is very messy. I can't believe I'm doing this."

"Come on, just write and stop thinking about what other people are thinking."

The teacher walked around as he continued to dictate. When he approached me he quietly told me that I had miss-spelt something.

"See; I knew that everyone could see what I was writing," I thought, feeling embarrassed.

Then the teacher passed around some handouts to put into our folders.

"You must be joking!" I gasped to myself. "I can't read any of these. Everything is so blurred that I can't even read the title. I'm going to have to ask the teacher for the CCTV book reader."

As the lesson went on the teacher gave us some more handouts and I became uncomfortable.

"I feel stupid, not being able to read anything," I thought.

He then asked us to write down the answers to the questions on one of the handouts.

"I'm not going to ask him to read them out so that everyone can hear. Some people might think that I can't read and I'm not ready to admit that I'm blind. I'm sure that the teacher has been told about me."

He didn't ask us to give our answers but I still felt out of place sitting and watching the other students completing the tasks. At the end of that section of the class, I asked the teacher about the CCTV book reader. He admitted that he was aware of my visual impairment and wasn't sure why the equipment wasn't available. Then he told me not to worry too much and that he would do what he could to help make the information easier for me to read. I then went to join the other students on our break.

When I got to the canteen, I looked at the mass of outlines of people who were in there.

"I'm not going to go in there and try and find my group," I thought, feeling disappointed. "There's no way that I can see clearly enough to find them. Everyone looks so distorted that they all blend in with each other. There's no way of me identifying my group. In the future I must remember to stay with them or I'll easily lose sight of them."

I stood looking at everyone wondering what to do.

"I wish that my eyes were clearer so that I could walk in there like everyone else and find people. I hate my eyes. No, I mustn't think like that, I'll get emotional. I'll go and find David, my brother in-law who works here."

So I went to David's room.

He's the Audio Visual Technician at the college and has worked there for more than fifteen years. He asked me about my course and offered to read the handouts for me and I stayed with him until the end of my break. This became my usual routine whenever I became separated from my group.

After break time the teacher gave out some more handouts. This time he had photocopied my sheets so that the text was twice as large. I was grateful for his efforts but my eyesight was still too cloudy and blurred to be able to read them. There was still no sign of a CCTV book reader or any other equipment for me so I sat and listened for most of that class. Then he used an overhead projector and asked us to copy the work. I explained that I was unable to read that too so I sat and listened some more! My frustration grew.

"This is so embarrassing," I thought. "What am I supposed to do? Sit here and listen while the other students write up the information that I'm missing out on? Sit here while the others get ahead of me? What's the point me coming in if the work isn't in a format that I can use? I'm going to get behind on completing tasks and then I'll probably be told to enrol next year again."

"Don't give up. You can do it. You want to be a Sports Instructor remember. Don't think about your problems. Think of something cheerful."

Then the teacher handed out another sheet that had diagrams on. It also had arrows pointing to certain muscles and we had to label them. But I had to sit there like an invalid and become further behind in my work.

"I'm going to have a lot of catching up to do at home," I thought to myself in distress.

Lunchtime came and I prepared to go home for lunch but the teacher wanted to see me after the class. Memories came flooding back and I became worried that he was going to tell me that I'm too difficult to teach and should enrol on another course.

"Here we go," I thought. "He's going to tell me that this course isn't suitable for someone with as much visual impairment as me. He's going to tell me to enrol next year again."

The teacher wanted to tell me that he would photocopy everything so that I would have the minimum amount of writing to do. He also assured me that he would have a copy of all the tasks on a disk for use on my computer equipment, which would be ready for my afternoon lesson. I was very grateful and went home for my lunch.

While at home I went on my computer and did a bit of work on my website. It had details of my interests and my Martial Arts classes. From my previous experience of computers I was able to design the website myself. I had also started writing a Martial Arts handbook, which would include the necessary criteria to pass exams up to the black belt level. I estimated it would be fifty pages long so I had plenty to keep me occupied at home.

As I walked through the classroom door for my afternoon lesson I saw some extra equipment in the room. My teacher said that it was a computer with a bright lamp, keyboard with large labels, magnifier, speech software and CCTV for my use. He apologised about there not being a printer but I was overwhelmed. He gave me a handout and I put it under the CCTV and was able to read it. Although my speed was slow because of the size of my text, I was able to see what the other students had. My eyes hurt from the bright light and degree of magnification but I still continued to read.

"It's great that they've finally remembered me," I thought. "The CCTV helps me read but now I stand out in the classroom. I feel good but also embarrassed. I hate having to read like this but at the same time, I appreciate it."

I became the centre of attention and students kept asking me what the equipment was for. My patience was tested.

"What's this?" a student asked.

"It's a CCTV for reading books."

"Why do you need it?"

"Here we go again," I thought to myself.

"I'm... registered blind and I need it to be able to read things."

"You don't look blind."

"What do blind people look like?" I thought to myself, not for the first time.

"I can see a little but I'm seriously short-sighted," I replied.

"How does it work?" they asked.

"It magnifies whatever is under the light."

"Can it magnify my hand?"

Before I knew it, he had put his hand under the magnifier and was moving it around.

"Hey! Look at my hand!" he bellowed to the other students.

More students came and gathered around.

"What am I supposed to do now?" I thought to myself.

"Wow! Look at his dirty fingernails. His hand looks massive under there," someone shouted.

"That will do," I said. "Can you all stop messing with it? It's a very expensive piece of equipment."

The teacher began to teach us about anatomy and physiology and I used the CCTV to follow what he put on the overhead projector. I still had to write down a few notes in my own handwriting because there were no spare disks for me to use and take home. The disk that he had supplied me with had some answers to the tasks and I had to return it after each class. I took my notes home and had to scan them into my computer along with most of the handouts so I was able to enlarge the text on my own screen to be able to read them. This made me much slower to finish the set tasks but I was determined to complete the course. Some handouts had spaces on them to answer the questions, but I was unable to write directly onto the sheets and had to retype them on my computer before answering the questions. I worked extra hard on the course to be able to have the same level as everyone else.

The next part of the course was participating in practical work. We sometimes took part in different activities in the sports hall but most of the time we stayed in the gym. The gym was different to what I was used to so I appeared to have even less sight because I couldn't guess what the machines were. We had to learn how to induct people into the gym as a Personal Fitness Instructor would. I found it extremely difficult because I had to learn how each machine worked off by heart, then instruct people on how to use them from memory rather than visually. The machines with digital screens were the most difficult. I couldn't see if people pressed the wrong button so I kept going through the routine of how to set them up.

"I can't see anything on these digital screens," I said to myself. "How am I supposed to set them up for people? Maybe I've chosen the wrong course. When I use my local gym, I guess the weight or count how many weights from the bottom I usually do. I can't do that when I'm giving someone else personal fitness training."

"Learn the different settings off by heart and ask them to press the buttons and hope that they follow your instructions properly."

The problem I had with the weight machines was putting the pin in the correct weight. I had to ask other people to do it for me. We also had to fill in forms; I signed them but asked them to fill the forms in themselves. Every problem that I encountered put me off the course and shook my resolve to complete it, but then I would fight my emotions to continue.

"There are too many things that I'm unable to perform efficiently. Gaining my Sports Coaching qualification is much harder than I expected."

"You want to teach other fitness activities don't you?"

"I look like an invalid on some of these machines."

"*You* can use them but you need to learn how to teach other people who may know nothing about them."

"It's too hard. I can't read the digital screens on the treadmill or the rowing machine."

"Think positive. You can do it."

"My eyesight is far too poor. I hate my eyes. They hold me back from learning things."

"Think of something happier to take your mind off your problems."

In the sports hall we were taught how to coach. We mostly did football because it's one of the most popular sports in England. Delivering the instructions wasn't too hard but when other students were coaching, I struggled to participate and sometimes I felt useless.

"Where has that football disappeared to again?" I thought to myself.

"Maybe you should sit at the side during these games."

"How am I going to dribble the ball and manoeuvre it around objects that I can't see?"

Every time I lost sight of the football that I was attempting to control, another student or the teacher had to retrieve it for me. I stood out like a sore thumb so I sat out several times and watched the others.

When they actually played a football match I was scared of the ball hitting me in my face and would sometimes leave the sports hall. I couldn't see the ball but I could hear it. When they kicked it hard, I kept thinking that it would smash into me.

"I'd love to be able to play football like them," I thought despondently. "To be able to run around so confidently and to keep my eyes on the ball. They're so fortunate to have that ability."

Sometimes we went on trips to participate in sports. I went on an army assault course and it looked like fun, but unfortunately I was unable to join in many of the activities. One of the helpers offered to assist and guide me around but I felt too frail and didn't like the feelings that it was producing in me. We did rifle shooting and I was able to hit a target that I couldn't see.

"Move your rifle a touch to your right," the instructor said.

"What am I trying to hit?" I asked.

"That target over there."

"Where is the target? I can't see it."

"It's on that large white board in the distance."

"Where's the white board?" I asked nervously.

"I've moved your rifle so that it should be pointing towards it."

"I think that I see the white board now. I hope that this hasn't got real bullets because I won't know where I'm shooting."

So I aimed for the middle of the small blurred white board and squeezed the trigger. After my target was retrieved, the instructor told me that I had hit the coloured area. I was ecstatic. How I was able to hit the target I'll never know.

There was also a wall to climb and abseil down. I would have loved to try it if I could see more clearly but I didn't want to risk getting hurt. I felt too uncomfortable imagining myself being guided during every step of the task. All I did was stand there and watch the rest of my group having fun.

"I wish that I could run around so confidently like them," I thought. "They walk like they know exactly where to step and they can see where to hold onto the wall. I can't even see the rope!"

"Don't worry about it. I'm sure there are things that you can do that they would struggle with."

"Maybe I should have a go."

"It's too risky and you'll probably slip over and make a fool of yourself."

"My eyes are holding me back from having fun."

"Stop thinking about it. You have plenty of fun with other things in your life."

There was one other person standing with me because they were scared of heights so I convinced myself that I wasn't alone.

We also visited several gyms to see how they were run. Most of the time I stayed near the back of the group, so that I could watch how the students in front of me manoeuvred around obstacles. I was unsure of lamp posts and didn't want to bump into any but I also didn't have my cane out in full. I tried a few times but I felt too fragile and vulnerable and I'm usually a confident person so there was quite a bit of a conflict going on in my head.

As the course went on I used the computer more frequently. The teacher had put most of the information onto a disk and I enlarged it on my screen so I was able to follow his teaching. We had to put all our tasks and assignments into a folder. Sometimes during a class, the teacher would relate his topic to a previous assignment and ask us to find it in our folders. He had to help me because I was unable to see what was written even though I wrote everything using my computer. This caused a few problems and I felt very uncomfortable. We also had to cross-reference everything with a list of criteria that we had to complete in order to pass the course. My teacher had to do that task for me too.

At the end of the course I was told that I had passed and I had also completed writing my book on Martial Arts and had created a website all on my own. Things were looking good for me now and I had a new direction in life.

Soon after passing the course, I started teaching Boxercise for a local gym. My first task was to prepare a CD for my class. I developed it at home and assigned the first few records to the synchronised warm-ups, so I was constantly listening to music and trying to time techniques for the warm-up. I'm pretty sure that I must have looked ridiculous to my children. They sometimes watched me jumping around in time with certain tracks, and then changing my routine to keep in time with the music. It was quite difficult, but it was fun to do. It also gave me something else that was positive to think about when I was having a few negative thoughts.

Prior to my first class, I plucked up the courage to ask an assistant to show me how to use the music studio. I had to memorise where all the relevant buttons were because I was unable to read anything – it was all too small for me and most of the buttons looked the same so I became very confused.

"Which one was the play button?" I asked for the second time.

After placing my finger on the play button I then moved my finger to the left and counted how many buttons there were.

"The play button is the third button from the left," I told myself. "Now make sure that you remember that. You don't want to keep asking for help all the time. That will make you feel useless so try to remember where all the buttons are."

At my first class, people placed their tickets in a pile on a table while I was setting up the pads and gloves. The lighting wasn't brilliant so I struggled to find pairs of matching gloves.

"Why didn't I buy all the gloves in the same colour?" I berated myself. "How am I going to find pairs of gloves when they all appear to be the same colour? Maybe I should use the spotlight over there to help me see clearer. Maybe that will be bright enough to see."

So I kept walking over to a brighter area of the room to organise the gloves. It was like magic how all the dark gloves revealed their colours under the spotlight. A mass of black gloves suddenly became blue and brown and purple. As I set them out, several thoughts flashed through my mind.

"This is embarrassing attempting to do this with so many people watching. Maybe I should organise myself and pair them up at home. Then put each pair in a separate bag."

This is something that I've continued to do. It speeds up the time it takes me to find a matching pair.

After all the gloves and mitts were set up I walked over to the table to count the tickets. Some of the tickets were little slips of paper that I struggled to see so they caused me a few problems.

"Shall I ask for help?" I thought. "No, I'm independent and I can manage. I'll brush my hand across the table and pick up whatever I touch. I don't mind telling people that I've got poor eyesight but I'm not telling everyone that I'm registered blind. I'll feel useless and I would prefer to go back home and become a recluse than feel that incapable."

After counting the tickets I then looked around to count the people.

"Whoops!" I thought. "I can hardly see anyone from here. I'm going to have to guess as usual."

So I looked around at all the cloudy ghostly figures and began to count. I could easily miss people who were standing very still because they blended in with the background.

"There are two extra heads," I thought to myself. "I hope that I've counted correctly."

"Can you *all* put your tickets on the table please?" I bellowed.

One person approached me and gave me their ticket.

"That worked!" I thought in satisfaction.

Then another thought flashed through my mind.

"Maybe I should shout for tickets all the time as though I know that tickets are missing, even though I can't see clearly enough to know for sure."

This is another trick that I use even today.

Then someone who knew me came to speak to me.

"Hello Vendon," the voice said.

"Who are you?" I thought to myself.

"Hello there and how are you?" I asked.

"I'm fine. I thought that I'd give your class a try," the voice replied.

"I still don't recognise his voice," I thought.

"So what have you been doing with yourself?" I asked, still trying to recognise the voice.

He told me about his job and then said, "You don't recognise me do you?"

"I've been caught attempting to guess who they are!"

"I'm sorry, but my eyesight is very dark and I can't see you clearly enough," I admitted.

"I know about your eyes," the voice said.

"What! He knows that I can't see yet he never thought to give me his name first?" I thought hysterically. "If he knows how does he expect me to recognise him?"

"Nice to see you again," I said calmly.

This is a situation that I'm faced with regularly. People know that I struggle to see yet they still expect me to be able to guess their names from the sound of their voices. I can do it but I sometimes get it wrong and I would appreciate it if people had a bit more consideration to realise the difficulties and frustration it causes me. I've asked my friends to treat me as though they're calling me on the phone. How difficult is it to say their name? Surely that's easier than having to consistently remind people that I'm registered blind.

The music started and I began to go through my routine with them. I was standing at the front of the class and everyone was in rows facing me.

"Everyone is so blurred," I thought to myself. "My friend has disappeared into the cloudy mist. Their ghostly images are too distorted to see if anyone goes wrong. I'll have to guess. I can't see anyone's face and parts of their bodies appear to be missing. I can hardly see anything. My eyes are too dark and I'm feeling really uncomfortable. I hate my eyes; they're so useless. Maybe I shouldn't look at them much. That way I won't feel so bad."

Sometimes I asked them to bend their knees, and then to bend them a little more so that people who weren't bending their knees much would think that I could see them and they would then try harder. It's another trick that I use when I teach Martial Arts too now. I also asked them to try and keep up with the music assuming that some of them would have slowed down.

The next section was boxing. They worked in pairs, one had to put a pair of gloves on and their partner needed some focus pads. The music was quite loud and I struggled to hear them speak.

"This isn't a pair," a student complained.

"Pardon? I can't hear you very well," I answered.

"I'm half deaf really and I can't see to lip read," I thought to myself.

After turning my good ear towards them I was able to hear. Then I attempted to find the other glove. On several occasions as long as they had a left and a right glove, I would ask them to keep them on even though they were of different colours. Then I showed them how to punch by hitting some focus mitts. It's very hard for me to see the small ones so I mostly demonstrated on a large pad. When I did demonstrate on the small pads I always moved them into position so that I knew exactly where they were, then proceeded to punch. The pads are very difficult to focus on because they appear so blurred to me but having already positioned them I knew where they were so I didn't really have to use my sight. I walked around close to people so that I could see if they were punching correctly. Unless they were directly under a spotlight, I wasn't able to see their faces or the faces of the pad holders. So I walked around guessing and memorising who the ghostly figures were. If I had to hold a pad while someone was punching they didn't realise that I was moving slowly towards a spotlight so that I was able to see them more clearly.

During the class, a few people spoke to me but I was only able to hear a few because of the loud music blaring in the background. Someone called me and I looked around but couldn't identify who they were from the distorted images I saw. I was getting confused.

"Who's calling me?" I asked myself. "I can't see clearly enough to be able to walk over to them. I'll have to walk slowly past everyone until I'm able to hear who's calling me. This is so frustrating not being able to see them clearer. I wish that I could see and hear people better so that I can communicate more efficiently."

Listening to the music cheered me up and stopped a great deal of sad thoughts from clouding my mind.

At the end of the class I asked them to pile all my pads up in a corner of the gym. This made it much easier for me to find them all and return them to my bag. Some of the pads belonged to the gym and I had more problems separating them.

"Look at this big pile of pads," I thought. "How am I going to find the pads that belong to the gym when they all look the same colour to me? My eyesight is really getting dark and I'm struggling a great deal in this light. I can't bring the pads to the middle of the hall to an area better lit by a spotlight. I'll have to put them all in one bag for now and sort them out after the students have left."

There were many challenges that I had to overcome in order to continue teaching Boxercise. On one occasion the sound system broke down and I struggled to use the cassette tape buttons. Sometimes I took my daughter Jasmine with me to help me out. She became so used to attending and helping me at my classes that she now joins in.

Once I had to rewire the sound system because someone had pulled out one of the wires and the previous teacher had been unable to move the hi-fi away from the wall to see what to do. They couldn't see where to put the wires so ended up not using music. I asked a member of staff to help me but when they were unable to find the fault, I did what I do best; I guessed! I turned the hi-fi off, then put my hands behind and pulled out all the wires. Then I slowly untangled them and put them in their correct sockets. I was unable to see what I was doing but not being able to see was something that I was used to! I was very proud of myself when I switched it on and it worked. This was one occasion where not being able to see was an advantage. It proved that most people used their eyes to complete most tasks. In situations similar to this I feel as though my hands are my eyes!

Sometimes my niece, Sinead, would join in and help me put out my equipment. Occasionally she would leave the room to fix her hair or something and when she returned and walked towards me I would say hello to her as though she was a new student who had come to join in. It made me feel so hopeless not even being able to recognise my own family any more.

Now I've told a few of my Boxercise students about the extent of my visual impairment and they've become my personal assistants. Lisa and Jenny help me to set up the pads and to separate the two bags at the end of the class. This is a great help and I appreciate it more than they realise. On a few occasions I've been tempted to give up teaching Boxercise because of the frustration it causes me at times, but with their kind consideration I actually look forward to teaching now. Knowing how much my students are enjoying themselves also keeps me going.

CHAPTER 27
FACING YOUR FEARS

"This feels great!" I thought to myself. "Teaching keeps me motivated and I enjoy helping other people reach their goals. I'm going to advertise myself as a Personal Fitness Trainer and start teaching people in their homes."

So without wasting any time I contacted my local newspaper to place an advertisement in their sports section.

"I'd like to advertise myself in your newspaper as a Personal Fitness Trainer," I said.

"Can you tell us a little about yourself?" the woman asked.

"It might be best if I mention that I'm registered blind," I thought, "so that people don't get any surprises when they meet me. This is going to be so difficult, admitting this. It's humiliating having to say it."

"I'm a registered blind Fitness Instructor and I'm interested in giving people personal training and I hope that my disability will inspire them," I said.

"How can you see to teach?" she asked.

"I've been teaching for a while and I'm fine."

"But how can you see them?" she insisted.

I became frustrated.

"I can see them but they're blurred," I answered.

"Don't you think that admitting that you're blind might deter people from using you?" she persisted.

"But I *can* teach. What's wrong with admitting that I'm blind?"

"I'm sure that you're a very good instructor, but people are easily put off. They too might wonder if you're capable enough to teach without being able to see."

A moment went by as I paused.

"That was so difficult admitting that I'm blind," I thought. "I hate saying it and now other people don't want me to say it. I may as well hide it as usual."

"What do you suggest then?" I asked.

"You would be better off saying that you're partially sighted. It doesn't sound as harsh," she suggested.

"It's bad that people might not trust a blind person," I thought sadly. "But then that's partly the reason I don't like to admit that I'm blind. Maybe she's right."

"Fine; advertise me as partially sighted then," I replied reluctantly.

I received a few phone calls and I went out to see my new clients. They filled in my questionnaire about their health, and then I asked them most of the same questions again because I was unable to read what they had written. I had memorised where to sign and gave them with a copy. Then I proceeded to get my equipment from my bag. There was a pair of boxing gloves and focus mitts that I used in my other classes. I also had a sit-up machine, an exercise mat and some small weights. A friend had helped me purchase the equipment from a shop, as I couldn't see clearly enough to select them myself.

I got into the habit of taking both a cassette tape and a CD with me so that I would always be able to play my warm-up music.

The client would put the music on and we would then begin the warm-up. I generally looked around at my surroundings to see which was the best area to stay in to be able to see the person I was training more clearly. Sometimes it became extremely difficult to see them but I would encourage them verbally.

"That's great; you're doing well," I would say, whilst trying to work out which way I should turn so that I could see them a little clearer. Their faces were often so dark and blurred that most of the time they appeared to be missing a head.

Another problem that I encountered was setting up the sit-up machine. Every now and then I would drop the little screw that was needed to clamp it together. It would fall on the floor and I would end up searching for it for a few seconds, which made me feel slightly uncomfortable and incapable but I enjoyed teaching too much to quit. Being a Personal Fitness Trainer made me feel good and was something else to keep me thinking positive.

Somehow I also got involved with a disabled activity group. They held weekly sessions at our local Sports Centre and had a choice of rifle shooting, bowling, pool, table tennis and swimming. My main interest was the swimming. I could only swim one length of a pool before my arms got tired. For years I had told people that it was because I was too muscular (wishful thinking!) and that made me too dense to float, but my new swimming tutor, Ben, told me that it was me who was dense in the head! He told me that I was swimming incorrectly and my style was all wrong so he began to teach me how to swim properly.

Swimming was fun and it was more interesting because Ben was also very funny and always made me laugh. During my lessons I removed my glasses and had serious difficulties seeing where I was going. Ben sometimes had to tell me when to stop because he thought that I was about to crack my head on the side. On many occasions I bumped into people and I got some mixed but hilarious comments.

"Please move out the way," Ben said.

"Can't he swim around me?" the person asked.

"No; he's blind and can't see you."

"He doesn't look blind to me."

"He can't bring his white cane into the swimming pool can he?" Ben muttered.

Some people didn't know what to say and others would ask me to wear my glasses. I've bumped into people and they've asked me if I was blind but I always saw the funny side and laughed as I replied, "Yes!"

After many weeks I'd improved a lot and could swim several lengths. Then Ben asked me to swim sixty lengths and at first I thought he was joking but I realised that he was serious. To my surprise I was able to complete the sixty lengths without stopping. There were a few times when I was tempted to stop because of cramp but I managed to work through it and completed the task set for me.

Another activity that I was put in for was to participate in a raft race. It covered about twenty miles but it felt more like a hundred because it took hours to complete. Most of our crew were disabled and there were two of us who were registered blind. We both struggled to get onto the raft and I was nervous because I kept thinking that I was about to fall into the water. It was difficult to see where to walk and I had to trust other people to guide me. After several hours I became desperate for the toilet and when we arrived at our destination, the toilet was the first place that I… ran to! We achieved second place beating other teams like the fire service. Ben asked me on many occasions to take part in other races but I always refused because of the length of time I had to survive without going to the toilet. I know that I should be able to control myself but I felt uncomfortable knowing that there were no toilets around for five or six hours.

In June 2002, my fun was cut short as I was given the shattering news of my sister Carline's health. She had been diagnosed with cancer some while before and had now been told that she had less than a year to live. All my family were devastated by the news. It seemed as though every time I tried to keep myself happy, something else would go wrong in my life.

My family appeared to be suffering with depression from the stress of it all – three of us registered blind and Carline with cancer. It was a lot for my other brothers and sisters to comprehend, all of whom, apart from Percy and Leroy, were suffering from some form of depression and Jennifer was becoming more delusional. (She lives alone in Ireland and regrets leaving her son Dyonn to fend for himself although she was suffering from depression at the time. She still can't come to terms with the loss of her mother while she was away on holiday.) June went to see a specialist for depression because she was worried about the effects the loss of my sister would have on Angela who was already depressed. Fergus tried to cover up his emotions by behaving very irresponsibly. This was the wrong way to go and now I wish that Fergus had went to seek medical help for his depression.

Fergus was quite a naughty lad right from when he was a teenager. We were all brought up with sound discipline but he seemed to ignore the good advice. He felt as though he was treated differently from the rest of us but he was grossly wrong – my parents loved and treated us all equally. I was given the nickname 'Daddy's son' because I chose to do more for my dad. Fergus chose not to do any favours for our parents so it was his bad choices that led him to self-destruction. Fergus got himself into a lot of trouble and became the black sheep of our family. Many of his friends called him a rat, but I feel that it was his bad choice of friends that helped lead him into disaster. On the 9th October 2002 Fergus was convicted of armed robbery and was given a five-year prison sentence. He took drugs like crack and one thing led to another. He once told me that it was his way of coping with his depression and his stressful life. He also said that he felt that there was no other way of putting a stop to his drug related life. It was as though he was trying to either kill himself or get locked up. If that was really his attitude then I'm glad that he was caught taking part in a robbery and I'm also very relieved that nobody got hurt. He's safer in prison and now has a chance to finally rid himself of his drug problems. We were all heartbroken from the news of his conviction at such an emotional stage of our lives. I'm embarrassed to admit to other people that we have an armed robber in our family after my parents tried their hardest to bring us all up with good morals.

Fergus has four wonderful children who won't be able to see him for a long time apart from visiting him in prison. He has also left Bev, his fiancée, behind, but she's promised to wait for him and I admire her for standing by him. Many people would move on and get on with their lives. I hope that Fergus appreciates Bev's patience and understanding.

Percy organised a family meeting and we discussed Carline's care. Many of my brothers and sisters were too busy with their own lives and occasionally visited her when they could find time. Percy was already looking after her everyday, cooking, cleaning, nursing and trying to help her become more comfortable. He asked us to share his workload because he was under a lot of pressure dealing with her mostly by himself. He even postponed a Social Economics course to dedicate more time to nursing her. I agreed to look after her every Thursday and hoped that it would also give Percy a rest from his stressful duties. June and Angela also volunteered for other days.

Angela became even more upset and depressed because she couldn't do more for her sister. For years she had enjoyed her independence and was looked up to as the older and wiser sister. She used to help everyone and was especially close to Carline. They did everything together but now Angela's eyesight had deteriorated to a much worse condition than mine, with no vision at all in her right eye and her left as blurred as mine. It seemed that the deterioration of her sight had accelerated and she was feeling frantic wondering when her left eye would become totally blind too. She so badly wanted to do more for Carline but was not physically or mentally capable.

On a Thursday I would look after Carline before and after teaching a Boxercise class. Cooking in someone else's kitchen was difficult for me. Sometimes I would cook at my home and take the food that I had prepared to her. One day I asked Carline what type of food she liked the most and would like more of. She told me that her favourite was Chinese food, and particularly liked pork fried rice with sweet and sour sauce, so I agreed to buy her a Chinese meal every Thursday. It felt good to be able to please her but I knew that part of my relief was due to not having to struggle to cook for her. It was stressful not knowing how many months I would be able to please her before she grew too ill to eat.

During Christmas 2002 Carline told everyone that she wanted to make it a special one because she knew that it was going to be her last. We all spent Christmas at my home and tried to make it very special for her – it was a very emotional time for us all. Carline bought special presents for all her nieces and nephews including my two children – she bought Jasmine her first Brats doll and car. (Jasmine now has over twenty Brats!) Carline also spoilt her son Hasani, who was then twelve years old. She tried her best to keep a smile on her face as she treated all the children but we could all tell that she was in a great deal of pain. She was also on a very high dose of morphine.

I found it difficult to hide my real feelings and emotions towards the situation. While I was caring for her on my Thursday evenings my mind would battle with the situation.

"Why is this happening to us? Hasn't enough happened to our family? Can't the problems stop now? It's hard enough dealing with going blind and wondering when my eyesight will deteriorate to the extent that I'm unable to see any movement at all, but I also have to deal with the fact that my sister and brother are blind too. I have to learn to deal with one of my brothers being in prison and now deal with another sister dying of cancer. This is too much pressure even for me and I'm supposed to be the strong one. People don't even know how much I'm suffering because I don't moan about life."

Although I hid the pressure I was experiencing from most people, I was unable to hide it from myself. I felt as though something else was wrong with me but wasn't sure what. After attending a doctor's appointment, he told me that I had high blood pressure so I was put on tablets to control that too. I felt like my body was falling apart under the pressure.

In January 2003, Carline became even worse. Percy was already staying overnight to look after her and he was struggling. His girlfriend, Colette, was a great help and supported him well but said that he needed more help so I offered to stay overnight on Thursdays too. We slept in the sitting room. I usually got the privilege of sleeping upright on a sofa chair, which caused me some back pains that I didn't need because of my teaching career but I was able to cope. Percy also began to suffer backache but his was more severe than mine. During this time I also experienced problems at home and had to sleep on my settee when I returned home. My emotions began to build up as time went on and my sister became worse. Sometimes I would sit there watching TV with tears in my eyes.

During a conversation with Carline she told me that she had suffered a small stroke and temporarily lost her eyesight. She tried to tell me that she felt fortunate not to be registered blind like her three family members. I became emotional, tearful and confused to a degree that tears were constantly in my eyes.

"How can she say that she's fortunate not to be blind?" I thought to myself. "I'm blind and it's incredibly hard, but I'm not dying from cancer. I should be grateful to be blind; I'm not the one who only has a few months to live. The problem with my eyesight is bad, painful and stressful but she's worse off than me. At least I have a chance to live my life. She has to prepare herself for death. That sounds scarier than wondering when I'll finally go totally blind."

We confused each other as I tried my hardest to get her to understand that I was the lucky one. She kept saying that she had enjoyed a good life being able to see everything she wanted. She told me how fortunate she was to have had the ability to drive, walk and see the world. Although I would have loved to do some of the things that she had done if I could see more clearly, I still wouldn't prefer a short life.

A few months went by and her condition continued to deteriorate. She was now struggling to eat, but she still insisted on having her weekly Chinese. I would teach Boxercise and try my hardest to keep smiling at my students. Then on the way to pick up her Chinese I became emotional and tearful. I knew that it was going to be a long night of worry and strain and I wasn't looking forward to sleeping upright in a chair. Percy was doing even more and was now nursing her every day and night with my help and that of the others who had chosen to look after her. Carline told Percy that she was afraid of what it might do to her son's mental health if he found her dead one morning, so we made sure that someone was always there with Hasani when he got up. There were a few helpers who also assisted her but she preferred her family. Carline also told us that she was afraid to fall into a deep sleep because she was afraid of dying and she wasn't ready to go yet.

Carline was strong willed but her illness slowly got the better of her and it got to a stage where she could no longer eat, talk or walk. We kept going to her house to nurse her and waited for the day when she would never wake up. Things were very quiet during my last Thursday night of nursing her. My nerves were on edge and I too was afraid of finding her dead but I had to be strong for the others.

On the Friday morning I prepared myself to leave her home. The doctor told Percy that he felt that she was about to pass away so Percy contacted every member of our family so that we could all be with her. We were all there, all together, waiting and worrying. During the afternoon we surrounded her bed to say our goodbyes. We watched as her breathing became fainter and she slowly slipped away from us. She had passed away with us all there. I cried that day.

For six months we had nursed her not knowing when she would leave us. She finally passed away on Friday 6th June 2003. The long-winded process had taken a lot out of all of us. Percy had promised Carline on her deathbed that he would look after her son Hasani, but he became a handful and caused a tremendous strain on Percy's relationship with Colette. They already had three children and were now overcrowded with Hasani so they had to live in two separate houses. Leroy had problems dealing with Carline's death and soon became depressed. He had been busy working and now wished that he had taken more time out to help her. He also had the added stress of his partner who decided to leave him just when he needed her most. June also continued to seek therapy for her growing depression and admitted that she was on the verge of a nervous breakdown.

I didn't have much strength to do anything constructive with my life. It was time for me to make a return visit to my therapist before I sank really low. I knew that I was beginning to feel depressed so I somehow persuaded myself to see her again even though I didn't feel like it. She told me that under the circumstances most people would feel the same and need time and space to grieve. We spoke about my feelings during the long ordeal of looking after my sister and then we slowly got back to talking about my personal problems.

"How are you coping with your eyes?" she asked gently.

"I hate my eyes. I can't cope with their deterioration and the things that they're holding me back from doing. I could have helped my sister much more if I could see more clearly. Even my sister Angela has become more depressed knowing that her eyesight prevented her from doing more for Carline. Being blind is a terrible strain on my life. Not being able to see affects me doing almost everything."

"Are your eyes getting worse?"

"Yes; they're continually deteriorating and I'm very scared of what will happen sooner or later. I had worse vision than my sister Angela and now her eyesight is worse than mine. She can't see anything through her right eye – nothing at all; no movements; no outlines; nothing. I'm scared of becoming like that too but it *will* happen one day. I have to just wait for it to happen and I'm very afraid. I'm worried that my strength will go and I'll end up not wanting to leave my home. Then I'll have to give up teaching everything and I can't imagine my life without teaching."

"Isn't there anything that they can do?"

"No; there isn't a cure as yet so I have to surrender to the fate of my eyes. The doctors keep telling me that I have special eyes but I don't think that they're special. I would swap them any day. If they perfected eye transplants, I would have the operation tomorrow and I wouldn't care what colour my new eyes were. I desperately want to see again, I don't want to be blind. The other day I saw a TV advertisement for laser treatment and I contacted the company. It would have been nice to at least have my short sight corrected so that I wouldn't have to wear glasses. My glasses affect me a lot when I'm teaching Martial Arts because I have to take them off when I'm fighting. It's so hard to see people's hands and legs when I remove my glasses. It really would have been a great feeling and I was very excited when I contacted them. But they too told me that I have special eyes. They told me that they're not allowed to operate on people who have RP eye disorder. I begged them to do it. I even said that I would sign a legal form to say that I couldn't take them to court if anything went wrong, but they refused and I'm so disappointed. My eyes are not special, they're a curse."

As I went on I realised that I had plenty to say. I wasn't holding everything inside like the last time I was depressed.

"How are you coping with the loss of your sister?" she asked.

"OK I guess; it hurts to think about it but I suppose we knew it would happen eventually. She was only forty-six years old, just ten years older than me. I don't understand the meaning of life. She thought that she was the lucky one – one of the family who had avoided the cursed eye disorder, yet she died first. How is she lucky? Her life was short. I might be registered blind but I'm still able to enjoy parts of my life. I've got plenty to moan about but even more to live for. I've still got a chance to enjoy my life so I think that my sister was the unlucky one."

"How are things at home?" she asked.

"I'm still struggling to keep my OCD under control. The worse my sight becomes, the more I become obsessed with having things in a certain place to cope with the deterioration. I feel as though I'm putting my family and friends under too much pressure looking after me and I hate that feeling. I don't want to be a burden on other people."

"You're a very independent person. Some normal sighted people ask for more help than you do so try not to think like that."

"People shouldn't have to help me at all. Why can't I have the ability to do things for myself?"

"Unfortunately you need your eyesight for many things."

"Why do we have to live in such a world that requires so much sight to be able to do things? Why is this happening to me? Why am I suffering so much? I'm not a bad person. I don't smoke and I hardly drink. I'm not a criminal. I'm a good person. I'm the one who helps everyone else, what about me? Who helps me? Sometimes I wish that I could duplicate myself so that I can help all my family and friends but then my lack of eyesight prevents me from doing more for them."

"Everyone has problems."

"I know; I just wanted to have a little moan. Most people don't even know how much I'm suffering on the inside. There have been loads of my friends who've said that I'm lucky not to have any problems. They don't realise that just because I walk around with a smile on my face doesn't mean that I have no problems. People look so blurred and distorted to me. They look like they're walking around in thick fog yet I have to dismiss the emotional feelings I have from seeing like that and get on with my life. Sometimes when I'm talking to people I'll blink vigorously a few times to try to be able to see them slightly better. While they're talking, I'm usually wishing to myself that I could see them more clearly. People probably don't see me constantly cleaning my glasses, but I do to try to see them more clearly or to rest my painful eyes from the constant straining. Some people have told me off for squinting but they haven't stopped to realise that I have to do that to see them slightly clearer. People don't hear me moaning though, I just get on with it by thinking of something else that cheers me up or I say that there are people suffering more than me out there."

After I finished talking so much, she gave me some positive news.

"You don't sound depressed to me."

"I don't feel depressed. I'm just stressed from the loss of my sister."

"I do think that you need a break. Is there anywhere that you would like to go?"

"Yes; France. My friend Jean-Seb is getting married to his girlfriend Estelle and he's invited me over to France for the wedding."

"Why don't you go?"

"I can't go on my own. I've got nobody who is willing to travel with me unless I pay for them. It would be far too difficult on my own."

"I think you really need a break and I'm sure that your friend Jean-Seb will look after you well."

I took a few moments while I contemplated. It would make me feel very uncomfortable but I knew that Jean-Seb would meet me straight off the Eurostar.

"Maybe I do need a break," I answered.

When I got home I went on my computer and emailed Jean-Seb. He was excited to hear that I would be attending his wedding and arranged where to meet me. There were only a few weeks to go so I promptly booked my ticket to France travelling by Eurostar again.

While booking it I told the Rugby Train Station that I was registered blind and travelling alone. Although I still felt slightly embarrassed having to tell other people, the train company seemed to be very understanding.

"Let's hope that I don't lose my ticket again," I thought to myself.

On the morning of my journey I awoke alone. My children had been up late the previous night and were still sound asleep although they'd told me that they would be up to see me off. After making sure that I had everything, I went into their rooms to say goodbye but they were fast asleep. I whispered goodbye and left them to their dreams. On my way to the train station, which was only a ten-minute walk from my house, some sad thoughts entered my mind.

"It would have been nice if my children had been awake to say goodbye. I'm scared of travelling alone and that might be the last time I'll see them. Maybe I'll never get to France. Maybe I'll be one of the unfortunate ones to be on the Eurostar when the Channel Tunnel collapses and I'll drown. Maybe that's how I'll die. Carline died young so maybe it's my turn."

It became too much for me and I couldn't contain my emotions; tears began to stream down my face.

"Why did my sister have to die?" I thought sadly. "Why is my family suffering so much? It was so difficult looking after her knowing that she could die at any moment. Nobody knows but I didn't want to wake up after looking after her and be the one to find her dead. I was afraid too but I had to be strong."

There were only a few roads to cross to get to the train station but as usual I was frightened every time I crossed. Although I had my white cane out in full, in my mind I kept thinking that I was about to be knocked over by a car that I was unable to see. Car engines are becoming quieter as technology advances, but the designers don't stop to think that it makes it more difficult for a pedestrian to know whether a car is there or not especially if they are visually impaired.

When I arrived at the train station I asked for assistance. Tears were still in my eyes as I spoke to the guard.

"Hello there, I booked some assistance for my journey to London," I said.

"Have you got your ticket?" he asked.

"Yes; I'll get it for you."

I passed him my ticket and then thought to myself, "I need to say that I'm blind. Even though he can clearly see my white cane, I need to make sure that he knows the extent of my visual impairment. This is going to make me feel very uncomfortable but it has to be done."

"I'm registered blind and travelling alone," I informed him. "I don't know where to go and will need assistance getting on and off the train."

"Can I see your registration card please?"

"He wants proof of my disability?" I thought to myself. "This is so embarrassing having to show people my registration card. I hate it because it constantly reminds me that I'm disabled and I hate having that label."

After the guard had looked at my card he walked me to the platform that I would need to board the train. I followed behind him so that I could copy his actions every time he changed direction. Then he left me sitting on a bench but told me that he would return when the train was due. So I sat there alone, lonely and emotional. Thoughts were still racing through my mind. I was scared of travelling but I kept telling myself that I needed the break and that Jean-Seb would look after me once I arrived in France. It was a continual battle to persuade myself that my dream of going to my friend's wedding was bigger than my fear of travelling alone.

The guard soon returned and told me to follow him because the train was about to arrive. As it pulled into the station, he asked me to follow him to the far end of the train. When we got there he told me that there was a step for me to take to enter the train. I became slightly scared because I knew there was always a gap between the train and the platform and I was worried that I would miss my step and fall into the gap. So I took my time climbing on board and then he told me to follow him again.

"Please sit here," he said kindly.

"This looks different to the last time I travelled," I said.

"We decided to put you in First Class so that you have a more comfortable journey."

"Thank you very much," I answered.

"We've also arranged for someone to meet you at London to assist you to the underground."

As he left more tears rolled out of my eyes at the man's kindness. I appreciated the help but still felt sad that I was incapable of travelling without assistance.

It was a quiet journey to London and as he said, as soon as the train arrived, there was someone to assist me to the London underground. He took me to the correct platform and waited with me. As the tube arrived he told me how many stops it was to Waterloo, where I was going, and said that someone else would be there to meet me. I knew that I couldn't read any names of where the tube stopped and was scared that I would miss where I had to get off.

As the tube began to move I carefully counted the number of times that it stopped. When it got to my stop, I carefully got off and waited for my assistance. Everyone left the platform and I was on my own, waiting for someone to approach me. I waited and I waited, but no one came to help me. I began to feel a bit hysterical because I couldn't see where the exit was, but I pulled myself together, took a guess and walked in the direction that most of the other people had gone. Using my cane, I felt for the steps and carefully made my way to the top. As I looked around I was surprised to notice that there was no one else in sight so I took another guess as to which direction to go in. As I walked and walked something told me that I was going the wrong way, so after a few more minutes I turned around and went the other way. After a while I came across some people and asked them if they knew where the guards were. They told me where to go, which wasn't far, so I walked alone and soon came across someone to help. As I explained what had happened, they apologised profusely and helped me to the Eurostar. Obviously I wasn't happy with their service but it was the fault of the underground and not the train line and I was too emotional to argue so I just boarded the Eurostar and took my seat.

The hardest and scariest part of my journey was over, I thought that I would be left stranded or not get off the tube at the correct stop but I did it and all alone. Now all I had to do was sit there for a few hours while the Eurostar travelled to France. It wouldn't be long before I would see my friend Jean-Seb again and I couldn't wait. A memory popped into my mind of a time when Jean-Seb had made me laugh. While he was living in England some years ago and training with me some French Martial Artists visited us. The instructor wasn't very good at English.

"My student Jean-Seb will translate for us," I said.

"Are you sure that he can?" the instructor queried.

"Jean-Seb is French but I'm not going to tell you yet," I thought to myself.

"Yes, he's good," I answered confidently.

The instructor began to speak in French and Jean-Seb translated it into English. Then I spoke and he translated my words into French. After a while of constantly translating, Jean-Seb began to laugh out loud.

"What're you laughing at?" I asked.

"The instructor told me that my French is very good and that I have an excellent French accent," Jean-Seb said in hysterics.

"Did you tell him that you're French?" I asked.

"Yes; I told him that I hope that I am good at French because I am French," Jean-Seb answered.

As soon as I stepped off the Eurostar Jean-Seb was there right by my side. Once again it was easy to recognise him because he towered over the rest of the people and he always said his name so that I wasn't confused with who he was. I nearly cried when I saw him because I couldn't believe that I had successfully travelled alone. I was an emotional wreck and very tearful. He linked my arm and we left to find his car that he had parked not far from the station.

He took me to his home where I would be staying for the week that I was in France. His car had the steering wheel on the left so I sat on the right. I was grateful for the difference in the side that the driver steers from because he was now on my left, which meant that I could hear him more clearly when he spoke. There was a big difference in volume and I could hear his speech clearly. We arrived at his home and he took my bag as he guided me around obstacles.

"There is a step," he said.

"Where?"

"Step up... now."

Jean-Seb looked after me well, maybe more than I expected. He gave me plenty of time to myself and sometimes I lay on my bed and cried for hours. It was only two months since the death of my sister and I was still grieving.

When we went outdoors, he guided me well, up and down steps, in and out of shops. I wasn't sure where any steps were or whether shops had glass doors but Jean-Seb helped me to feel more comfortable. He took me literally everywhere he went. There were lots of preparations to be done for his wedding and I was always asked to stay by his side. When his family began to set up the wedding hall, I asked if I could help. I didn't like standing around like an invalid because it made me feel useless. I helped set up the tables by following other people who were also rolling tables into position. I also helped with the chairs and inflating the balloons with a pump.

Then I was given the biggest surprise of all, which made me tearful. Jean-Seb said that I was his special guest and told me that I would be sitting on his table by his side. This made me feel as though my scary journey by myself was well worth it. As we continued with the preparations in the wedding hall some of his friends and family introduced themselves and helped make me feel welcome. Most of them were very proficient at English and I enjoyed listening to their French accent. It sounded so sexy and always brought a smile to my face.

At the wedding Jean-Seb fetched my meal for me because I was unable to see any difference between the various foods. It tasted delicious, but through my eyes it was a mass of integrated colours. He kept topping up my glass of wine because he knew that the glass was invisible to me. I also preferred red wine because it gave the invisible glass colour again so that I was able to see it but every time my glass became empty it also became invisible again. Most of the time I would leave a bit of wine in the bottom of my glass so that I knew where it was. It was also difficult eating food that looked like grey mist. It wasn't clear what to cut with my knife or pick up with my fork. I couldn't enjoy the true beauty of the food by sight but I sure ate it all up. During his speech, Jean-Seb made reference to me and stated that I was registered blind and had travelled alone from England to be at his wedding. I felt like I belonged there. He made me feel so special. After that, many of his family and friends visited our table to help make me feel welcome.

His friends made me feel too welcome and began to fight over who would take me home one afternoon. When I got into a car that belonged to one of his friends and settled myself on the seat, I was startled by the sudden appearance of a large dog that had been reclining peacefully in the back. It kept sniffing me and I began to laugh to myself wishing that I had chosen another car to travel in but I enjoyed the entertainment, really!

During my stay in France I learnt that French people really do like their cheese. They seem to have a different choice of cheese for every day of the year. I wasn't too keen on cheese before I visited France but now that I've eaten so much of it, I must admit that I love it. Sadly my holiday in France came to an end and it was time for me to return to England. Jean-Seb drove me to the station and asked if he could park his car very close to the station because he had a blind person with him. Then he walked me in as far as he was allowed and asked for an assistant to help me onto the Eurostar. They were very helpful and guided me to my seat. My long return journey started and I began to feel lonely again. I closed my eyes for most of the journey because I didn't know where to look. Sometimes I would be looking at people without realising it and I never wanted other people to feel uncomfortable. Most people were too blurred and distorted for me to tell the difference between them and the background.

When I arrived in England and stepped off the Eurostar, my adventure began once more. There was no guard in sight so I followed the crowd instead of helplessly waiting for someone who might never come. When I got to the exit, there were a few assistants standing around so I asked for help. One of them took me to the correct platform and saw me onto the tube in the London underground. After counting the number of stops once more, I carefully got off the tube. Once again there was nobody to help me. I was scared because I didn't know which way to go but I followed the crowd again rather than waiting for help. When I got to London Euston, I slowly walked around until I spotted a guard. He took me to an assistant at the information desk and left me there. The woman was busy giving details to other people about the times of various trains, so I just stood there waiting. After half an hour or so, she called another assistant to help me onto my train. I felt so helpless having to rely on so many people. My new helper took my bag and walked with me to my train, but I felt as though this person had no training of how to deal with disabled people. I clearly had my white cane out in full so he knew exactly what my disability was yet he walked as though I could see without problem. He walked too fast and didn't seem to care whether I could keep up. Then he climbed ahead of me onto the train without turning around to make sure that I could manage the step. I felt humiliated and disgusted with his attitude. He showed no compassion towards me and I struggled to stop myself from giving him a mouthful. Then he walked through the train until he came across a seat. The first seat that he saw had someone's bag on it and there was a family with a small child taking up the other seats. He picked up their bag and told them that the seats were for sitting on, then he told me to sit there. I sat down and ignored him. I didn't want to say anything because I didn't trust myself. Then he walked off and disappeared out of sight. I apologised to the family and told them that he had a bad attitude and no experience of how to treat people with respect. Then I closed my eyes for the rest of my journey and tried to think of something cheerful to prevent me from dwelling on what had just happened.

When I arrived in Rugby I stood up and walked over to the door. There was nobody else getting off and I was unable to see which button to press to open the door. There is Braille on the buttons but I, along with many other blind people, am unable to read Braille. Slowly I began to panic thinking that the train was about to pull off again. So I pressed both buttons and hoped for the best. The doors opened and I hastily left the train. There was nobody to assist me out of the station but fortunately I have made train journeys before and found the exit from memory.

Then I made my way back home, worrying every time I crossed the road, thinking that it may be my last. I've often said that I'll probably die by being knocked over accidentally. When I got home I was happy to see my children again and they were just as happy to see me. The break away to France helped me to deal with the loss of my sister. Although I had gone to France feeling sad, I returned feeling happy.

CHAPTER 28
BUMP IN THE NIGHT

A young lady called Sophie kept watching her child train with me. Somehow I was able to notice her – maybe it was because she was very attractive. Sometimes she would come and talk to me after the class and other times I would be distracted by her and approach her during my lesson. Slowly our friendship grew and we became good friends.

"Why don't you go and sit in the bar while you're waiting for my class to finish?" I asked.

"Because I like watching your bum in the mirror," she answered.

My interest in her grew rapidly and I asked her out for a drink. We had a great night out and ended up having sex. She told me that she was in an unstable relationship but wasn't ready to leave her partner so we remained friends. She became a special friend to me, someone who I could open up to and share my problems with. We didn't use each other; we mostly talked and were there for each other with a shoulder to cry on when needed.

In November 2003, we decided to go on holiday together to Barcelona. It was another aeroplane journey for me, but I was getting more used to flying and although I was still nervous, the thrill and excitement of a holiday was far greater than my fear. Sophie knew about my eyesight problem and guided me around Barcelona. It was a beautiful place, but there were a lot steps that were unmarked with a strip to help poorly sighted people. I did use my white cane to get around but I still struggled because the surroundings were unfamiliar to me.

At night Barcelona looked stunning. Most of the buildings had small spotlights shinning onto them at different angles and it made them look amazing. Sometimes I would stand and stare at brightly lit buildings for ages, admiring the view. The famous architect, Gaudi, who designed many parts of Barcelona, sure had good taste. I would say that Barcelona is quite a romantic place to take someone who you care about. You can stand outside bars and listen to the music in the night air or go for walks by the water fountains. I enjoyed the four days that we stayed there.

Sophie and I still remain special friends and we keep in touch regularly.

The Spanish life caught my heart and I returned in May 2004. This time I travelled to Benidorm in the Costa Blanca with my sister June and her family. There were five of us and we all stayed in the same apartment. I was getting even more scared of going completely blind by this time and was forcing myself to enjoy my life while I was still able to see. The world is a beautiful place and many people seem to take it for granted. If other people knew that they were about to lose their eyesight maybe they too would learn to appreciate the wonders of the world.

My sister and her family had to look after me while we were in the apartment and out and about. The kitchen was a completely new layout for me and I was finding it difficult to do simple things like turning on the tap for water. I decided to take a back seat and leave most of the usual household chores to them (lazy!) so that I didn't accidentally break anything. They had to show me where literally everything was and how to use them. Knowing where the soap or toothpaste was with so many people around created a challenge so I used my own and kept them in my room in the same place so that I was able to find them each time without having to constantly ask for help.

Someone always came with me to the shop that was across the road. There was a lift to get downstairs and I couldn't see clearly enough to use the buttons in it. When we got down and had to walk out through the door, I couldn't tell whether it was open or closed because it was a large glass door. The handle was also invisible to my eyes. When we got across the road to enter the shop I would be told where the steps were. Then I would follow whoever I was with around the shop while they named many of the items. I didn't touch or look at anything – it was all too blurred. All I could do was walk around feeling like my eyes were closed. Not being able to see anything clearly frustrated me and was sometimes difficult to deal with.

"This is ridiculous," I thought to myself. "Everything is so blurred and cloudy through my eyes. What's the point of me looking at anything? I can't work out what the different items are and there are too many things in the shop for me to be able to pick them up and hold them close to my face to see what they are. I wish that I could see clearer and be able to see the milk and the bread and the drinks. Life isn't fair! Oh well, I won't think about it or it will make me feel incapable. I'll think of something cheerful."

Sometimes I felt so hopeless that I preferred to stay in the apartment and let my family go to the shop for me.

When we went out into town or sightseeing, I found myself memorising my surroundings as usual. Lamp posts and boulders were in awkward positions, different to where they might be back in England. After a day or so my sister told me that I seemed to know how to get around better than she did. As long as it was a route that we used regularly I knew the pavements and obstacles in my path and also where most of the steps were. After a few days I found myself walking around much more confidently.

Most days the weather was beautiful and the sun shone brightly, but the light was so dazzling that I had to use my sunglasses. They were prescription sunglasses so I could still see and they helped a lot when I was on the beach, but when I went into shops the goods became so dark that they disappeared completely. I found it frustrating trying to work out whether I was better off seeing everything blurred but being in pain from the unbearable sun, or seeing most things as shadows but being relieved from the pain of the glaring sun.

"The sun is too bright," I complained to myself. "Why can't I have better eyes to be able to appreciate everything? I had better not think about it much because I don't want to concentrate on my disability. I want to enjoy my holiday."

My niece and nephew loved to play on the beach, but when they took a few steps away from me I had difficulty in identifying them from the rest of the people around. Levante Beach is very busy and I was confused with where to walk. Sometimes my sister would make reference to what her two children were doing and all I could do was wonder in my mind.

"I wish that I could see my niece and nephew," I thought. "I would love to be able to see their faces as they play and enjoy themselves. They're just a few metres away from me and yet I can't see them. I would love to be able to run around the beach and join in but I would bump into everyone. Never mind, I can walk carefully along enjoying the beautiful weather and feel the warmth of the sun."

I even missed out on the beautiful view of the surrounding buildings that June enjoyed looking at.

"Look at that beautiful building over there," June marvelled.

"I bet it looks amazing," I answered.

"I wish you could see what I see Vendon. There are so many tall buildings around and I can even see our apartment block from here."

"Our apartment is about half a mile away," I thought. "It would be so great to have the privilege to be able to see so clearly, but I'm having problems seeing what's directly in front of me."

"Is it an exciting view?" I asked.

"Yes, and the beach is wonderful. The sand is very fine and there are lots of people around and they all look so happy. My children are running along the beach and you should see the sea, it's beautiful," she answered.

"I have to miss out on most of the excitement because of my fading eyesight," I thought sadly. "I wish I could see the children running along the beach."

As we walked along the path beside the beach we came across something in the sand.

"Oh wow! I wish you could see this," June said.

"What is it?" I asked.

"Someone has built a large castle in the sand and it has lots of detail, and there's also a drawing in the sand of the twelve disciples of Jesus and their faces are really clear. It must have been done by an artist because it must have taken hours or even days to complete," June said.

As I looked down all I could see was a mass of sand that was so bright in the dazzling sun that it hurt my eyes to look at. There were no details for me to marvel at through my eyes. When I put my sunglasses on, the sand became a dark shadow but at least the sun stopped hurting my eyes. As I looked, I knew that I was missing out on something amazing.

"Can you see their faces in detail?" I asked.

"Yes; you can see their eyes, noses, mouths and even the food on the table," she answered in amazement.

"I wish I could see them," I thought. "I bet they're all beautiful to look at. June is very lucky being able to see the different designs in the sand. I'm better off thinking of something cheerful than wishing for something that I will never see."

At the end of the path there were lots of rocks that led down to the sea. It was very hot and David told me that he could see lots of cats lying on the rocks enjoying the sun. Although I'm not a great lover of cats, it would have been nice to be able to see them. David asked me to take some photos of him near the seafront. I guessed where to direct the camera and took a few photographs. David looked at the photos on the digital camera and told me that I should become a blind photographer because I'd caught him perfectly.

Then we went shopping to look for gifts. David showed me a shop that sold mainly glass ornaments. He had to describe them to me. Some of them had colourful lights on but I was unable to see. They sounded beautiful so I bought one.

"I would have loved to be able to see them for myself," I thought. "The way David described them sounded so impressive. Most of the things in this shop are invisible to my eyes so I'd better be careful not to break anything."

At night it became even harder for me to see. The nights seemed to be getting darker the worse my eyes became. Sometimes I would walk in the road so that I wouldn't bump into any lamp posts that I was unable to see. My sister and her husband David helped me well and even pulled me out of the way of lamp posts just before I collided with them but they were unable to save me every time. I managed to bump into a few lamp posts but I was fortune to only hit them with my shoulder. I also bumped into a few people on our way to the nightclubs. The clubs and pubs were very impressive. They allowed children in until 1 am so we were able to stay as a family. June told me that there were many different coloured lights illuminating the names of the clubs, but all I saw were bright blurred lights that I was unable to read. Sometimes I could see the different colours and I would stand and stare as I admired something that I hardly ever had the pleasure of seeing.

In the clubs I felt disorientated because I wasn't used to where things were so it took me a while to work out what each blurred object was. It was easier for me to let David and June get my drinks at the bar because I wasn't sure when the bar staff were asking to serve me. Their faces were too dark and distorted for me to see their facial features. Finding the toilets was also difficult and I had to be escorted by one of my family to the door of the men's toilets. They then waited for me and took me back to the others. I don't feel comfortable being guided all the time and that's why I usually drink in the same pubs back in Rugby. I know where the toilets are and can manage to get around by myself.

My holiday to Spain with my sister's family was great. Fortunately I enjoy being on holiday so much that I can cope with the problems I experience getting around. Although I can't see clearly, I feel as though I can see enough to enjoy myself. Not being able to see is a constant battle to face but I think that I'm more fortunate than my sister who can only see through one eye, but then she's more fortunate than my brother who can't see through either of his. My vision at night scares me more than the constant grey mist that I see throughout the day. It usually takes a while for my friends to persuade me to go out for a drink at night in Rugby. Sometimes I make up excuses not to go but my real fear is not feeling comfortable seeing so little in the pubs and clubs. My eyesight does hold me back from going out and having fun but I do try my best to enjoy myself.

My friend Nij convinced me to join him for a drink one night. On the way into Rugby Town Centre Nij constantly guided me so that I wouldn't bump into anything. We were chatting and he forgot to tell me that there was a bin in my way; I bumped straight into it and knocked it flying. Then Nij said; "Oh, watch out for the bin."

"It's a bit too late to tell me now," I answered as we fell about laughing.

Then we walked on towards a road and everything was dark so I couldn't tell if there was a cyclist coming. It was too difficult for me to work out whether it was safe to cross the road so he dragged me by my jacket as he hastily led me across the road. As I walked along my eyes darted from left to right trying to find the best part of my eyes to focus with. Sometimes when I looked straight ahead I couldn't see anything, not even shadows, but when I looked to my side and used the side part of my eyes to see the same place, I can see shadows or even more sometimes. Using the side of my eyes I can sometimes see people approaching me but when I look straight again, they seem to disappear like magic. I noticed that some of the roads we used to get to the pubs were looking much darker to me but when I asked Nij he said that he could see fine and the thoughts would rush through my mind.

"My eyes are getting noticeably worse. People seem to appear from nowhere just before I'm going to collide with them. I'm a hazard to other people these days. Maybe I shouldn't come out during the evening. I'm so afraid of walking into lamp posts and parked cars that I can't see. It's like I'm living in a black and white world at night. It's so difficult to see most colours."

As we walked into town and came across the brighter lit areas, I had some more mixed thoughts.

"I can see the bright lights from the shops but the people walking past are like shadows – ghostly figures without faces. Most of them appear to have distorted masks on and I bet some of them are good-looking people. I wish I could see their faces in more detail whether they're attractive or not."

Then I suddenly stopped as I remembered that there should be a boulder nearby and I didn't want to bump into it. Carefully I walked on. Then I stopped again because I thought that a shadow was a person I was about to crash into. Then I walked on. Although I had Nij to guide me, I wasn't ready to put all my trust in him or anyone else. People make mistakes and although I found it quite funny walking into a wheelie bin, it could have been a lamp post that would have left its mark.

A few months ago I went to visit a friend during the daytime. I thought that I was walking carefully and I was also using a route that I was very familiar with. The layout of the road was in my head, memorised from years of use but suddenly I bumped straight into a post and within seconds a large lump appeared on my forehead. When I looked up to see what the post was, I saw that a builder had put up some scaffolding around a building without any obvious markings to indicate that something was there. Fortunately it didn't hurt me but my pride was hurt as I hastily walked back home to nurse my poorly head. It's at times like that when I sometimes wonder if I would be better off staying indoors and out of harm's way.

As Nij and I made our way into Rugby Town Centre, we passed the clock tower. I used to be able to read that huge clock, but when I look at it now, I can only see the white circular shape. The numbers and the hands of the clock have disappeared. It's a constant reminder of how much my eyes have deteriorated over the years.

Just before we got to the pub someone walked past me and said hello.

"Who was that?" Nij asked.

"I don't know!" I replied.

We laughed and walked on. If it was someone who didn't know about my disability then they wouldn't know that I was unable to identify them. If it was someone who knew about my difficulties, then they should have thought before they spoke. The obvious way to communicate with someone with a serious visual impairment is to identify yourself by name first. That way the person with the visual impairment doesn't have to guess the name of whom they are speaking with.

There was a step to enter the pub.

"Mind the step," Nij cautioned.

I lifted my leg high and took a step into the pub. It wasn't clear to me whether it was a small step or a large one so by assuming it was a big step, I shouldn't trip up. The only problem was that I probably looked stupid lifting my leg so high but I've learnt to deal with it positively. My glasses steamed up as I walked in. Most of the time I leave them to clear by themselves because I can't see much anyway. There were shadows of ghosts everywhere and I was unable to identify anyone. Their faces appeared to have very dark masks on. There are parts of pubs that have spotlights and it's sometimes brighter near the bar, so this is where I prefer to stand. When I'm talking to someone I try to position them so that the light reflects off their face. This helps me to see them clearer and I feel more comfortable talking to people who I'm able to see a bit. Most of the time people appear to have dark masks on that cover their eyes, nose and mouth. When I talk to someone who appears too dark to see anything more than their outline, I get confused with where to look. In these situations I try to estimate where their eyes would be from the size of their shadowed head! Then I look towards the centre of the shadowed head and I've been told that people can't tell that I'm not actually looking at them. I also constantly look away from them to see if they look any clearer from the sides of my eyes. When I'm near a spotlight, I can see their head more clearly but I struggle to see their facial features in detail, so most of the time I can see their eyes and mouth but not clear enough to see what colour their eyes are. This is why I stay in the brighter areas of places I go. Even if I visit someone else's house, I normally stay in the brighter areas. I appreciate seeing people because I don't get much chance to see them clearly and the darker they appear, the more negative thoughts I have.

"This pub is full of people yet I can't see anyone clearly," I thought to myself. "Everyone appears to be so badly distorted that I can't tell if they really are people. I'm having problems seeing the person directly in front of me. Sometimes they look like they haven't got a head. Sometimes I can see them clearer using the sides of my eyes. I don't know where to look when I can't see the face of the person I'm speaking to. I'm sick and tired of seeing dark shadows for people."

My babysitter, Josie, was in the pub and she approached me. She has beautiful big green eyes and long red hair. Sometimes when I'm out in the bright sunlight I can see that her hair is red but I can no longer see the colour of her eyes. Even under the spotlight in the pub she appeared to have long dark hair. We chatted for a while before she left with her friends. Josie has been looking after my children for ten years and has grown very close to my family. She inspires me and helps me deal with my sight disorder. I feel as though she's worse off than I am because she has a rare illness and doesn't know how long she has to live. Her heart is lying sideways and this is causing many problems including slowing down her rate of growth. She's only twenty-seven years old and has been having injections on a daily basis to keep her going. She reminds me of me and gives me more strength to carry on. She always has a smile on her face and tries her best to get on with life and I admire her greatly for that.

We went to the bar to get a beer and I decided to try to get served. It was very difficult to know when the bar staff were ready to serve me. I couldn't see their facial features clearly enough to see them speak and I could hardly hear them because of the blaring music and my deafness in one ear. When I did get served I noticed that Nij was talking to someone. I had ordered two different beers for us but couldn't tell the difference so I asked the bar person.

"Excuse me, but which one is the Stella?" I asked.

"The one that has the name Stella on the glass," he replied cockily.

"Thanks for that, but I'm registered blind, so which one is the Stella?" I repeated.

I could feel his embarrassment.

"Sorry, I'm really sorry but I didn't think. This one is the Stella," he answered as he pushed the glass slightly nearer to me.

"Thanks," I said giving him a slight smile and I walked over to Nij.

We spoke for a while before someone else approached me.

"Hello Vendon," a voice said.

"Who's that? I don't recognise their voice," I thought to myself.

"Hello, but I can't see you, who are you?" I asked politely.

"You know who I am!" the voice said.

"You look like a ghost to me," I thought. "I can see your face but I can't see any features."

"Actually I'm blind and I struggle to see at night," I replied.

"You do know who I am!" the voice repeated.

"I give up," I thought to myself. "I don't care who you are now. I've told you that I can't see and you still mock me. How difficult is it to mention your name?"

We had a conversation and as time went on, I learnt that the person I was speaking to was already aware of my disability, yet they refused to give their name. I didn't get upset from this ordeal and put it down to them being too drunk to realise that they were ignorant.

After a few beers my bladder became full and I suddenly needed the toilet. I mostly drank in pubs where I knew where the toilet was so I slowly made my way through the crowd of people. I could only see the person directly before me so it was difficult for me to know whether there was a group of people in front of me. Basically I just walk and make my way through the crowd. I have occasionally gone the wrong way and ended up facing a table or wall but I put that down to being blind drunk!

When I got to the toilet door I tried to touch it on a part that I thought other men would hardly touch. Then I went inside and used the toilet before washing my hands. I prefer to use automatic taps that you don't have to touch to make the water come out. I dried my hands as I waited for someone else to come into the room, then I made a sudden dash for the open door so that I didn't have to touch the door handle. Although I'm still suffering from OCD, I'm slowly learning how to control it. I made my way back to where I had left Nij. If he had moved I would struggle to find him so as I approached he called out to me to let me know that I was in the right place.

After a short while of chatting and drinking, a young lady came over to me. She had long blond hair but I was unable to see her face very clearly.

"Excuse me, but can I have your autograph please?" she asked.

I chuckled, "Who do you think I am?"

"You're the man from the Halifax Bank commercial on TV."

"No, I'm not him, sorry," I answered.

"You look just like him! Can you come over and meet my friends?"

"Just tell them I said hello," I answered in embarrassment.

Several of my friends had already told me that I look like Howard Brown from the Halifax Bank advert on TV. Although I disagree, since I've had my hair cut shorter than usual, several other people have stopped to ask me the same question. I was once approached by a very old lady who couldn't wait to shake my hand and I didn't want to disappoint her so I didn't correct her mistake. I enjoy the attention from the ladies but several men have also stopped me and that spoils my fun!

We left that pub and went to another one that I'm familiar with. Once again I passed someone who appeared to know me.

"Hello Vendon," they said as they casually walked on.

"Hello," I replied.

"Do you know who that was?" Nij asked.

"Nope," I answered.

We began to laugh again. Once again I was unable to identify someone but we saw the funny side of it.

We entered the pub and had a few more beers. I stood in the brighter part of the pub so that I had a better chance of seeing people who I knew. My nephew Dyonn said hello as he hastily walked past. He forgot to mention his name first.

"Was that Dyonn?" I asked Nij.

"Yes," he replied.

Then Nij told me that Natalie was in the pub close to the bar. He directed me to her and I walked over by myself. When I got to someone at the side of the bar where Nij said she was, I checked for her outline. When I decided that it was her, I began to speak.

"Hello there, I didn't know that you were coming clubbing," I said.

"Hello, I love clubbing!" she answered.

"Who're you with?" I asked.

"Just some friends," she said.

"Are you well?" I asked.

"Yes thanks," she answered cheerfully.

At that moment a worrying thought rushed through my mind. "Oh-oh, that didn't sound like Natalie."

"Err, sorry," I said. "I thought you were someone else. You're not Natalie are you?"

"No, but don't worry, people think that I'm someone else all the time," she answered nicely with a smile.

Just then someone tapped me on my shoulder from behind and I turned around and saw Natalie. She had been talking to someone else and had her back to me.

"That was definitely not Natalie then," I thought in amusement, "but she seemed to enjoy the conversation as much as I did."

Later on, a young lady with very long dark hair said hello as she was passing. There were several people in my mind that she could have been but I wasn't sure. Her facial features weren't clear enough. Although I thought that I could identify her, the truth is that I will never know. Long dark hair is easy for me to see because of its length, which is probably the reason I prefer long hair on ladies. It catches my eyes more easily!

Nij and I then had a dance on the dance floor (but not with each other!). We seemed to attract more attention when we wore Addidas aftershave. It was mine but Nij always borrowed it when we went out to have fun. Sometimes we also buy a cheap bottle of champagne each and people ask us if we're getting married or if they can have some. It all adds to our fun!

At the end of the night when the lights were turned on, I looked around at the way people's clothing changed colours. It always feels great to see any colour other than black and white. After we finished our drinks, we went to have our usual curry. We were a little drunk and started singing our usual song. You can always tell when Nij and I are drunk because we start singing the same song and it doesn't take much to get me drunk. It starts off with these words: 'If you like a lot of chocolate on your biscuit, join our club'.

I know that we sound sad but we do have a laugh when we go out.

So we went to have a late night curry which is something we do on a regular basis. It's very difficult to avoid the lamp posts and other obstacles when I can't see but it's even harder when I'm drunk. I tend to walk slowly so if I do hit anything, it normally doesn't do any damage to me. I appear to be a clumsy drunk person to other people and I'm fine with that. It feels great to be able to have fun despite my disability.

I followed Nij to where he wanted to sit and looked for the brightest place but I also had to take my hearing into consideration. Sometimes I might sit somewhere that is slightly brighter but where I will struggle to hear or sometimes I might sit somewhere that is slightly darker but I will be able to hear better. It confuses me too! Sometimes I take a few seconds to decide where the best place would be to sit.

The waiter brought over some menus.

"We only need one menu," Nij said.

"Why?" the waiter asked.

"Because my friend is blind and can't read the menu," Nij replied.

Although it makes me feel slightly useless, it's a situation that I'm learning to accept. I have to sit there looking around trying to identify things on the table or trying to work out where Nij's head is. Sometimes I can see his outline and other times I can't. It depends on where we sit and the lighting. It sometimes feels uncomfortable talking to a headless body so most of the time I don't look at people so that I don't feel emotional. I also think of happier things to take my mind off what I can't see. Nij read out the menu to me. Most of the time I have the same meal anyway. I sometimes get confused with the amount of choice on the menu and Nij has to read it again. We ordered our meals.

We usually have water to drink with our curry even though it's a bad choice for me. I can't see the glasses very well and when they have water in, they're still almost invisible to my eye. Nij tells me where my glass is and I slowly pick it up, trying not to knock it over, then I put it in an easy place where I can't accidentally knock it over. Sometimes I put the glass in a position where it may be easier to see but it's not always possible. When I need more water Nij pours it for me because if I did it I would probably pour it over the table! I hate not being able to see glasses. It's like my eyes are closed when I'm reaching for the glass but that's another thought that I try to dismiss regularly. I know that I would be better off with a dark drink but I usually need water after having beer.

When I got my meal, I searched around for my cutlery. I had a bit of difficulty because the knife, fork and spoon had blended into the table as if they had become transparent. Having found them I used my fork to work out where the food was on my plate. What I see on my plate depends upon the different contrasts of food. If the plate is bright and the food is dark, then I will see that there is food on my plate but I won't be able to see the details. If the food is also bright like potato or salad, then I won't be able to see it so using my fork to feel where it is becomes a great help. The opposite happens when the contrasts are swapped. If the plate is dark then meat and other darker foods become invisible but I'm then able to see potato or salad. For this reason, when I eat out I usually refrain from having salad even though I like it. Most plates are bright, causing the salad to disappear before my very eyes. Eating without seeing is a stress that I'm used to and try not to think about, much. There's nothing that I can do about it so I constantly battle in my mind, trying not to get distressed.

During our meal, another young lady approached us.

"Hi there," she said.

"Hello," we answered in unison.

"Are you Gos from the Big Brother TV show?" she asked looking at Nij. "And are you the man from the Halifax advert?" she went on looking at me.

We broke out in laughter.

"Yes we are!" we answered jokingly.

"Can I have your autographs for my friend who's waiting outside?"

We looked outside but I was unable to see anyone. Nij told me that he could see another lady waiting by the door. I became jealous and wished that I had his clear vision.

After we had finished our curry, we walked home in the dark. Most of the streets appeared to be darker than usual. I asked Nij if it was dark to him but he said that he was still able to see things. The darkness slightly scared me because I couldn't see the pavement, the parked cars, trees, lamp posts or people walking towards me. I felt disorientated, but then that could have been the alcohol. Most of the time I walked behind Nij and hoped that he wouldn't move without telling me or I might walk straight into someone or something.

My house is slightly to the left of a bright streetlight. The light guides me to my house and as long as I'm on the right side of the road and not too drunk, it's quite easy to get to my front door. A few weeks ago I was out with my family and we got a taxi home. Maybe I was a little drunk because when I got out of the taxi and headed for the left of the streetlight, they called to me and told me that I was trying to go into the wrong house. I hadn't realised that I had got out on the other side of my road but thought that I was going towards my house from memory. They found it funny and laughed at me crossing back over to the other side. I felt very disorientated but that could have been the alcohol too!

CHAPTER 29
I'M BLESSED TOO

On the way to my next eye appointment in April 2004, vivid thoughts began to cloud my mind.

"Here we go again. It's taken me a year to build my confidence back up by learning to get on with my life and cope with my visual impairment, and now I'm off to another eye appointment to knock my confidence right back down again. I must be mad. Why am I putting myself through this punishment? Is all this really worth it? There's nothing they can do to help me so why am I punishing myself for other people? They're only using me as a guinea pig. I suppose it will help find a cure for my children and other innocent people, so I guess it'll be worth it."

Sometimes I feel like missing appointments because as time goes on since the previous appointment, I grow stronger and more positive towards life even though I know that my eyes are still deteriorating. When the doctor informs me of the degree that they have deteriorated then it knocks the confidence right out of me. I already know that I'm about to have bad news so maybe I should avoid appointments!

This time my two children went along with me for moral support. They kept me happy prior to my first test by being their usual funny selves and it wasn't long before I was called in. As before, the first test was to read the letters on the chart. Obviously my eyesight had become more blurred and the chart appeared even more distorted. With my glasses still on, both my eyes were unable to read any lines on the chart, not even the huge letter at the top on its own – the one that I always thought that I would have to be blind not to be able to see. The doctor used another large card with a single letter on and slowly walked towards me until I was able to read it. He was almost upon me before I could see the letter clearly enough.

"He's even closer to me than last time," I thought to myself. "He must be only a metre away. When will this suffering stop? I guess it will stop when I'm totally blind in both eyes like my brother. Everywhere looks very distorted as though my short sight is becoming worse yet there are no new prescription glasses to help me. How am I supposed to get around if everything looks like this? I guess my future really is to be guided around by other people."

My vision had deteriorated and everywhere and everything was more out of focus. My cloudy vision made it much harder to see things. It felt like I was in a car and it was travelling through thick fog, but this mist never goes away, it only thickens.

The next test showed that more of my vision had become covered with blind spots, which meant that there were more areas in which I appear to be totally blind. I could be looking straight at someone and not see them. When they're closer to me then the blind spots take up less space on the area I'm looking at and sometimes I see them.

Everything was already blurred but then the doctor administered the eye drops to dilate my eyes. These made my already blurred view even more distorted and visually disturbing. Once again I sat and watched as what little vision I had was taken away.

"I suppose I should be grateful that I don't see like this all the time," I thought. "How am I going to cope when it happens? How do other blind people cope who have less vision than this? This is a cruel way to punish someone – taking away my eyesight, something that most people value the most – it makes me feel completely useless."

The tears started and I became emotional.

"It could be worse," I told myself, "there are people worse off than me so I should count myself lucky. At least I still have a chance to appreciate things."

My specialist gave me the results of all the tests. It was nothing that I wasn't expecting but it still hurt to be told. The results showed that my eyesight was slowly continuing to deteriorate and they confirmed that I was suffering more from night blindness, which explained why roads appeared to be darker when I was out at night. I was also told that I had to continue taking my eye drops to relieve the pressure of the glaucoma and that the cataract was slowly growing.

"Have any cures been developed yet?" I asked.

"No, I'm afraid not. It will be many years before a cure is found because the eyes are very complicated."

"What about my children?" I asked, feeling very worried for them.

"It's possible that they may develop RP, as could your siblings' children. The strain of RP that you have can affect 50% of a family.

It can remain dormant then be passed along to children. We don't know who will develop it."

"My poor children," I thought. "They could get it too. Life isn't fair. What have they done to deserve this evil punishment?"

"Is it worth having them tested?" I asked.

"Yes, but it's difficult to detect at their young age."

"I don't want to put them through vigorous tests if there is no certainty that you can do a correct diagnosis," I said.

"It's your choice."

"Can they correct my short sight with laser treatment?" I asked.

"Your eyes are too delicate and no specialist would touch them because we still don't know enough about RP."

"Life isn't fair," I thought again. "It would have helped a great deal if I could have had laser treatment. People look ridiculously blurred when I take my glasses off, which is so frustrating when I'm teaching Martial Arts and fighting with my students. Maybe it's time to give up fighting altogether."

When I was asked if I was experiencing any more discomfort, I replied that the floaters in my eyes appeared to be growing and there seemed to be more of them. This causes me to think that I see something when it's actually my eyes playing tricks on me.

Floaters are clumps of dead cells that move around the eyes at random. They seem to speed up when I look from left to right and can sometimes look like shadows so I often think that someone or something is in front of me. Then I will suddenly stop because I think that I'm about to collide with something that isn't even there. This distresses me and causes me much confusion. Sometimes they look like small rats and I feel as though I'm seeing things.

My darker vision also adds to my confusion and it creates more illusions in my visual field. Sometimes I think that it's because my glasses are dirty and so I clean them. Removing my glasses also relieves some of the pain from constantly straining to see. There are no stronger glasses to help me see so all I can do is watch my world fade away. There are times when I think that cleaning my glasses makes a difference but after a while I become confused with what I see again. My next idea is to blink vigorously or close one of my eyes for a few seconds. The best way for me to cope with my dark eyesight is to constantly use different parts of my eyes to see with but I feel very uncomfortable doing so.

When my specialist had finished, someone assisted me back to where my children were waiting patiently. They jumped up to greet me and then guided me out to the car park. I felt helpless.

"Why does my eyesight have to be so blurred that I can't walk around unaided?" I thought in distress. "I know that there isn't anything that they can do for my dark sight but surely there must be stronger glasses to help focus my vision. I'm sick of seeing like this. I'm sick of seeing as though I'm looking through foggy rain that doesn't become clearer when I wipe my glasses."

As I went outside, the blinding rays of the sun hurt my dilated eyes so I put my sunglasses on.

On the way back to Rugby I became tearful; again.

"Why did I come?" I thought to myself sadly. "Why do I keep putting myself through this pain and suffering? It's not like they have a cure that can help me. I'm not sure if I can take any more bad news about my eyes. Why can't they hurry up and discover a cure for RP? Other people are so lucky being able to see the world. I'm learning to deal with it but I really don't want to go totally blind. I'm so scared of losing my vision completely. Why does it have to be so blurred? Why does it have to be so dark and cloudy? Please let it stop."

Tears streamed down my face throughout the journey home. My poor children sat in silence not knowing what to say to me. What are you supposed to say to someone who is known to be strong and yet looks like an emotional wreck?

The next day my eyes were still slightly dilated so I didn't do much, but my day of misery was over and I knew that it was time to put my appointment behind me and start building up my confidence again. I knew that my eyesight was getting worse and that there wasn't much difference between what I saw with my glasses on or off. Soon I would no longer need to wear my glasses so I felt like I was now in a rush and running out of time to be able to see things. It was time to learn to deal with my sight loss.

The changes started with brushing my teeth. I often missed the toothbrush when trying to squeeze the toothpaste onto it, so I started spreading the toothpaste on one of my fingers, and then I smudged the toothpaste that was on my finger onto my teeth. Then I brushed them as normal but I washed the toothpaste off my finger first! I stopped looking in the mirror so that I didn't see a blurred image of myself as that usually created negative thoughts. There were many things that I avoided so that I didn't have so much chance to feel hopeless.

Somehow I learnt to control my OCD to a certain degree. I ignored most of the mess my children left. By avoiding looking at it or thinking about the problems it caused me by having to manoeuvre around toys, it slowly became easier to cope with. When I ate I tried not to look at my food unless I was using other parts of my eyes to see it. When I made a cup of tea, I held my cup over the sink. This way any spilt water went in the sink and not on the worktop. When I had toast and butter, I put the lid of the butter down somewhere that was a completely a different colour to it. It was a regular problem that I had because the lid seemed to disappear on the worktop, as it seemed to be of the same colour.

Most of the time I began to avoid eye contact with people because if I don't look, I don't think so much about my visual impairment. Sometimes I missed looking at people and would look at them using my central vision when the lighting was better. When I spoke to people I looked at them from the side of my eyes more because I seem to have more vision from the side. So when I appeared not to be looking at someone, I probably was and when I looked directly at them using my central vision in poor light, I couldn't actually see them. It feels cool sometimes because it's amazing how much more people look at you when they think that you're not looking at them.

Using my computer was still causing me stress. The keyboard began to look more cloudy and distorted so I found that I was pressing the wrong keys more often. Large text on my screen also became very difficult to see so I began to use magnification and speech software more regularly. Sometimes I amazed other people, especially my children, who could be struggling to manoeuvre around the computer screen and then I'd come along and do it with greater speed. I've switched off the screen and impressed my children by finding saved work solely using the speech software. It helped but I still struggled with the Internet so I hardly used it any more – most websites are not visual impaired friendly. Printing was another challenge. It was difficult for me to see if my work had printed correctly and colour prints were my greatest problem because I couldn't see colours like yellow, so my children agreed to check them for me. There have been many occasions when I thought that a coloured printout looked fine, but when my children checked it, they said otherwise.

When I went out at night for a drink I usually gave my money to a trusted friend to purchase my drinks from the bar. This prevented both hearing and eyesight confusion especially when there was blaring music in the background. I avoided going to the shop when there were other people around. I was slowly asking for more help; my friends read my letters for me and dealt with paperwork that I was unable to see clearly enough to deal with myself. My children wrote my cheques and I admit that they sometimes signed them for me. I also asked my friends for more lifts when I felt uncomfortable walking but I still wasn't asking as much as I should. It wasn't easy; it's never easy – I knew that I had a choice to become sad or to become strong. I knew that I couldn't become a recluse because there was too much for me to do for myself and other people like my students.

My Martial Arts club was asked to take part in the Rugby Carnival. With all the problems that I was experiencing with learning to cope with my deteriorating eyesight, I thought that it wouldn't be a good idea to take part in a demonstration. I felt that it would be too difficult to perform in front of a crowd of people without sufficient sight, but as usual my students persuaded me to participate. I didn't like to let my students down because taking part in these kinds of activities helped to build their confidence.

The carnival first travelled through Rugby Town Centre and we walked along with the procession. There were crowds of people everywhere, waiting to see a quick but effective Martial Arts demonstration. When I looked towards the crowd of people they looked similar to lots of coloured dots drawn on a piece of paper. I was unable to see anyone in detail. They were so distorted that they almost blended in together but I knew they were there.

"There are hundreds of people out there and I can't identify one person," I thought to myself. "I'm sure that there are many people out there who know me and can see me and I wish that I could see them. My children are in the crowd somewhere and they're going to have to come up to me or I won't be able to see them. Life isn't fair. Oh well, it could be worse."

The less I observed the distorted crowd of people the happier I felt so I kept avoiding looking into the crowd.

Most of the time I walked along in my own little world, leaving most of the demonstration to my students who I had prepared in the run up to the event. I walked behind everyone leaving plenty of space between us so that there was little chance of me colliding with one of my smaller students who constantly seemed to disappear out of my sight. When I was ready, I stopped a student and put a pad in his hand and stood back knowing that the pad was now almost invisible to me and proceeded to kick a blurred pad that seemed to keep disappearing.

"This is very difficult," I thought as I continued to kick. "I'm kicking a pad that most of the time I can't see. Hundreds of people are watching me kick and hardly any of them realise that I'm blind."

I preferred to kick a pad because my students always left me room to kick. Some of them were walking around and kicking at random but I was unable to do that because I wouldn't be able to tell if a student was in the way. The last thing I wanted to do was kick my own student because I was unable to see them so I didn't do as much as I would have liked to.

As the procession continued through the town centre, I heard my name being called.

"That sounded like my children calling me," I thought anxiously. "Where are they? I wish I could see them but everyone looks too distorted to be able to identify anyone."

They suddenly appeared at my side and I spoke with them for a short while before continuing on my way.

Then we had to put on a demonstration in a park. Although I left most of it to my students and made them look good, I also had to perform. Everyone was waiting in anticipation to see the black belt's skills. I did a weapon demonstration and hoped that I wouldn't drop it or I might have difficulties finding it again. Then I kicked a pad a few times, which was hard because it kept disappearing and I didn't want to kick the person holding it with so many people watching. I normally kick fast but have been told that I'm pretty powerful so if I miss the pad, I could end up hurting the person holding it. Then I jumped very high to reach the pad – maybe about eight and a half feet. As I started running towards the pad, I thought, "Nobody knows that I can't see the pad until I'm about to jump off the ground." Then I focussed very quickly and hit the pad.

The hardest thing to do was to fight one of my students because I was always afraid of accidentally hurting them due to my low vision. Most of the time I slowed down my techniques to prevent accidents, but I usually fought without my glasses and that made it even harder to see my opponent. The worse my eyesight became, the more blurred the image of the person I was fighting became. Another problem that I experienced was seeing which students to pick to perform techniques.

However, all the difficulties that I experienced paled into insignificance when I thought about the benefits that my students received. It felt great to watch a student who was once shy perform confidently in front of people. My students looked so happy and enjoyed the demonstrations as much, if not more, than I did.

A few weeks after the demonstration, I had to collect my sister from the airport. I have two half sisters, Mavis and Alberta, who were from a previous relationship of my mother and they live in Jamaica. We'd never met but kept in touch on a regular basis and after Carline passed away, we were all quite eager to meet them. Since they hadn't much money I offered to pay for one of them to visit England. Alberta came over in August 2004 and I travelled by car to collect her from the airport. She walked straight past me and went to the information centre to call me on their loud speaker, then I remember walking past her too but then we both turned around and recognised each other.

She stayed at my house and I introduced her to all her family here. I even took her to meet her brother Fergus who was still in prison. Everyone seemed very pleased to finally meet her but there was still sadness amongst us from the loss of Carline. I showed Alberta where my parents used to live and I also took her to our mother's grave. She soon got used to guiding me across some of the roads and thought that I got around well for someone who couldn't see.

Alberta was used to going to church and somehow persuaded me to take her one Sunday morning. I was like a lot of people, used to go to church for years, then grew up and experienced too many problems and blamed them on the easiest target; God. Then we stop attending church. I'd thought about it for a long time but I'd never returned. I blamed God for my eye disorder and hearing loss and the rest of the troubles in my life so I had a few words to say when I got into the church.

Things turned out a little differently to how I'd planned it though. We sat in the same church that my parents had brought me up in – they'd taken me to church on a regular basis for sixteen years then they had given me the choice. I was busy working and doing all the other excuses we use not to be able to go to church, but it had crossed my mind on many occasions to return. I never did, well, until now. The church is called the New Testament Church of God, and it's on Oliver Street in Rugby. It's not an old fashioned church where the congregation sit still in silence, it's a typical Jamaican church where you see people expressing themselves and experiencing the spirit. The preacher doesn't talk calmly; they show their emotions while they speak the word of God. I sat and observed everyone for a while.

Some memories crept into my mind of when I used to attend with my parents and I could almost feel them there. Then Alberta began to get into it and sang and danced to the many songs; I only remembered a few from when I was young. Most of the time I stood clapping my hands while everyone else sang. Alberta seemed to know all of them and the music relaxed me and made me feel good. After all these years of not attending church, I found myself beginning to miss it and suddenly I wanted more.

The next part of the service was for prayer. I listened to a few other people praying first before I started on God, but I was surprised by what I heard. Most people were praying for the same thing – they were asking Got to keep helping them through their problems. I heard some of the problems that they were asking God to help them with and it was at that moment that I realised that I wasn't alone; I wasn't the only one who had problems. There was even a blind woman praying and thanking God. I reflected for a few minutes and thought that maybe I should ask God to help me and thank Him for what I had because I could be worse off than just being blind. So instead of blaming God I ended up thanking Him and I felt as if I was given more energy. I had felt low and drained before I entered the church but now I felt as though my batteries had been recharged. It was a mind changing experience that changed me for life. I was reminded that there were people worse off than me out there in the big bad world. It made me think about my sister Carline who had passed away from cancer and I realised that she had been worse off than me. There are many more people with incurable illnesses who are also worse off than me. Their lives could be very short whereas I have the chance to learn to live with my disabilities and enjoy life. Just then I realised that I too was blessed.

Alberta stayed in England for a month and after she left, I returned to church by myself and have being attending regularly ever since. A week of stress goes by; most of the time I'm strong enough to cope but as the week progresses I feel more drained and find it much harder to deal with some of my problems. Sometimes I feel so alone as if God has stopped helping me but I continue to pray and attend church. When I get there I feel like someone has given me more energy and strength to cope. I realise now that God carries me when I give up and that He hasn't given up on me and never did. I now believe the moral of the story called 'Footprints in the sand', where there are two sets of footprints and then there is only one. This is where we think God leaves us but it's actually where God carries us through our problems. I attend church and listen to every word to see if I can learn something and each week, I do.

My family continued to experience difficulties. In November 2004, my brother Percy came to my house to ask for my help. He was on the verge of a nervous breakdown and wanted me to look after Hasani. Percy had been looking after Hasani since his mother, Carline, had passed away but he was becoming quite a handful. Percy was on tablets to relieve him of some pains that he was experiencing in his back, which he claimed had been brought on by constantly lifting Carline when he was nursing her. These tablets weren't having any effect on his back pain and seemed to be giving him side effects, such as delusions. I looked after Hasani as Percy continued to struggle with his health, but after a month Hasani ran away from me and returned to Percy who was still unwell. I don't think that I was too hard on Hasani, I just taught him some discipline. We asked for help from Social Services but they seemed reluctant to do much.

During this period I was asked to be a bodyguard for a friend who was experiencing problems with a drug addict. He was on heroin and had threatened her many times so I defended her. I even ended up sleeping on a settee again, waiting for him. It was clear to me that she was on a path of destruction by choosing to be with a drug addict. Sometimes I would lay there on the settee wondering what I was doing in this situation. Here I was trying my best to avoid these kind of negative people but now my life was being threatened by defending someone else. I was told that he was going to stab me with a knife if he saw me. Being a bodyguard and putting my life at risk took a lot of energy out of me and I was thankful to return to church each weekend to be recharged once more. After a few weeks of sleeping on her settee waiting to confront him, her problem slowly faded away and I never had to use my Martial Arts. I found that after this episode when I went out I was always watching over my shoulder and always on my guard, just in case. One of my problems faded while another appeared to be escalating out of control.

Over the next few months Colette pleaded with the various services for help with dealing with Percy's deteriorating health but to no avail. She got in touch with his doctor, a specialist at the Rugby Hospital and with Social Services. Colette tried everything she could to help Percy but nobody seemed to take the matter seriously and it started to frustrate her. She only had good intensions – all she wanted was for Percy to receive the correct medication for his depression, which had escalated to paranoia and schizophrenia. Percy was hearing different voices in his head telling him what to do. It was clear that he needed medical help and fast.

On Thursday 3rd February 2005, Colette told me of her desperation and I went to visit her first thing in the morning. She explained what had been happening with Percy's delusional behaviour and I was startled by what I heard. It was clear that Percy was now suffering from some sort of personality disorder and was accusing Colette of not looking after their child, Theolantia, but to me it was clear that she was doing a brilliant job of bringing her children up. I offered to try and help by visiting Percy to convince him to seek medical help, but when I arrived at his house he refused to speak to me. Colette then joined me at my house and we contacted the hospital several times. I'm a very patient person and even I was becoming frustrated now. Nobody seemed to take her seriously and she ran out of ideas. After a few hours we gave up and Colette returned home.

At about 7 pm that day Colette called me on the phone and told me that Percy had just been to her home and she admitted that she was becoming scared. I didn't know what to do because I was just about to go out to teach Boxercise as usual but I also wanted to do something to assist her. The only thing that I could think of was to advise her to lock her doors and not to let him in again but to ring me later if she needed me.

She never called again but my brother-in-law, David, did. He told me that Percy had stabbed Colette with a knife and she had been taken to the hospital. He said that Percy had been arrested. He didn't know the extent of her injuries so I called the hospital, but they wouldn't give me any information. I went to see who was at Colette's home and to make sure that her children were taken care of.

I arrived to see that her street had been cordoned off and a lot of police were present. I became worried and felt that she must have been seriously hurt for that many police to be called. The police wouldn't give me any information so I waited until after I took my children to school at 9 am Friday morning and then I went straight to Colette's parents' house to ask how she was and to see if I could visit her in hospital. Her dad told me that she was dead.

Apparently Percy had stabbed her in the back and she had died at about 9 pm Thursday evening – two hours after she had asked me to help her. Then I phoned one of my sisters and she started crying and said that I was the strong one and should inform the rest of the family. She was wrong on this occasion about me being the strong one. Colette had been with me for most of the last day of her life and I started to feel as though it was partly my fault for not having come up with a solution to help her. During all my phone calls to my family I cried out loud in hysterics over the loss of Colette. The tears were streaming down my face and still I contacted everyone. Then I broke down and cried on my settee. I cried so much that I was given sleeping tablets to calm me down. All I kept thinking was that maybe, just maybe, if I had gone to help her instead of going to teach Boxercise, she would still be alive today.

Late that Friday evening the police came knocking on my door. They were trying to retrace Colette's steps on the day of her murder. She had been with me for a good part of the day so I had a lot of information to share. They asked me if I would make a statement and this is my view of what happened:

Percy was a happy person with a great personality. He always had a smile on his face. He was always giving positive advice to me and other people. He had a great personality that people would always remember.

Then, after looking after my sister Carline in 2002, his personality began to change. Our sister had cancer and was told that she was dying. We helped to nurse her at home because she chose to be mostly at home with her family rather than be in a hospital away from us. Somehow Percy began to do more for her than the rest of us did and he ended up being her main carer looking after her on a daily basis.

Percy cooked, cleaned and even slept on a settee at my sister's house. He looked after her son, Hasani, and took my sister wherever she wanted to go. He was a great help and my sister really appreciated him. As my sister came towards the end of her life, Percy even took over her nursing duties like taking her to the toilet and other difficult private duties. He was prepared to do what he could to make her happy before she died. I helped once a week but Percy would be there to assist me too.

When our sister finally died of cancer on June 6th 2003, I saw Percy's personality change once more. He was no longer the outgoing person who was always smiling. Instead he was suffering the most from the loss of our sister. He went to a few counselling sessions but struggled to attend due to transport. He was happy to take on board looking after Carline's son, Hasani, because he didn't want Hasani to end up in care. It caused Percy's family with Colette Lynch to grow and Percy had to move out with Hasani because of the lack of space in their house.

A few months later Percy's health began to deteriorate and he experienced pains in his back. He went to his doctor and was given special tablets. His personality seemed to change further and he became delusional and very paranoid. It worried us to the extent that we referred him back to his doctor in July 2004. I even made an appointment with the doctor, Doctor Knight, as he is my GP too, and told him about my concerns.

Percy was taken off the tablets for the pains in his back but I felt that there was already damage to his mind and I thought that he was now seriously depressed.

By October 2004 he went around spreading his paranoia. He would say:

- The Government is covering up a problem about yellow fever.
- He has yellow fever and we have yellow fever.
- The Government is covering up a serious problem with sugar and it's going to kill us all.
- Most of our illnesses are due to having too much sugar and it's bloating up our stomachs.

He began to avoid sugar and drank several litres of water everyday.

After experiencing many problems with Hasani's behaviour, Percy agreed to have a break from looking after him. He was quite upset having to do so because he had promised Carline that he would do his best to look after him after she died. He didn't want to let her down but I told him that he was heading for a nervous breakdown and desperately needed a break. Percy agreed that he had problems and I then looked after Hasani.

After a few weeks of me looking after Hasani, he ran away and went back to Percy. I told Percy that Hasani would add to his stress of not having a chance to grieve over the loss of Carline, but Percy said that Hasani just wouldn't leave him alone and only wanted Percy to look after him. I was worried about Percy's health and got in touch with Social Services to see if they would convince Hasani to stay with me because of Percy's deteriorating health but Nicky Hall from Social Services said that Hasani would be fine. I strongly disagreed but couldn't change their minds.

Percy still had many medical problems that were unresolved and I felt that his depression was getting worse. He was still paranoid and went to see his doctor several times to have various tests. He told me that he still became bloated when he had sugar and he avoided many foods. He told me that he even had an MRI scan. He was convinced that he was seriously ill and thought that he was dying. I kept telling him to see his doctor because I thought that he was depressed and might be going mad.

Then at the beginning of 2005 he appeared to take a 180-degree turn. He no longer thought that he was ill and was now talking to himself. His sugar problem had also vanished and he was having more sugar. He started drinking lots of Lucozade. His girlfriend, Colette, told me that Percy said that she was trying to kill Tia, their two-year-old child, by not giving her enough sugar. It was obvious to me that my brother Percy was still ill and needed medical attention. I spoke to Percy several times about his condition. He told me that he could hear different voices in his head that were not his voice but he felt fine. He went on to say that he had received information from his ex-girlfriend who has two children of his. He became emotional as he told me that she was planning to move to Canada with her husband and Percy's two children and Percy thought that he would never be able to see them again.

I had several conversations with Colette in January 2005 about Percy's mental state. She told me that she had contacted his doctor and the local mental hospital for help and support and was getting nowhere. At the end of that month I was told that Percy had gone to the Rugby Council and acted inappropriately. My sister June told me that there were even police officers called to the premises. This made me much more sure that he was heading for a nervous breakdown so I visited him on several occasions to offer him support. He told me that Hasani had problems with his school and kept being sent home to him. It was obvious to me that Percy was under serious stress and was still having delusions. Percy told me that he kept hearing voices in his head. I became worried and urged him to seek medical help but he continued talking rubbish as if he was losing his mind.

On the morning of Thursday 3rd February, I went to see Colette at 16 Garath Williams Close. I arrived at about 11 am. I spoke with

Colette and her mother and was told that Percy had broken her window on Wednesday night. Colette told me that the police had gone with someone from the hospital to see Percy. She said that she wanted Percy to be taken away to the hospital to undergo medical tests for his mental state. She was very upset when she told me because she said that the police and the medical officer saw Percy and decided to leave him to sleep. She told me that she had ran out of ideas to help Percy because she wasn't getting the medical support that she was desperate for him to have. I told her that I would try and encourage Percy to attend an appointment at the hospital that had been booked with Sandra Bell.

At about 1 pm I arrived at Percy's home at 6 Newland Street and tried to convince him to seek medical help but he refused to talk to me because he was paranoid that I was trying to get him sectioned. My other brother, Brian, was there so I spoke to him very loudly so that Percy could hear. I advised him to seek medical help and to stay away from Colette's home until he did so. I also told him to stay away from my sister Angela's home because she is already registered depressed and didn't want Percy to keep walking to her home, especially after midnight like he had done a few days ago.

I got back to my home at 1.30 pm and Colette joined me to call the mental health team at the hospital. We spoke to Sandra Bell and told her that we couldn't persuade Percy to attend the hospital for an appointment and insisted that they come out to assess him at his home. Later on in the day they even left a message on my answer machine asking me if I was able to convince him to attend the hospital for an appointment. We kept asking them to come out but they wouldn't.

Colette and I spoke until 3 pm at which time she left to collect her children from school. We were very upset from the lack of support we were receiving from the doctor and the hospital. We told the hospital that we were very worried about his mental state and told them about Percy's behaviour. He was walking the streets for hours; talking to the radio; taking light bulbs out because he could hear messages coming through them; he had destroyed his mobile phones because he thought that he could hear strange messages; he was hearing voices in his head telling him what to do; he thought that messages were coming through his television and was paranoid about everyone. Colette told me many things about Percy's behaviour and I too became seriously concerned about his state of mind.

At about 7 pm Colette called me on the phone and said that Percy had just visited her home at 16 Garath Williams Close and was acting weird. I asked her if she was sure that he had left and she said yes. I told her to lock her doors and not to let him in. That was the last time that I spoke to her. A few hours later she was dead.

I feel that Colette never gave Percy any reason to murder her. She only wanted him to get medical help and she cared for him very much. She will be sadly missed.

After I signed my statement, the police left. Since then I have gone over the events of that day in my mind hundreds of times, wishing that I had done things differently. Sometimes I even think that it could have easily been me who got stabbed. I was the one who backed up everything that Colette was trying to do. It's as though the curse of our family continues and we're all feeling more superstitious now. Even though Percy is my brother and I'll always love him, I can't help thinking that all Colette wanted was to help him and there was no need for her to suffer such a cruel death. The last thing I wanted was for Colette to die. She was loved by everyone. She was always smiling, even when she was trying to tell someone off, she would still have a happy smile on her face. We're all shocked and disturbed by her sudden death. Her poor family are shattered by it. She was only twenty-four years old, so young, so innocent – her life taken away from her for trying to do the right thing. All she wanted was for Percy to seek medical help. I hope that he'll now receive the help Colette lost her life fighting for. Maybe one day he'll realise that she did love him and wanted the best for him.

Our next battle was to protect their homeless children. Although several members of our large family were willing to take the children in, Social Services stepped in and gained custody of the three little children. They told us in a letter that Hasani was better off staying with us, but we totally disagreed with the way that they handled this complex situation. The last thing that any of us wanted was for the children to end up in care. Theolantia Wright is only two years old and by the time Percy is released from prison she'll be a teenager. It's unfair to the children to be in care when there are family who love them and are willing to look after them. I think that the way things were dealt with may send a sign to the children saying that nobody wanted to look after them, and this could affect them in their later life and cause them unnecessary stress.

Attending church regularly gave me the strength to cope with the traumatic situation. I prayed and asked God to help me and my family with the problems we were experiencing. Sometimes I had a personal prayer where someone prayed for my family and for me. I have also been blessed by the preacher and it was a very moving experience, the energy from the preacher seemed to revitalise me. People say that I'm the strong one and should look after the rest of my family; I'm not afraid to say that I feel as though I get my strength from believing in God. Death comes to us all, we cannot hide from it so we need to accept it. We should all be given time to mourn, but then we have to learn to get on with our lives.

As a sign of respect, I'm now continuing where Colette left off and I'm constantly fighting for Percy to receive the medical help he should have had a long time ago.

CHAPTER 30
NOW I CAN SEE

For quite a while our friendship has slowly become stronger. Pat and I have been friends for some time and see each other on a regular basis; she has become a close friend who I sometimes share my problems with. We speak about all sorts of things and not just about our personal problems – I don't like being a burden on other people and don't like moaning to them. When people moan to me I normally think of something cheerful in my mind so that I don't feel as though I have their problems to worry about too. I have enough of my own! We sometimes go out for lunch or generally have a laugh.

One day we played a truth or dare game and she asked me a few general questions about myself. It was fun and I asked her a few things about her too. Before long we diverted our questions onto our private lives, which is when our game became interesting.

"Have you ever had feelings for a friend that you shouldn't have had?" I asked.

"Yes," she answered.

"This is cool," I thought to myself. "I wonder if I can find out who she secretly fancies?"

"Have you?" she countered.

"That's cruel," I thought, "I wanted to know about her and not to open up my dark secrets. I wonder what her dare would be? Maybe I should tell her for now."

"Yes I have," I answered.

We began to laugh nervously as I prepared myself for my next question.

"Have you got any feelings for anyone at the moment?"

"Yes," she answered, looking slightly embarrassed. "Do you have any feelings for me?" she asked, suddenly sounding more confident.

At that moment I burst out laughing, not knowing how to answer.

"Maybe I should try the dare now," I thought to myself.

I giggled for a while before I plucked up enough courage to answer.

"Yes," I answered.

"That's all I'm telling her," I decided. "She's very fast to get from having feelings for anyone to me having feelings for her. Maybe I should stop being so shy and ask her some direct questions too."

The game began to get very interesting.

"Have you got any feelings that are more than just friendship for me?" I asked hesitantly.

"Yes," she answered.

"Well I *am* a typical man then," I thought to myself. "I didn't see any obvious signs. I always thought that we were just good friends. This is a cool game for discovering secrets. I'm going to ask some more direct questions before she does."

But it was her turn to ask the next question.

"How long have you had feelings for me that are more than just good friends?" she asked.

"I can't believe I'm about to share this," I thought to myself.

"I've had feelings for you for several months," I answered shyly.

"My turn again," I thought triumphantly. "Maybe I should ask her something that she can't answer so that I can get her to do a dare."

"Have you ever had any sexual thoughts about me?" I asked.

"I can't believe you just asked that!" she said looking even more embarrassed.

"Well you don't have to answer it. You can always do a dare," I suggested cleverly.

"I don't trust you and your dares, so I will say yes."

"For how long?" I continued eagerly.

"It's not your turn so you're going to have to wait!"

The game began to warm up as the questions got more personal.

"Have you ever fantasised about me?" she asked.

"This is getting serious now," I thought. "Maybe I should forfeit a dare because I'm about to share one of my most secret thoughts."

"Yes I have," my voice said.

"Really? Give me some details!"

"Hey, it's my turn!" I replied.

"Go on then ask your question."

"Did we kiss?" I asked nervously.

"Yes," she answered.

"I'm beginning to like this game now," I thought.

"Have you fantasised about me more than once?" she continued.

"Yes," I admitted.

"I can't believe I've just told her that!" I thought. "This is getting deep so I'm going to ask her a big question."

"Have we had sex in any of your fantasies?" I asked eagerly.

"I'm not answering that question!" she replied.

"You'll have to do a dare for me if you don't!"

"I'll do a dare," she replied.

"Oh wow!" I thought. "I've done it. I've forced her to do a dare. What should I ask her to do?"

"I dare you to kiss me," I said.

"We've kissed before so what kind of kiss do you want?" she asked coyly.

"A sloppy French kiss," I answered hungrily.

"Are you sure?" she responded.

"Yes!"

We laughed and giggled nervously as we slowly got closer. Our faces were almost touching as we smiled at each other. Then I touched her lips with mine and kissed her. We kissed some more and it felt good. I didn't want that moment to end so I held her face with both my hands and sank deeper into her lips. My heart began to beat faster as I grew eager for more. We kissed and cuddled for a while and soon forgot about the titillating game.

We'd created an awkward situation where we both wanted more, but we had issues to sort out first. My eyesight plays an important role and I know that my days of holding onto what little vision I have left are drawing to a close and part of me doesn't want anyone to have to look after me. The possibility of one day getting together still enters my mind and helps to bring a smile to my face when I'm feeling low.

Most days now I'm finding it harder to persuade myself to go out. During the day my eyesight is very cloudy and out of focus; as time has gone on I've seen how objects slowly blend into each other and then disappear. I constantly see as though I'm looking through thickening fog and it becomes more noticeable as each month goes by. I'm finding it difficult to see the difference between the pavement and the road, the colours of most cars, lamp posts and boulders. Now people seem to have blended into the background to such an extent that I can hardly notice that someone is there unless they're moving close to me. Most of the time I'm now using every last part of my eyes where blind spots have yet to take over. This means my eyes have to dart around from left to right and in all directions to help me focus on something. While I'm doing this I'm also trying my best to constantly dismiss the thoughts from my mind that will lead to me feeling emotional.

"Where does the path end and where does the road start?" I thought to myself in confusion one day. "This consistent foggy vision is getting worse. The lamp posts and other obstacles are becoming more difficult to see. Maybe I shouldn't be walking anywhere any more because I'm worried about being knocked over much more these days. It's a pity that I'm not a great lover of dogs or I would get a guide dog. Maybe I should trust and rely on other people, but then what about my independence? I have to keep doing some things for myself because I'll have to rely on other people more as my eyesight slowly fades away forever. I've got to fight this feeling and keep active or I'll whittle away to nothing."

A friend called Daniel came to see me and he told me that we are strong and can cope with the stresses of life. He told me that I should carry on teaching Martial Arts because if he was blind, he would too. I told him to imagine that he was in my shoes and couldn't see.

"Close your eyes and try to imagine what it really feels like to be blind," I said.

"It would be hard but I think I could cope," Daniel said.

"How would you get home? Or cook for yourself if you couldn't see?" I asked.

"I would rely on other people of course."

"Would you?"

"Yes."

"Do you trust other people with your money?" I continued.

"No, but I would have to get used to it," he said.

"What about going to the shop when nobody is around to help you or what would you do if you dropped something?" I asked.

"I would wait for someone to visit then ask them to help."

"So you would wait another day or two for someone else to do it for you? You're independent at the moment but you would rely on other people. Are you telling me that you wouldn't feel any different?" I asked.

"Yes I would, but you have to accept that you can't do it for yourself any more."

"Could you still do your job?" I asked.

"Yes; I would ask other people to help," he answered.

"Now imagine that you can never open your eyes again. How do you feel now?" I asked.

"It doesn't feel good, but I could still do it. If I was you I would still teach," he said.

"The feeling of closing your eyes for a few minutes is much different to closing them forever. You would have emotions that you would struggle to control."

Then I told him to open his eyes and look around at everything in the room.

"Now put my sunglasses on and tell me how you feel."

He put my glasses on and the comments flew out of his mouth.

"This is what you see?" he asked incredulously.

"I see similar to that," I answered.

"I can't see anything! Everything is blurred!"

"Now look around at the things you saw without the sunglasses on," I instructed.

"Some things have disappeared. I can't see the glasses any more. Nothing looks real. How do you cope?" he asked.

"Look at the trees and flowers outside the window, look at your reflection in the mirror," I continued.

He looked and commented more.

"It doesn't look like a tree any more. The flowers have lost their detail and I can't see myself in the mirror."

"That's why I've been telling you to appreciate the little things because one day you might not get the chance again. What people look like is no longer important if you can't see them. Imagine never being able to see your loved ones, like your children?"

"It must be so hard to deal with," he said sorrowfully.

There was one more question that I had to ask him.

"Daniel, I want you to tell me the truth."
"What?" he asked.
"If you saw like that, permanently, would you keep teaching?"
There was a pause as he gasped.
"No," he admitted.

It was the answer I was expecting. I knew that if I could get him to experience what it really feels like to be blind then his opinions would change. He admired me for still teaching as a registered blind instructor.

Getting out of my bed is getting more difficult as my eyesight deteriorates. Sometimes I have to force myself to attend the gym. After ten minutes or so of exercise, the energy inspires me to want to carry on. I usually train at 9 am because it gives me energy to get through the day. I have developed many friendships with other people and they help convince me to train.

I try to train three times a week. When I use the machines with weights it causes me a few problems and thoughts rush through my mind.

"Is there anyone already using it who I can't see? I'll walk slowly past it until I'm pretty sure nobody is there. I shouldn't have to guess. Think of something positive."

Then I sit at the machine.

"Where's the pin? It's very difficult to see. I'll sit here for a few seconds and see if it appears, it sometimes does."

Then I brush my hand down the centre of the weights where the pin is inserted. Eventually my hand comes across the pin.

"Now I have to struggle to insert it in another hole."

It's too difficult to see the hole where the pin fits into and I can't read the amount of the weight that I want so I will count how many weights down I normally have or put the pin in where I think I usually have it. If it's wrong then I sometimes remove it and put it somewhere else. Sometimes I leave it where it is because I'm not allowed to lift heavy weights because of the pressure it puts on my eyes. Sometimes I feel as though I'm a wimp as I watch other people lifting heavy weights like I used to.

One day a young lady came to speak to me while I was on a weight machine.

"Hello," she said.

"Oh, it's Nicole from Boxercise," I thought to myself.

"Hello; sorry I was miles away and I didn't see you – I was thinking of some different techniques to use during my Boxercise class," I said.

"I didn't know that you taught Boxercise."

"You've attended one of my classes," I thought.

Then a weird sensation came over me. "Whoops! I don't think that this *is* Nicole who I'm talking to."

She wasn't aware that I had made a mistake and I somehow diverted our conversation to a different subject.

After a while a blond lady rushed into the room and took some small weights before rushing back out.

"I'm pretty sure that was Sarah," I thought to myself. "Who else rushes around like that? I'll speak to her when she returns the weights."

Sarah is a friend who I see in the gym on a regular basis. She's a gorgeous blond with very long hair and green eyes. I can't see her clearly and have never had the pleasure of being able to admire her green eyes for myself but she has described them well enough to give me a pleasant picture of her in my mind. Her long blond hair is easy to see but I have made a few mistaken identities.

Sometimes I try to be clever and say hello to her before she sees me. As I entered the gym once she was standing near me talking to someone.

"There's Sarah," I thought.

So I tapped her on her shoulder.

"Hello," I said.

There was no answer so I walked on and tried not to disturb her. She normally wears a red top and the top was red! After about ten minutes someone with long blond hair approached me, but she had a black top on so I didn't say anything to her. I suppose I shouldn't have been looking anyway!

"Good morning Vendon, it's Sarah," she said.

"If she is Sarah then who was I speaking to ten minutes ago?" I thought to myself.

"Did you change your t-shirt?" I asked her.

"No; why?"

I explained the mistake and we laughed.

There have been other times when I've thought she was someone else too. She was on the treadmill once and I got on the one next to her. I took a quick look but it didn't look like her outline and also she was wearing a different t-shirt. Why I was looking again, I don't know! Sarah normally jogs and this person was walking.

"Hello Vendon, it's Sarah," a sweet voice said.

"Hello Sarah," I answered.

"I don't believe it," I thought. "She doesn't appear to have any of the characteristics that she normally does apart from her blond hair. She was standing right next to me and I didn't know who she was. My eyesight is definitely bad."

"Am I on the right side of you to hear me?" she asked.

"Yes but I couldn't see you. I was expecting you to be wearing a red t-shirt and be jogging," I said with a smile.

"I've hurt my knee but I'll wear a red t-shirt for you next time," she said compassionately.

The digital clock on the treadmill is too hard to read. To use it I press the start button twice and it automatically starts with a setting of ten minutes. I use it for twenty or thirty minutes so I press the start button again when the first set of ten minutes have finished. It would be great to actually see what I was doing but that's how I've adapted to still be able to use the equipment.

It feels very peaceful and relaxing walking on the treadmill. It's during this time when I gain inspiration. Many thoughts rush through my mind and I choose which ones to build on and try to dismiss the rest. We tend to be controlled by our automatic thoughts and reactions but we can learn to control them and control our actions. If I have a negative thought in my mind then I battle to create positive ones to fill my head so I hardly think of the negative one. The more I think of something else rather than my original thought, the easier it becomes. It's a habit that I've created and it seems to work well.

We can choose what to think and we have a choice of what path we take. We all have problems – that's life. There are always other people worse off than us and I think about that all the time. Maybe if we stopped being so selfish and thinking that we are the only one with problems we could all learn to enjoy life more.

A friend of mine once told me that he had serious problems and moaned about them a lot. After a while I told him to thank God that his problems were not as bad as other people's. I also told him to try and enjoy his life while he could and not take anything for granted. He then asked me what I knew about problems because he didn't think that I had any. He had forgotten that I'm registered blind and don't advertise the problems that blind people experience, every minute of everyday so... I reminded him. After my short lecture on some of the obstacles I have had to get over on the way to dealing with my disability, he apologised. Just because people go around with a smile on their face and refrain from moaning, doesn't mean that they haven't got problems. I'm a good listener when someone has a serious problem, but I admit that I don't like listening to people moaning about trivial things. It causes me unnecessary stress and I normally switch off. I wasn't born strong or born able to cope with problems; I have persistently and consistently worked at it and shaped my personality.

Sometimes I ring up friends and force myself to go out for lunch or something to distract my thoughts from my fading eyesight. At lunch we eat and I may see the chips as one jumbled mess.

"I can't see the individual chips because my eyesight is too blurred."

Then I quickly think of something else and not dwell on my problem.

"I'll use my fingers and pick up the chips," I compromise. "I mustn't look at the chips then I won't feel so emotional and I'll try to keep talking about something funny to force that negative thought out of my mind."

Sometimes my drink might seem to disappear.

"Where has my drink disappeared to? Stop thinking about what you can't do. Things could be worse. At least you have the ability to get out and enjoy yourself. There are other people who've been in hospital for long periods of their lives and are not able to get up and go out for lunch like you can."

Once I arranged to meet someone for lunch and they were late. Although I had a mobile with me, the battery was low and it wouldn't work well enough for me to ring them. I can't see clearly enough to use a telephone booth so I went back home to call them. They then told me that they had left me a text message on my mobile and thought that I would have read it. That friend has known that I have been registered blind for ten years and should have known that I can't read text messages. It's a thought that still makes me laugh!

When I'm talking to someone I'm constantly trying to manoeuvre my head into the best position to see them more clearly.

"I need to be slightly closer to them to see their facial features clearer," I think to myself. "It feels great to be able to see them. Although they're not exactly clear, I can see them well enough from this position to be able to appreciate what vision I have left."

Sometimes the person I'm with might comment on someone's facial features and a thought passes through my mind.

"They don't know how lucky they are being able to see that clearly. Maybe if they temporarily lost their sight they might appreciate that person for their personality and not their appearance."

It's in situations like this that I realise that I *can* see. I see when someone is kind and helpful or has a great personality – I can see people for who they truly are.

There are times where the lighting is great or the sun reflects off someone's face so that I'm able to see their features slightly clearer. It's at moments like these that you can catch me staring at people. It could be a male or a female friend, it doesn't matter, I'm just grateful to be able to see them. It doesn't matter how attractive they are or not, I'm thankful to be able to see them at that time because I know that most of the time I see people's faces as shadows. It's like a blessing for me to have these brief moments.

"Why can't people appreciate what they can see instead of constantly judging people on their appearance? Maybe we should all close our eyes so that we judge people for their personalities and not their images. Maybe if people had limited vision like me, they would appreciate what they can see. I wish that I could see the colour of people's eyes but I'm grateful to be able to see their blurred faces in the bright sunlight."

Appreciating what I can see extends to other things, such as my children. I have never been able to see them in great detail. School photos and other pictures are too blurred or too dark for me to see them clearly. It would have been nice to see them properly and I do miss having the ability but I have to settle for my imagination. I don't need to see them in detail to know that my children are beautiful. They are funny and keep me happy, that is beautiful to me. I have drawn a detailed photo of them in my mind and they are perfect and bring a smile to my face when they're around me. I find myself constantly wanting to please them. Sometimes they ask me to take them to the cinema and although getting to my seat is difficult, and seeing the huge screen is difficult, I still go to the cinema to please them. I do have fun there sometimes – there have been times when I've laughed at some action that I thought I saw or concluded in my mind after building a picture of what's going on in my head.

"What are you laughing at dad?" they asked.

"That man just collided with the table."

"No he didn't! The little boy put some toys on the table when his dad was coming."

"Oh well, my version was much funnier," I concluded.

This adds to the excitement of the movie and happens quite often, especially when I watch TV at home. Sometimes my children make me laugh when one of them is in my way.

"Can you get out of Dad's way? He can't see the TV through you."

"He can't see it at all!" the other one replies.

It's funny but true. Unless I'm sitting inches away from the TV, my vision is too dark and blurred to see details well. If you paused a picture on my TV, the background would look similar to the people and I wouldn't be able to tell what was human and what was the background. People are constantly moving so that's how I work out where the people are but I make up the details of what they look like in my head. Everyone is attractive in my mind! Sometimes I get tired of listening to other people moaning about people's appearance. It really isn't that important as long as they have a good personality so maybe people should try closing their eyes when people speak. You might admire them for who they truly are and not for how they look.

Sometimes I get tired of guessing what people are doing on TV and I lay down on my settee while watching, or should I say listening, to the TV. Most of the time I don't look at the screen, I pick areas of the room to stare at or sometimes just close my eyes. I've noticed that I get fewer negative thoughts when I have my eyes closed. Although I do a good job at dismissing my negative thoughts, they are few and far between when my eyes are closed.

When I'm on my own I'll have the radio on or music channels on the TV. Anything that uses less sight to understand creates fewer thoughts in my confused mind. Music is beautiful and generally encourages positive thoughts in me. I listen to music a lot. One way that I flood out negative thoughts in my mind is to imagine that I'm listening to my favourite tracks or artists. Michael Jackson, Bounty Killer and Sanchez are my favourites, but there are many more musical artists who I admire. I sometimes get emotional when I listen to Stevie Wonder, but I really do admire him because his achievements have far surpassed mine and he has less vision than me. Compared to him, I can see. With the correct lighting I can see the difference between black and white. I can see red and sometimes yellow in bright light. I can see people's eyes, nose and mouth if the lighting is right. When I think of Stevie Wonder I realise how lucky I am.

There are many more people who are worse off than me and I think of them to motivate myself when I'm feeling low. Joyce unfortunately passed away a few months ago. Joyce was a happy, cheerful lady who always said something positive to make you laugh or smile. Sadly she had leukaemia, but to her last days she kept smiling and kept giving me positive advice on how to deal with the pressures of going blind. She had similar thoughts to mine; she was known as the strong one but she too had bad days like me. She had days when she refused to ask for help and assistance so that she wasn't a burden on other people. If you closed your eyes when she spoke you would never be able to tell that she had one leg or was a few months away from dying. She was amazing and her positive spirit will always live on in my mind. We had a laugh once when we were out with her family and friends. They were all engrossed in conversation and left her in her wheelchair to find her own way into a pub. So I pushed her and she guided me because I couldn't see where I was going.

There have been other incidents when I've shocked a few people. These are some of the thoughts I have to cheer me up and bring a smile back to my face. I was standing waiting to use the pedestrian crossing when I sensed that the man next to me was struggling more than I was to cross the road. I listened carefully and realised that he was blind.

"Would you like some help crossing over the road?" I asked.

"Yes please," he replied.

"Hold onto me," I said.

"Thank you; you're very kind."

"You wouldn't trust me if I told you my little secret," I said jokingly.

After we got across to the other side he turned to me and asked; "What's your secret then?"

"I'm blind too," I answered.

"I couldn't tell," he said.

"I don't tell many people and I follow where other people walk so that it appears as though I can see," I replied.

"How are you able to get around so well?"

"I force myself to come out regularly so that I learn where most of the obstacles are."

He seemed to know where he was going from there so I left him. My friend who I was with was in hysterics.

"Well that really was the blind leading the blind," he said.

That wasn't the only time it happened. There was also another elderly man struggling to cross a road. I wasn't sure whether he was blind or not and I was going to pass him but decided to observe his movements a little more closely.

"Can you help me?" he asked.

"Yes, of course I can," I replied.

"Most people see me struggling and walk right past me."

"I was going to do that too," I thought to myself jokingly.

"They are inconsiderate people," I said.

"Can you guide me to the bank please?" he asked.

"I struggle to find the glass door too," I thought to myself.

"Yes, no problem," I answered.

He was very grateful and I never told him that I was registered blind too. I thought that maybe he would have run a mile and not trusted me to guide him.

There was another incident that sometimes makes me laugh when I think about it. I was out using my white cane (properly) and a car pulled up beside me.

"Excuse me, but can you help me?" a voice asked.

When I stopped to see what the problem was, I was surprised to hear that they were lost and were asking me for directions. The funniest thing was that I managed to point them in the right direction. I will always be confused with why they would select a blind person to ask for directions.

When I'm out on my own, walking slowly and manoeuvring around difficult obstacles, I feel blind, vulnerable and helpless. Then when I go shopping with my sister Angela who is more severely blind than I am, suddenly I feel as though I can see again and I end up guiding her around.

My friend Zack guided me once and we ended up in hysterics. It was at night and in an area that I wasn't used to so I felt disorientated. There were few streetlights and I kept thinking that I was about to bump into something. Zack kept telling me that I was nowhere near a lamp post but I felt unsafe. He then linked my arm as though we were married and he led me towards the restaurant. Zack told me that several cars stopped and the drivers and passengers were having a good long look at us, obviously thinking that we were gay. Zack is a muscular man (like myself!) and together we appeared to be two big strong gay blokes. We laughed in hysterics as people continued to wonder in their sick minds.

People's opinions can sometimes hurt and I think that we should try to keep our opinions to ourselves, especially when they're about people's appearance. None of us are perfect and we all have something that we'd like to change. Why then do we comment on other people if anything looks abnormal? People might appear to walk with a waddle and some may find it amusing but that person may have severe arthritis and be in a great deal of pain which is what causes them to walk differently. A child may appear to be naughty, yet they might have other underlying problems like being autistic.

I have an autistic child in one of my Martial Arts classes and I've learnt to adapt my teaching to make it flexible enough to allow him to fit in. He has a short concentration span and I've developed plenty of different activities to keep him busy. He's only seven years old and is a lovely child – it's not his fault that he has a problem so I try my best to continue helping him. His parents watched him take an exam with me and watched me as I adapted to help him complete his one-hour exam. His mother became very emotional with me and I had to hold back my tears. She told me that he wasn't able to be taught in mainstream education because nobody could cope with him and here I was teaching him and getting on with him very well. His parents told me that they mentioned me in a governor's meeting – they made me feel very special just because I gave their child a chance to fit in. Helping other people helps me continue to teach despite my difficulties. His parents told me that they were surprised to see that he was making eye contact with me and he smiled most of the time. He wasn't known to make eye contact with people but then I wished that I could have made clear eye contact with him. I felt deep down that he knew that I couldn't really see him. He is very bright and a gifted child so it isn't fair for him to be labelled as a naughty, disruptive child when he is actually crying out for help.

Adapting my teaching techniques to help other people seems to come quite easily. Why should people miss out just because they're not considered to be normal? If my instructor had done that with me then I would never have achieved my black belt. I have many students with different abilities and disabilities but I try my best to help them all. It feels great to know how much I'm helping other people. Through my eyes, they are all normal and have the ability to achieve great things.

After twenty years of Martial Arts I have come to the point where I hardly ever kick. This is because I have many young students and I can hardly see them so I don't want to accidentally kick them. When I teach I try to have fun. I like to see how many times I can talk to students thinking that they are someone else! It happens all the time and after a while I realise that they are not the person I thought they were. It mostly happens with new students because I'm not yet used to their voices and their outlines. Sometimes I've assumed a student is training and then I call them by their name and wonder why they failed to respond. When I walk closer to them I then realise that it's someone else and I laugh to myself. A mistake that I make often is with their payments.

"Here are my training fees," someone would say.

I take a look at the money and see that they have given me a £20 note.

"Couldn't you give me something smaller? I'm not sure if I have enough change for this."

"It's not £20, it's only £5," they respond.

"Oh, I'm sorry, I couldn't see it clearly… as usual."

It feels great to encourage and inspire other people in achieving more. My students get a badge for doing well. The badges become sweets over the Christmas season. It's an incentive that I use that seems to work well, especially with my younger students. I can almost magically get students to try harder. What I do is purposely give a badge to someone and then I watch all the rest trying harder as they attempt to gain a badge too. They receive badges for being disciplined, trying extra hard, kicking well, becoming flexible and fighting with effort. I watch shy people become confident and people with introverted personalities become outgoing and great leaders. I encourage students to believe that they are better than they think they are. I try my best to pass on my positive attitude and after a while they believe it too and become more confident. I change the lives of many people and that makes me feel as though I'm doing something worthwhile.

Life is too short and we need to find ways to enjoy it because we never know when our time will be up. Stop looking for Mr Perfect when you already have Mr Right. We all have something we would like to improve about ourselves so we need to think differently about people. Don't let your thoughts control you. Try to control your mind. I do have emotions but I've learnt to control them well. Sometimes it's nice to cry but I don't stay emotional for long – I avoid things that make me feel too emotional. Recently I've found out that I'm not the only blind person with a positive attitude. I contacted the RNIB for some advice on equipment for the blind and the receptionist cheered me up. Her name is Pauline and she told me that she was also suffering from RP. After speaking to her for a while I felt as though I was talking to myself – she was as happy and as positive as I am.

Sometimes I listen to music and come across my sister Carline's favourite tracks. I have my moments of thought and am reminded that I miss her. If it makes me feel too emotional then I change the music and think of something cheerful again.

Thinking of my children usually cheers me up. The other day they were listening to different musical tracks that they thought I should use at my Boxercise classes. They started punching and jumping and dancing in time with the different beats and I laughed as I watched them.

Getting food out of my freezer is stressful but cooking it is fun. When I'm on my own but too hungry to wait for my children to return, I attempt to cook things by myself. I'm pretty good at it because I've worked out that as long as I'm using a deep fat fryer, everything takes six minutes to cook. I can't read the label so I guess. Fish, chips, sausages and chicken portions all take six minutes! (Yes they do, or they do for me!) Sometimes I cook things from frozen and I don't know what it is until I bite into it! Well I'm still here so I must be doing something right.

Laughing is something that I enjoy very much. I love to laugh. It cheers me up. If I don't laugh then it means that I'm having a *really* bad day. I need to laugh and smile every day. When I'm shopping and hear a mother telling her child off in public, I usually laugh. I laugh when I hear parents talking in strange ways to children but I admit that I used to do the same thing when I was speaking to my small children. Sometimes I watch shows on TV just for the jokes to make me laugh or smile. Hearing a woman speaking French makes me smile. I think the French accent is very sexy. When my eyes are closed I can imagine that it is whoever I like. I think that Catherine Zeta Jones and Julia Roberts are beautiful and I can see that they are because of the interesting characters that they play. When I hear their names it brings a smile to my face and makes me laugh. My favourite is Sandra Bullock – her voice is very sexy and I always smile when I hear it. Maybe I'm easily pleased but at least I'm enjoying my life – it isn't easy but I'm enjoying life despite my problems.

For years I've been used as a guinea pig for postgraduates who may become doctors. I've sat there while so many of them look into my eyes using their ophthalmoscopes and I hope, I hope and pray that one of them will look into my eyes and see their way to discovering a cure. It might not be for me but at least the next generation of RP suffers may have a cure. It might happen one day but I'll not wait. I can enjoy my life with what little vision I have left.

My low vision has opened up my eyes to see people for who they are and not for what they look like. At long last I understand what my father meant when he told me that I *would* be able to see. He didn't mean with my eyes.

You only have one life. Life is the greatest gift, so cherish it instead of wasting it.

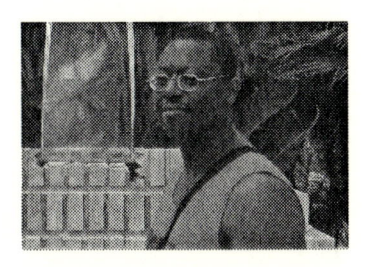

Background

My name is Vendon Aston Wright. I was born on the sixth of August 1966 in a small town called Rugby in England, where I attended Fareham High School. Generally, people think that the most interesting aspect of the town is that it is the home of the game Rugby Football.

I have two children named Michaela and Jasmine. Their ages are fifteen and ten respectively. I'm one of eleven children consisting of six girls and five boys. I'm registered blind and have a rare genetically developed eye disorder called Retinitis Pigmentosa (RP) and at present there are no known cures. So far one in three thousand people suffer from RP. My full-time job was a Computer Technician. After over ten years of computers I was forced to give up due to my failing eyesight. Now I teach a Martial Art called Taekwondo, which is a sport that is featured in the Olympics, and am also a Personal Fitness Trainer.

I attained a 4th Degree Black Belt Master of Taekwondo and I was the first registered blind person in England to achieve this level of excellence. After studying Taekwondo for over twenty years, I now teach many classes of my own to help inspire others and at present have twenty Black Belts. I hope that I can show others that disabled people can still achieve great things. This book shows some of the challenges that visually impaired people have to overcome to live a normal life. I explain what it feels like to see the world through a blind person's eyes. Hopefully it will motivate people to see a positive side to their problems and it may also encourage people not to take what they see for granted. The inspiration to write a book came from persistently helping my friends with their problems. Now I would like to help other people by passing on my strengths. The story of my life could be used as a motivational tool for other people. It shows how to cope with a wide range of emotions. There are many visually impaired people that could benefit. The positive thinking market could also find use of my book as it shows a positive way of coping with the challenges of life.

About the book

When I was six years old I started wearing glasses to correct my short sight. My perception of my low vision changed when I was twenty years old and found out that my brother had suddenly gone blind. He was told that he was suffering from Retinitis Pigmentosa RP), a disorder that slowly destroys the pigment cells in the eyes. There are three different strains of RP and the one my brother has runs in the male line of a family. So far, there are no known cures. My brother's eyes deteriorated quickly which confused us all. I soon became curious and convinced myself to attend an eye appointment to determine whether there was more wrong with my eyes than just being short sighted. At the age of twenty-one I was also diagnosed with RP. Since then I have been slowly going blind, not knowing when my world would finally fade away forever. Finally at the age of twenty-eight I was also registered blind. Then to everyone's surprise, my sister was registered blind two years later.

Despite the problems it has caused me, I have managed to keep a positive attitude towards life. I hold a 4th degree Black belt in Taekwondo and I was the first registered blind person in England to achieve this level of excellence. After studying Taekwondo for over twenty years, I now teach many classes of my own. At present I have twenty Black Belts.

The inspiration to write a book came from persistently helping my friends with their problems. Now I would like to help other people by passing on my strengths. The story of my life could be used as a motivational tool for other people as it shows how to cope with a wide range of emotions.

Printed in the United Kingdom
by Lightning Source UK Ltd.
107897UKS00002B/37-102